Theory for Midwifery

Theory for Midwifery Practice

Second Edition

Edited by

Rosamund Bryar

and

Marlene Sinclair

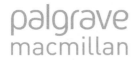
palgrave
macmillan

First edition 1995
Second edition 2011

Published by
PALGRAVE MACMILLAN

Palgrave Macmillan in the UK is an imprint of Macmillan Publishers Limited, registered in England, company number 785998, of Houndmills, Basingstoke, Hampshire RG21 6XS.

Palgrave Macmillan in the US is a division of St Martin's Press LLC, 175 Fifth Avenue, New York, NY 10010.

Palgrave Macmillan is the global academic imprint of the above companies and has companies and representatives throughout the world.

Palgrave® and Macmillan® are registered trademarks in the United States, the United Kingdom, Europe and other countries

ISBN 978–0–230–21192–6

This book is printed on paper suitable for recycling and made from fully managed and sustained forest sources. Logging, pulping and manufacturing processes are expected to conform to the environmental regulations of the country of origin.

A catalogue record for this book is available from the British Library.

10   9   8   7   6   5   4   3   2   1
20   19   18   17   16   15   14   13   12   11

Printed and bound in Great Britain by
CPI Antony Rowe, Chippenham and Eastbourne

Contents

List of Tables, Figures, Boxes and Illustrations

Tables

Figures

Boxes

Illustrations

Foreword

The difference between this second edition and the first (1995) edition of this book is striking. That difference reflects, in many ways, the developments in midwifery thinking and theory during those 16 years.

This new edition has a wealth of contributors from a number of countries. The topics covered are many, and all of them important. The diversity of the contributions reflects different midwifery systems and, most importantly, a fascinating variety of midwifery approaches and philosophies.

The range of Part II of this book is impressive and encouraging. It is great to see contributors from other parts of the world whose work I have long admired. It is also good to see issues addressed that are worrying, such as bullying and the rising caesarean rate.

If 'theory provides the tools for the job' (Chapter 1), then we have here a splendid tool chest upon which midwives can draw when practising our craft. It deserves to be well-used. It is the central contention of the book that 'thinking affects practice', and the conditions of practice are such that much thinking is currently needed. The last chapter is an appropriate analysis of a concept we hold dear and tend to accept without thinking; it shows how much thinking we need to do.

I recommend this book to my colleagues.

MAVIS KIRKHAM
Emeritus Professor of Midwifery
Sheffield Hallam University, UK

Acknowledgements

I would first like to thank the many people who supported the development and writing of the first edition. The original book arose out of a project undertaken at Queen Charlotte's Maternity Hospital (1979–82) initiated by Margaret Adams, Grace Strong and Elaine Ward. Some years later, Emeritus Professor Jo Alexander suggested to Macmillan that the first edition should be written and kindly suggested that they approach me to do that. At the time of writing the first edition, I had moved back into the world of primary health care, where I have remained. This has made the preparation of the second edition even more challenging. I have been given particular help and encouragement over the several years that it has taken to produce this edition by two people. Dora Opoku, formerly Head of the Midwifery and Child Health Department, City University London constantly encouraged and kept me motivated to complete this edition for midwives and midwifery. Lynda Thompson, Senior Commissioning Editor for Nursing and Health at Palgrave, initiated the work on the second edition and provided much needed support throughout, before handing over early in 2010 to Kate Llewellyn. My colleagues at City University London in the Public Health, Primary Care and Food Policy Department, while mystified at my involvement in the world of midwifery, have always been supportive. Quentin, Siobhán, Saoirse and Laurence, my brother and his family, have provided support in a multitude of ways while Bounty, Pookie and Alfie have put up with shorter walks than they would have liked.

RB

I acknowledge the many people who have made a contribution to this seminal work including my long-suffering and loving husband, Terry, and my children, Mark and Jane. They offered support in their intercessory and special loving way. Mary Rose Holman of the Learning Resource Centre, University of Ulster, Belfast and Mary Dharmachandran of the Royal College of Midwives, London undertook literature searches to identify midwifery theory literature; their help and expertise was invaluable. Living life without a librarian would for me be unthinkable!

MS

Rosamund and Marlene would like to thank, in particular, Kate Llewellyn, Project Editor at Palgrave Macmillan, for steering this book to completion. Without the contributors, this book would be nothing and they would like to thank them for their patience over the time that it has taken to complete this project and for their stimulating chapters.

The authors and publishers would also like to thank the following for granting permission to reproduce their material: Professor D. Silverman for Figure 3.5, originally from Silverman, D.: *The Theory of Organisations: A Sociological Framework* (London: Heinemann, 1970); Cambridge University Press and Jean Ball for Figures 3.8 and 3.9, originally from Ball, J.A.: *Reactions to Motherhood: The Role of Postnatal Care* (Cambridge: Cambridge University Press, 1987); Mark Hakansson/Panos Pictures for the picture of the Himba Woman and Child (Illustration 6.5). Every effort has been made to trace and contact all copyright-holders, but if any have been inadvertently overlooked the publishers will be pleased to make the necessary arrangements at the first opportunity.

Notes on the Contributors

Rosamund Bryar is Professor of Community and Primary Care Nursing at City University London, England, UK. She is also co-editor (with Professor Sally Kendall) of the journal *Primary Health Care Research and Development* and co-chair of the charity International Conferences on Community Health Nursing Research (www.icchnr.org).

Kenda Crozier is a Senior Lecturer in Midwifery at the University of East Anglia and a Research Fellow of the Royal College of Midwives, England, UK. She has a deep interest in the theoretical underpinning of midwifery, and is currently involved in research capacity building.

Kathleen Fahy is Professor of Midwifery and Head of Discipline at the University of Newcastle, New South Wales, Australia. Kathleen's current theory and research work is focused on understanding and changing maternity care practices in order to optimize women's psychophysiology, which necessarily enhances birth outcomes.

Maralyn Foureur is Professor of Midwifery for the Northern Sydney Central Coast Area Health Service and the University of Technology, Sydney, New South Wales, Australia. Maralyn's research interests have gradually evolved into a focus on the impact of the birth environment on the physiology of women and babies and, more latterly, the impact of the birth environment on the epi-genome.

Patricia Gillen is a Lecturer and Academic Coordinator of Post Registration Education at the University of Ulster, Northern Ireland, UK. She is currently undertaking a systematic review on the interventions that are available to reduce the incidence and the impact of bullying in the workplace, and the effectiveness of these interventions.

Carolyn Hastie is a Senior Midwifery Lecturer at the University of Newcastle, New South Wales, Australia. She has written on the workplace culture, horizontal violence and doctor–midwife interaction, and maintains a blog: *Thinkbirth* at http://thinkbirth.blogspot.com, where she highlights issues and ideas that are of interest to midwives and birthing women/couples.

Billie Hunter is Professor of Midwifery at Swansea University, Wales, UK. She is well-known for her doctoral study: *Emotion Work in Midwifery* (University of Wales, Swansea, December 2002), which was the first study to focus explicitly on the emotional aspects of midwifery work.

Lynn Jones is Head of the National School of Furniture (High Wycombe) and Course Leader of the MA in Furniture Design and Technology at

Buckinghamshire New University, England, UK. She is known for her external collaborations with industry, other academic institutions and her postdoctoral research at large NHS hospitals, and the breastfeeding chair she designed was awarded *Parenting Product of the Year* in 2006.

Michelle Kealy is Research Fellow at Mother and Child Health Research, La Trobe University, Melbourne, Australia. She is an Investigator on a number of studies including vaginal birth after Caesarean section, postnatal care and perinatal outcomes associated with older maternal age at Mother & Child Health Research, and her research interests include methodological issues and Caesarean section.

Sally Kendall is Professor of Nursing and Director of the Centre for Research in Primary and Community Care at the University of Hertfordshire, England, UK. She is co-editor (with Professor Rosamund Bryar) of *Primary Health Care Research and Development* and the co-chair of International Conferences in Community Health Nursing Research (www.ichnr.org).

John Keller is Professor of Educational Psychology and Learning Systems at Florida State University, Florida, USA. During his career, he has made major contributions to development of approaches to designing motivational systems, and contributed to design of performance improvement and systematic training design processes. He is best known for the motivational design process he created that is called the *ARCS Model* (http://arcsmodel.com).

George Kernohan is Professor of Health Research at the University of Ulster, Northern Ireland, UK. His primary interest lies in research methodology applied in nursing and midwifery, with associated interests in health technology assessment, evaluation of innovation in health, health informatics and computing.

Katharine Kolcaba is Associate Professor Emeritus at the University of Akron, Ohio, USA. Her presentations and workshops are focused on the application of Comfort Theory for improving the work environment and the patient experience. She has published extensively on the patient outcomes of holistic comfort, including an award-winning web site called The Comfort Line (www.thecomfortline.com).

Pranee Liamputtong is Personal Chair in Public Health, at La Trobe University, Melbourne, Australia. Pranee's particular interests include issues related to cultural and social influences on childbearing, child-rearing, and women's reproductive and sexual health. Pranee is a qualitative researcher and has published several research method books.

Rosemary Mander is Emeritus Professor of Midwifery, School of Health, University of Edinburgh, Scotland, UK. Rosemary has until recently continued regular practice as a midwife, both in the health service and independently. Her research has focused on a range of aspects of decision-making related to childbearing.

Jenny Parratt is Conjoint Senior Lecturer at the University of Newcastle, New South Wales, Australia. Since 2001, Jenny has been researching women's experiences of their changing embodied self during childbearing, and writing midwifery theory. Her methodological expertise is in feminist interpretive work with a post-structural philosophical foundation.

Sam Porter is Professor of Nursing Research at Queen's University, Belfast, Northern Ireland, UK. Sam has written many papers, book chapters and several books that focus on qualitative research, realist philosophy, and social theory and health, and is currently involved in the development and application of innovative research methods using musicology.

Carolyn Sampselle is Carolyne K. Davis Collegiate Professor of Nursing at the University of Michigan School of Nursing, Michigan, USA. Carolyn's research spans more than 20 years in the field of women's incontinence prevention and self-management. Through her research, she has also addressed health care disparities among women of different race/ethnic and economic backgrounds.

Kerri D. Schuiling is Distinguished Professor and an Associate Dean and Director of the School of Nursing at Northern Michigan University, Michigan, USA. She is the senior staff researcher for the American College of Nurse-Midwives, and is on the editorial board of the *Journal of Applied Nursing Research*. She was also recently named as the co-editor of what will be the official journal of the International Confederation of Midwives, the *International Journal of Childbirth*.

Marlene Sinclair is Professor of Midwifery Research at the University of Ulster, Northern Ireland, UK. Marlene has over twenty years of experience in higher education and is Ireland's first Professor of Midwifery Research. Her ambition is to develop clinical midwifery researchers at doctoral and post-doctoral level, and to build research leadership and capacity of midwives, locally, nationally and internationally.

Janine Stockdale is Lecturer in Midwifery at Trinity College, Dublin, Ireland and a Research Fellow of the Royal College of Midwives, England, UK. Her primary research interests include the psychology of breastfeeding, the role of motivation, development of women-centred interventions and the psychology of learning. Janine maintains collaborative research interests with colleagues at the University of Ulster and in the USA.

Denis Walsh is Associate Professor in Midwifery at the University of Nottingham, England, UK. He lectures and runs courses for midwives internationally on evidence and skills for normal birth, and is widely published on midwifery issues and normal birth. Qualitative research methods – in particular, ethnography, phenomenology and metasynthesis – are his areas of methodology expertise.

PART I

Theoretical Basis for Practice

Signposting Future Developments in Midwifery Theory, Practice and Research

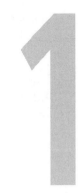

Rosamund Bryar and Marlene Sinclair

Introduction

Midwives have been challenged by Kirkham to develop and understand the theory base of midwifery practice:

> Beyond this there is much that needs to be done in midwifery research and the subsequent development of midwifery concepts and theory. There is little time to do this, for the majority of midwives are now vastly limited in their practice by the nature of their setting. But midwifery researchers drawing upon the knowledge of those midwives who still retain a degree of autonomy in their practice could feed much of value into midwifery education, as well as raising our consciousness by showing us the nature of our own practice. (Kirkham, 1989: 136)

This book is part of the response to this challenge. In this first chapter, we set the scene for the discussion of theory development in midwifery, identify the issues considered in the two parts of the book, outline the structure of the following chapters and introduce the interactive nature of the book. We hope that, by working through the activities at the end of each chapter, when you return to the final activity at the end of this chapter you will feel that your understanding and excitement about theory for midwifery practice will have been challenged, deepened and developed.

Midwives and midwifery

The word 'midwife' means 'with woman'. We are all very familiar with this definition – but what does it mean? Descriptions of midwives' activities with women identify midwives' empathy; their openness; their awareness of the feelings, thoughts and processes that a woman and her family are experiencing. Skills of observation are acute: the midwife watches patiently and with love; palpates and touches with sensitivity and kindness; listens with attention and time; smells with understanding and concern.

Midwives are described as special people with special attributes, wise women; in some cultures, only women who are mothers themselves can become midwives. To be a midwife is to use the self, the person who is the midwife, in the practice of midwifery and the care of women and their families. Being a midwife becomes an inextricable part of who the person is: dependant on individual personalities, experiences and beliefs but all, if they are 'good' midwives, will have, as part of their nature, the empathetic, intuitive, 'with woman' approach to midwifery practice. Midwifery identifies clearly that the practice of midwifery is dependent on the use of the self by the midwife.

Descriptions of midwifery practice and discussions with midwives emphasize the intuitive, the empathetic nature of the midwife's care, rather than the theoretical underpinnings to their practice. The sensitive midwife, who listens and hears, palpates and understands, observes and comprehends, uses her personal attributes but is able to collect and interpret information through the use of skills acquired through midwifery education and practice, to compare the information collected with knowledge and experience acquired through life, midwifery education and practice.

Midwives have been provided with a surfeit of midwifery textbooks containing both experiential and research-based knowledge that describe the knowledge base of midwifery practice. Both Ina May Gaskin (2002) and Elizabeth Davis (2004), two empathetic and experiential midwives, emphasize the knowledge required to support women during childbearing in their respective books, which can be categorized as textbooks of midwifery practice. Textbooks describe, for example, physiological theories of labour and the production of breast milk; psychological theories of attachment and loss; sociological theories of social roles, and many others. If the day-to-day practice of midwives is observed, they can be seen, for example, explaining the process of foetal development to parents, based on their knowledge of intrauterine growth, or helping a woman decide on the appropriate method of pain relief, based on their knowledge of the physiology of labour.

The ability of the midwife to 'be with' the woman and her family may be based on personal, empathetic, intuitive qualities, but the ability to help is based on the use of these qualities in combination with knowledge, with theory and with thinking about practice. In fact, this is the great achievement of the skilled, intuitive midwife: to be able to use the extensive knowledge base of midwifery and, at the same time, to care for the woman, her family and community in a sensitive, loving way. These midwives are the skilled, knowledgeable craftspeople who care for and love the tools and the medium with which they work (Sennett, 2008).

Knowledge and theory at first appear to be anti-empathetic, anti-intuitive, anti-, in Elizabeth Davis's (2004) term, being open. Anti- all those attributes that midwives see as being central to midwifery care and anti- all the personal attributes that midwives feel they demonstrate in their care; that is, anti- our image of ourselves as people. This attitude says that you can either be empathetic, intuitive and 'with woman', or you can be a theorist, use models and thus be distant, detached from women. In fact, those midwives who are intuitive, empathetic and who love and care for women are probably those who are most concerned to gain new knowledge, to read, to question, to undertake research. They have such concern for the women and families with whom they are involved that they feel that the care they give must be based on the most up-to-date knowledge. This may be the most recent midwifery research about information needs in labour, physiological research about foetal blood circulation, or it may be knowledge about complementary therapies that may relieve depression and stress in pregnancy. Whatever the discipline or source of knowledge, these midwives are concerned to provide the most effective evidence-informed care for women.

These midwives are also concerned to develop knowledge. Through their empathetic observation of women throughout the childbearing process, they build up a huge stock of knowledge about the process of childbearing and the needs of women and, through this process, develop practice theory. Through reflection, further observation and more reflection, they are able to make predictions about the type of care that will be most suitable, for which women, under what circumstances, and can put forward theories of practice. They are able, in research and theory-building terms, to make statements about causal relationships between concepts. They can make statements, for example, about the relationship between immersion in water in the first stage of labour and dilation of the cervix and pain relief. Their close observation and concern makes it possible for them to make such statements which they, and others, can then test and develop into models or theories of midwifery care (see Chapter 2).

Skilled midwifery care results from the combination of the personal qualities of the midwife with knowledge, theory, reflection and thinking about how theory and knowledge can best be used in the care of the individual woman (Mander and Fleming, 2009). Theory provides the tools for the job. Theory provides a structure within which midwives can compare the present experiences of the woman they are caring for with the responses identified in the theory. Theory for practice sensitizes midwives to the things that they should be watching for, and helps to identify those factors that are central from those that are less important. The use of theory involves the comparison of the experiences of the woman with knowledge and theory from midwifery practice and from a range of disciplines. Midwives make this comparison through thinking about women, and thinking about the theories they hold about the behaviour and needs of women. This thinking leads to the development of practice theory and theories for practice. The quality of the thinking that midwives undertake will have a direct effect on their actions, their care of the woman, her family and the community.

This book is about understanding theory generation, theory testing and theory in practice. Midwifery care is essentially practical, and much of the learning about midwifery focuses on the development of practical, interpersonal skills. These skills are developed through a process that must include thinking. Less attention has been paid to the process of thinking, the need for reflection, and the development of midwifery theory, than to the actual doing of midwifery. Socrates, the son of a midwife, in Plato's *Theaetetus* describes himself as a midwife of ideas, helping others to bring forth ideas, but not himself giving birth to ideas, in the same way that a midwife helps a woman to give birth:

> My art of midwifery is in general like theirs; the only difference is that my patients are men, not women, and my concerns are not with the body but with the soul that is in travail of birth. And the highest point of my art is the power to prove by every test whether the offspring of a young man's thought is a false phantom or instinct with life and truth. I am so far like the midwife, that I cannot myself give birth to wisdom; and the common reproach is true, that, though I question others, I can myself bring nothing to light because there is no wisdom in me. The reason is this: heaven constrains me to serve as a midwife, but has debarred me from giving birth. So of myself I have no sort of wisdom, nor has any discovery ever been born to me as the child of my soul. (Cornford, 1946: 26)

Working with the book

The aim of this book is to help midwives to value the contribution that theory can make to midwifery knowledge and practice. Midwives need to clarify 'where they are coming from', to make explicit to themselves and to others the basis for their practice: the values, attitudes, skills and knowledge that combine in midwifery care. This book is an aid to this process. It aims to help midwives think about the basis of their practice and the conditions that are necessary for midwifery care; to help in the thinking about the underlying concepts or theories of practice and to consider the use of those concepts or theories in the tools they use in their everyday practice. Much of this underlying theory and the concepts of everyday practice are generally hidden from discussion and from view, sometimes even hidden from the person who holds them! If these theories, concepts and models can be identified and discussed, they form a way of aiding communication between midwives, the childbearing woman and her family, and other practitioners, helping to identify shared meanings and values. One way of clarifying the meaning of midwifery is to examine the basis and context of care. In Box 1.1, we have identified a number of questions that might help you and those you work with begin to explore these issues.

In this book, the aim is to discuss these and other questions, to work towards an understanding of the context of midwifery care, to consider the need for shared meanings or, at least, the discussion of different meanings and ways of putting these shared meanings into practice through the utilization of models and theories of caring and practice.

Box 1.1   Questions to start the process of theory development

- How do I think about women and about myself?
- What are the needs of women in the process of childbearing, childbirth and, later, in child rearing?
- Do I consider all the needs that women and their families may have, or do I tend to focus on one area of need?
- If I focus on one area, why is that?
- What knowledge do I use in caring for women?
- What constraints do I experience from day to day In caring for childbearing women?
- What is the contribution of other members of the multidisciplinary team to the care of the childbearing woman and her child?
- How much responsibility do I want?
- How much responsibility do women want?
- How do I help women exercise control in their care?
- Do I have polemic views on normal and technological birth?
- What are my views about care, empowerment, choice, holism, equality and continuity?
- What are the views of my midwifery and other colleagues' about these concepts? Do we share the same views? Have we ever discussed them?

You need to make this book work for you. We want to make you think intuitively, theoretically and critically about the art and science of all that is 'midwifery'. We do not know the values that you hold: you have to bring them to the surface yourself. We cannot reflect on your practice for you: you have to do that. We cannot know the context within which you practice midwifery: you have to identify the supports and constraints there yourself. We cannot know the theories that you have developed from your own practice: you have to describe them yourself. All we can do is bring together contributions from a wide range of people and sources that we hope will help you in your thinking about midwifery practice (or action), and the theory/theoretical research contributing to that practice. This material will help you to consider the theoretical tools that you use in your practice, and may contribute to making these theories more coherent to yourself and to others. Your thinking about these issues will then contribute to the wider debate within midwifery and the search for a language or languages for midwifery practice.

The central contention of this book is that thinking affects practice: that the mental pictures that we each hold affect our practice, and that the mental pictures underpinning the organizations within which we work and provide care (and which we may or may not share) have a profound effect on the care experienced by childbearing women. This book seeks to help clarify the questions: How do I care? How do you care? What impact does that have on the woman's experience of care?

Organization of the book

There are two themes that permeate this book: the role of the midwife, and the needs of the childbearing woman. It is the premise of the book that a clearer understanding of the concepts, theories and models that inform midwifery care will result in a better understanding of the role of the midwife, the type of care that women need and provision of that care. All the chapters are therefore concerned with the process of clarifying and identifying these concepts, theories and models. The exercises at the end of each chapter may be undertaken by individuals or groups as part of this process of clarification and theory building.

The first edition was published in 1995 and since that date there has been a huge expansion in the amount of work on the development and application of theory to midwifery practice. There has been an increase in the amount of midwifery research that has tested and developed theory, and a focus on theory is now central to the initial preparation of midwives and their development at master's level. The content of this book reflects these developments.

The book is organized in two parts. In Part I, following this chapter, there are three chapters that provide the context for Part II of the book. In Chapter 2, some of the terms – such as theory, philosophy, models and concepts – are explored and defined. The central concepts that inform the practice of midwifery are also considered with the process of developing theory and the question: Where does theory come from? The chapter concludes by examining two theories that have a considerable impact on practice: the medical model, and the model of pregnancy as a normal life event. Chapter 3 focuses on a number of midwifery theorists and theory development work by a number of midwives. In the first edition of this book, the theorists considered were all, apart from Jean Ball, from the USA. In this chapter, we could have included now the work of a number of midwifery theorists from the UK, Australia, New Zealand and other parts of the world, many of whom have written chapters for the second part of the book. This chapter roots the book in theory development from the 1940s onwards, and includes the current theory development work of Soo Downe and colleagues and the work that led to the first edition of this book by Rosamund Bryar. Theory, as outlined in Chapter 2, may be developed deductively or inductively. The value of theory from other disciplines to midwifery practice is illustrated in Chapter 4. This chapter, the final chapter in Part I, introduces motivational theory, a psychological theory. Janine Stockdale and co-authors provide a detailed examination of the concepts that form this theory, describing the potential application of motivational theory in the work of midwives in supporting women to breastfeed.

Part II consists of 10 chapters illustrating the development and application of theory to midwifery practice, written largely by midwives. This section demonstrates the enormous growth in theory development in midwifery over the past decades – in particular, in the middle-range theories. The first chapter in Part II, Chapter 5, is written by Janine Stockdale and co-authors, and provides a description of the research that she undertook to test the application of motivational theory to the support of women breastfeeding. The utility of this approach, and the potential that use of this theory has to enable mothers and midwives, is amply demonstrated. With Chapter 4, this chapter illustrates the utility of theory from other disciplines and one approach to applying such theory to practice issues. Chapter 6, by Lynn Jones and Sally Kendall, may seem rather challenging, as the theory base used moves away from more familiar sociological or psychological theories to theory involved in furniture design. Lynn Jones is a furniture designer and undertook her PhD, supervized by Sally Kendall, on the development of a chair to facilitate breastfeeding. The chapter illustrates the value of combining qualitative research with knowledge from other disciplines and, in this case, has resulted in the manufacture of a chair making use of these different theory bases.

The development of theory and models for practice often involves research activity and the research experience is often presented in publications as being a non-contentious activity. Billie Hunter, well-known for her work in developing our understanding of normal birth, provides a description in Chapter 7 of the reality of undertaking research concerned with examining emotion in midwifery work. She explores the many dilemmas, from her anxiety at challenging received wisdom concerning emotional labour, to her questions about the relevance of research methods and her conclusions about the need not to be afraid to ask questions of every aspect of the research process, as only by doing this will theory be tested and refined.

The subsequent three chapters are concerned with exploring the concepts that support and facilitate the birth experience. In Chapter 8, Denis Walsh illustrates the development of theory concerning the centrality of the concepts of caring, nesting and matresence through detailed qualitative research using observation of birth in a birth centre. This chapter also provides evidence of the importance of environment in the context of birth, a theme reflected in a number of the subsequent chapters. In Chapter 9, Kerri Schuiling and co-authors explore the concept of comfort, demonstrating the use of quantitative methods to test the Comfort Theory developed by one of the co-authors, Kathryn Kolcaba (1994). While a number of the chapters in Part II are concerned with naming concepts, this chapter describes research into testing the evidence of the relevance of the concepts in a theory, Comfort Theory, to women in labour, the next stage of the theory development process. Chapter 10 presents a developed theory of midwifery practice, Birth Territory Theory, developed by a group of midwives in Australia (Fahy et al., 2008). The chapter introduces the concepts that combine to form the theory, and the development of the theory through observation of care is illustrated. This chapter demonstrates the wide range of knowledge that theories may draw on and, while some of the ideas may be unfamiliar or challenging to some, this presentation illustrates the range of theoretical positions held by midwives that will influence and inform their care.

Kenda Crozier and Marlene Sinclair, in Chapter 11, also demonstrate the work of building on and testing theory, extending the theory developed by Marlene Sinclair in her PhD work. In this chapter, these authors demonstrate the need for, and the range of methods that are helpful in testing and refining theory. They demonstrate the use of the Hybrid Method of Concept

Development in studying the roles of midwives in supporting women in labour who need technological interventions (Swartz-Barcott and Kim, 2000). The three models of midwifery practice that emerge from this work relate closely to the discussion of the impact of the elements included in the action approach to organizations discussed in Chapter 3, and are reinforced by Billie Hunter's work reported in Chapter 7.

The process of examining practice through interrogation and synthesis of evidence from the literature, from pre-existing theory, is demonstrated in Chapter 12, in which Michelle Kealy and Pranee Laimputtong consider issues related to decision-making around the need for Caesarean section. They present a challenging analysis that has the potential to stimulate thinking about everyday practice and questions for research.

Throughout this book, the concern is with the practice of midwifery and the self of the midwife is identified, in this chapter and in Chapter 2, as being central to the care that is given. Chapter 13 is concerned with the environment that supports or undermines the individual midwife. Patricia Gillen and colleagues have examined the experiences midwives have of being bullied in the workplace. They demonstrate the use of Walker and Avant's (2004) concept development framework to examine the concept of bullying and the process of research undertaken that led to refining the definition of bullying (Royal College of Midwives, 1996), and identification of additional attributes of the concept from the research. As these authors conclude, bullying has a profound impact on the individual midwife and, potentially, has a profound impact on the type of care she is able to provide for women.

Chapter 14, by Rosemary Mander, concludes Part II and provides an analysis of concepts that are held dear by midwives: 'with women' and 'partnership'. She examines the partnership model developed and implemented in New Zealand, and shows that theory building, theory testing and use are not neutral activities but, rather, may be very political. This chapter provides another and different perspective on the utility of theory in and for practice, and suggests the need for close examination of the origins of theories.

A point needs to be made about the use of language. Midwives may be female or male, and efforts have been made to refer to midwives in the plural to avoid identification of midwives as female or male. The identification of midwives as female has only occurred when discussing midwifery practice in periods or countries where it is, or was, an exclusively female activity.

The process of building midwifery theory

Theory building is incremental. To provide an idea of the current extent of literature on midwifery theory, we undertook a database search in 2010 of papers on midwifery theory generation and midwifery theory testing. To do this, we contacted the chief librarian at the Royal College of Midwives and the subject librarian at Ulster University to support us as we undertook a comprehensive and systematized review of the literature on midwifery theory, midwifery concepts, midwifery models and midwifery theorists. We were advised to use three electronic databases: CINAHL (Cumulative Index to Nursing and Allied Health Literature), Medline, and the British Nursing Index. We discovered 'midwifery theory' was not a medical subject heading (MeSH) in any of the databases. Papers were selected if the abstracts indicated that they were likely to provide relevant data on applied, tested or developed theory within the context of midwifery practice.

CINAHL

'Midwifery' was not a MeSH or a subject heading. Searches for key words 'midwifery theory', 'midwifery concepts' and 'nurse-midwifery theoretical constructs' produced no results; this did not change using smart searching techniques. We also undertook a key word search using 'theory generation' combined with 'nurse midwife', and the result was zero. MeSH 'nurse midwives' was a subject heading in CINAHL and produced 1292 papers. Theory was added and exploded to include all terms resulting in 76,000 hits that were reduced to 58 when we added 'theory testing' and 'theory genera- tion'. The abstracts were downloaded and read, and it was found that 10 papers were relevant to midwifery practice.

OVID Medline

'Nurse-midwifery' was a MeSH, but 'midwifery' was filed under 'nurse specialties'. The search was replicated and a potential pool of 5407 papers was identified. This was reduced to 82 when the key words 'midwifery theory', 'midwifery concepts' and 'nurse-midwifery theoretical constructs' were added. This was further reduced to 37 when 'theory generation', 'theory develop- ment' and 'theory testing' were added.

British Nursing Index

'Nurse midwifery' was not a MeSH, and a key word search revealed no papers under this umbrella term. A key word search for 'midwifery' and 'nurse- midwifery' revealed 189 papers. The terms were exploded and a pool of 2472 papers became available. However, when 'theory generation' and 'theory development' and 'theory testing' were added, this was reduced to 29.

Although this search generated a small number of papers, it was encourag- ing that many have been published in recent years – demonstrating, as do the authors in this book, the continuing growth and development of midwifery theory building and testing. As many of the authors of the chapters here acknowledge, they are often building on or challenging work undertaken by others. In Chapters 2 and 3, in particular, we have deliberately reminded the reader of the contribution to our knowledge that has been gleaned from the work of early researchers in the field. It is extremely important to do so, as we need to be reminded of the value of research or reference materials that are over 10 years old. These may be more difficult to source by means than through Internet searches, but they provide a foundation for our current work, helping the process of incremental building and thus the future stability of our knowledge building for midwifery practice.

In this book, we provide a solid foundation for the future development and testing of midwifery theory. We believe that the art and science of midwifery must be equally valued and evidence-supported for post modern "Y" generation women to make truly informed choices about their birthing experience, in partnership with midwives and doctors. This poses considerable challenges:

- asking answerable and appropriate questions about our knowledge base
- keeping our focus on searching rigorously for the 'truth'
- assembling new knowledge into meaningful explanations and laws or theories
- applying, testing and evaluating these theories and their relationships to practice education and research, prior to building foundational models for 'midwifery'.

A concrete foundation needs to be built with proportionate amounts of the right ingredients and, in midwifery, we require three key substances: education, research and practice. Each of these must be equally balanced and carefully monitored in order to produce the desired outcome – a solid evidence base on which to build midwifery practice with pillars of knowledge. The evidence in the book demonstrates theory derivation, theory generation, theory application, theory development, theory testing, theory evaluation and theory synthesis. However, it is important to remember the purpose of a theory and its limitations. A theory should provide auditable and transparent data on its concepts, attributes and empirical referents, as well as proposed tentative relationships or theoretical assumptions. Describing a theory and its application is similar to the production of a map in which the cartographer helps the navigator to visualize the journey and see the dimensions, connections and boundaries. This is very helpful, but it is mostly of 'extrinsic 'value. It is only after experiencing the journey equipped with your own personal knowledge, skill and attitude that you really know and understand the 'intrinsic' value of 'doing' and move more towards becoming enlightened. It is our hope that, through your experience of doing, of engaging with this book and the exercises, you will develop your abilities in the critical analysis and evaluation of theory, and be confident and competent to question the value, relevance and 'fit for purpose' contribution of any theory for midwifery practice.

Conclusion

In this chapter, some of the issues have been raised that need to be considered in any discussion of theory building. It has been argued that midwifery theory needs to be thought about and placed centrally in any discussions of midwifery practice. The interactive nature of this book has been presented: when you reach the end of the book, if you have undertaken the activities you should have a clearer idea of your own models and theories of and for midwifery practice. The structure and content of the book has been described. This book is not a prescription for 'doing' or 'applying' theory. This book is a challenge to you and your thinking about midwifery theory, research and practice. Our message to you is: 'Change the world of midwifery care that you live in by changing the way you think'.

ACTIVITIES

To be undertaken when you begin this book

Undergraduate

Consider the content of this introductory chapter and, before you proceed to the next chapter, challenge yourself to answer the questions in Box 1.1.

Postgraduate

Imagine you have the freedom to create a strategy for developing the knowledge, skills and attitudes of midwives with regard to theory. Using the seminal work of Bloom (1956) and Marzano and Kendall (2007) design a plan of activities to inspire and encourage them to move from simple knowledge acquisition to evaluation and creation of new knowledge.

Bloom, B.S. (1956) *Taxonomy of Educational Objectives, Handbook I: The Cognitive Domain.* New York, NY: David McKay.

Marzano, R.J. and Kendall, J.S. (2007) *The New Taxonomy of Educational Objectives*, 2nd edn. Thousand Oaks, CA: Sage.

To be undertaken when you finish reading the book

Having read and worked through the chapters, we suggest you re-read this chapter and undertake the following activities.

Undergraduate

Undertake a systematic search of current electronic databases from 1950 to the present and search for: 'midwifery theory'; add 'models and theories in midwifery'; add 'testing midwifery theory'; add 'generating midwifery theory' and combine.

Save your search strategy and creatively explore other possibilities – such as the inclusion of 'nurse midwife' and 'nurse theorists', use non-academic search engines – to develop an awareness of the challenges involved in searching for relevant literature from both academic and non-academic Internet-based resources.

Postgraduate

Consider the contribution of this book to knowledge development and ask yourself: 'How can midwifery make the necessary connections between the knowledge shared in these chapters to produce a solid foundation for building the future of midwifery?' Read the short editorial by Sinclair (2007).

Sinclair, M. (2007) 'A Guide to understanding Theoretical and Conceptual Frameworks', *Evidence Based Midwifery*, 5(2): 39.   *cont.*

Also, consider the following key questions:

- What do I know about the phenomenon that I want to study?
- What types of knowledge are available to me (empirical, non-empirical, tacit, intuitive, moral or ethical)?
- What theory will best guide my midwifery practice?
- Is this theory proven through theory-linked research?
- What other theories are relevant to this practice?
- How can I apply these theories and findings in practice?

Finally, we suggest you revisit the seminal work of Silva (1986). In this paper, Silva publishes unique data from a systematic exploration of American literature from 1952–85 (62 published papers) in which research had been used to test theories. Although these were mostly nursing theories, the approach and the selection criteria used are relevant and replicable for midwifery today. We propose that you repeat this literature search for 'midwifery theory' from 1952 to the current year, applying the following inclusion criteria:

- papers in which the research determined the validity of the assumptions/ propositions in a theory
- theory as an explicit framework for the research
- whether the relationship between theory and the study hypotheses is clear
- whether research hypotheses were deduced clearly from the assumptions of the theory
- whether research hypotheses were tested in an appropriate manner
- whether research provided indirect evidence as to the validity of the assumptions/prepositions of the theory
- whether the evidence was discussed in terms of how it supported, refuted or explained theory.

Silva, M.C. (1986) 'Research Testing Nursing Theory: State of the art advances', Nursing Science, 9(1): 1–11.

References

Cornford, F.M. (1946) *Plato's Theory of Knowledge*. London: Kegan Paul/Trench, Trubner & Co.

Davis, E. (2004) *Heart and Hands. A Midwife's Guide to Pregnancy and Birth*, 4th edn. Berkeley, CA: Celestial Arts.

Fahy, K., Foureur, M. and Hastie, C. (eds) (2008) *Birth Territory and Midwifery Guardianship*. Edinburgh: Elsevier.

Gaskin, I.M. (2002) *Spiritual Midwifery*, 4th edn. Summertown: Book Publishing Company.

Kirkham, M. (1989) 'Midwives and Information-Giving during Labour', in S. Robinson and A.M. Thomson (eds), *Midwives, Research and Childbirth, Volume I*. London: Chapman & Hall, ch. 6: 117–38.

Kolcaba, K. (1994) 'A Theory of Holistic Comfort for Nursing', *Journal of Advanced Nursing*, 19(6): 1178–84.

Mander, R. and Fleming, V. (2009) *Becoming a Midwife*. London: Routledge.

Royal College of Midwives (1996) *In Place of Fear: Recognising and Confronting the Problem of Bullying in Midwifery*. London: RCM.

Sennett, R. (2008) *The Craftsman*. Harmondsworth: Penguin Books.

Swartz-Barcott, D. and Kim, H.S. (2000) 'An Expansion and Elaboration of the Hybrid Model of Concept Development', in B.L. Rogers and K.A. Knafl (eds), *Concept Development in Nursing*. Philadelphia, PA: Saunders, ch. 9: 129–60.

Walker, L.O. and Avant, K.C. (2004) *Strategies for Theory Construction in Nursing*, 4th edn. Norwalk, CT: Appleton Lange.

Conceptualizing Midwifery

2

Rosamund Bryar and Marlene Sinclair

Key points

- Theory building terms are defined
- Different approaches to theory building outlined
- Comparison made between the 'medical' and 'pregnancy as normal life-event' models
- The models of practice midwives hold are important for the care they provide.

Introduction

The purpose of this chapter is to consider some of the words and ideas used in thinking about theory and practice:

- What is meant by the terms 'philosophy', 'paradigm', 'conceptual model', 'theory' and 'concept'?
- How do these terms relate to each other?
- Where does theory come from and how is it described?
- How can an understanding of these terms contribute to understanding of the day-to-day practice of the midwife, and how can this enhance the experience a woman has of midwifery care?

The process of theory development is then outlined. The chapter concludes with a comparison of 'the medical model' (birth as normal, in retrospect), and the 'pregnancy as normal life-event model', and the consequences of these models for midwifery care.

Thinking underpinning practice

Fundamental to this chapter and the whole book is the view that individual and collective beliefs held by midwives influence the care that they provide. As Wessell and Ellis comment:

> In all his writings, Grantly Dick-Read spoke not of a 'method' of childbirth, but of a philosophy of life, of which birth is just a part, although a most essential part. He believed that the quality of the birth experience influenced (for good or ill) not only the child, but the family into which he or she was born. He stated that the childbirth practices of a nation were reflections of that nation's beliefs concerning the integrity and dignity of life, and influenced that nation for good or ill, and that ultimately the world itself is affected. (Dick-Read, Wessel and Ellis, 1987: 2)

When a midwife undertakes any activity and provides care, that activity is undertaken in the light of the midwife's personal understanding, knowledge and theories. First, the midwife has to have an understanding of the need or problem that requires attention. This understanding will be based on previous experience of such needs and what has been previously learnt about such needs (the knowledge base). The midwife will be able to state or define the need. Next, the midwife will have an understanding of the action that might alleviate the problem or reduce the need. Midwives will also have an understanding of their ability or the ability of their colleagues to meet the need.

For example, if a woman is experiencing a primary post-partum haemorrhage, she will have a range of physiological needs relating to sudden blood-loss. She will also have psychological needs relating to anxiety about her own safety, and concerns for her newborn baby and partner. It is known that immediate action has to be taken to halt the haemorrhage and restore fluid balance. Midwives also know that they will need the assistance of obstetric colleagues to care for the woman in this emergency situation. At the same time, the woman and her partner must be provided with support and information.

The actions carried out in this situation are preceded by thought that brings together the knowledge needed to meet and to respond to the situation. If one of the elements is omitted in the actions, the care provided may be less satisfactory. For example, if the haemorrhage is stopped but no attempt is made to restore fluid balance, the woman may suffer further complications or, if treatment is provided without adequate reassurance and explanation to the woman or her partner, one or both may suffer long-term anxieties.

This thinking and reflection about the action provides a theory about the best way of meeting the need (practice theory). Thinking about the outcome of the actions – how quickly the woman recovered, the way that different members of the health team worked together, or the woman's reaction to her care – can lead to modification and development of the theory, which can then be tested and developed further in other practical situations where haemorrhage occurs. In this way, a practice theory becomes a theory of or for practice. The thinking and reflection on this recent incident, combined with information from earlier incidents, may help to overcome one problem about this approach to theory development, which is the influence of more recent events or experiences on practice. More recent events will be clearer in the memory, and the theory developed following these events may be applied to the present experience of haemorrhage. However, it may be that the present haemorrhage might be more similar to other haemorrhages experienced some time ago, and the theory developed following these experiences may be more appropriate to the present care. In-depth reflection, which brings together theory from past experiences with theory developed from the present experience, will integrate the knowledge from this range of experiences and ameliorate the effect of recency.

In this example, the midwife has brought together pre-existing knowledge combined with previous experience to provide a theory of what action should be taken to enable immediate, appropriate care to be provided. This combination of knowledge with experience is one of the characteristics of the expert practitioner (Hardy et al., 2009) and demonstrates skills in reflection (Gibbs, 1988; Cronin and Rawlings-Anderson, 2004). Agyris and Schön (1974) describe this type of theory as a theory-in-use, and it is this type of theory (practice theory) that Benner and Wrubel (1989) seek to expose in descriptions of exemplars of nursing practice. Luker (1988) describes these models as 'working models' that the individual nurse or midwife uses in their own practice. Theory, in this sense, is intimately bound up with practice being developed from the articulation of the practice of midwifery or nursing, and is termed 'practice theory' (Pearson, 1992). This description demonstrates the use of two types of theory in practice: the use of knowledge from other disciplines; and knowledge derived from practice, practice theory or theory-in-use. This description excludes reference to another type of the theory: that derived from the general or grand models of nursing.

In 1991, Chinn and Kramer proposed there had been a shift in nursing theory towards the development of practice and research-based theory, away from the more general or grand 'theories' (conceptual models) of nursing. This differentiation of two forms of theory development is important for an understanding of the development and role of theory in midwifery. In their most recent book, Chinn and Kramer (2008) restate the value of theory to practice and refer to a summary of the development of nursing theory that includes descriptions of the general or grand 'theories' (conceptual models) of nursing developed by theorists including Roy, Orem, Wiedenbach, Neuman and many others. Alligood and Marriner-Tomey (2006) and Marriner-Tomey and Alligood (2006) have similarly examined the work of a range of nurse theorists, including that of Ramona T. Mercer (see Chapter 3), and demonstrate the value of these theories and models.

Midwives and nurse-midwives have concentrated on understanding practice, and midwives have called for theory that is based in practice (Kirkham 1989; Price and Price, 1993). Midwives and nurse-midwives have focused on developing and testing middle-range predictive theories of aspects of midwifery practice that have considerable potential utility (Lehrman, 1989) (see Chapter 3 and Part II). It is interesting to speculate why midwives may have taken this approach to theory development in contrast to their nursing colleagues. Midwives may have always been more concerned with the practice of midwifery, rather than theorizing about that care. The grand or general models of nursing, because of their very generality, may appear to lack immediate practical relevance, which may also have deterred midwives from developing models for midwifery along similar lines. Midwives, in this sense, may be seen to have leapfrogged the grand-model development stage and moved to the stage of developing or, in Smith's (1991) term, discovering practice theory that, in recent years, has become central to nursing theory development (Benner and Wrubel, 1989; Rolfe, 1996).

Defining terms

Philosophy

Philosophy is a discipline concerned with exploring and postulating explanations for reality (Chinn and Kramer, 1991). There are a large number of philosophical approaches to this thinking about reality, including religious traditions, Marxism, existentialism and phenomenology (Pearson and Vaughan, 1986; Rhodes, 1988). In relation to thinking about midwifery practice, the need is for each midwife to identify their personal philosophy or philosophies of life and midwifery practice. These philosophies will be based on wider philosophies or ways of describing reality found in the general community as the midwife is a person, as well as a midwife, and the attitudes, values and beliefs that midwives hold result from their membership of a particular community and society, as well as from their secondary socialization into the world of midwifery practice. Pearson and Vaughan describe a philosophy as both the pursuit of knowledge and a description of personal beliefs:

> So philosophy can be interpreted as the pursuit of wisdom or knowledge about the things around us and what causes them. A philosophy is an explicit statement about what you believe and about what values you hold. These values and beliefs will, in turn, affect the way you behave. (Pearson and Vaughan, 1986: 8)

There has been a great deal of activity in midwifery units and teams to generate ward, unit or team 'philosophies'. Downe commented on this and urged midwives to avoid the simplistic notion of devising a 'philosophy for midwifery' that is forgotten once it is filed in the procedure book and, instead, to think honestly about their beliefs and values, their philosophy, and the consequences of their philosophy for care:

> It [the midwife's philosophy] must be an expression of our honest thoughts about what midwifery means to us. For example, if we use a medical model, what are the consequences for the women we serve? Are they different if we use a midwifery model of care? (Downe, 1991: 3)

Downe (1991) emphasizes the need to make beliefs about midwifery practice explicit. One way to do this is to consider the types of knowledge that combine to make up the philosophy that the midwife might hold of midwifery care. Carper (1992) (in an article originally published in 1978) describes four types of knowledge that underpin the practice of nursing: empirics, nursing science; aesthetics, the art of nursing; personal knowledge; and ethics, the moral component.

Nursing science is described as the knowledge and theories about nursing that explain and inform nursing care. This knowledge is in the process of being developed, so it is not possible to say that nursing shares one common world view or paradigm to explain nursing practice. Carper (1992) uses the example of the change in the definition of health – to a definition that sees health as more than the absence of disease – as an example of a radical rethinking of health, which is now thought of as a process or continuum rather than a static state. This way of thinking about health then leads to new possibilities for interventions by the nurse (or midwife) to support people in moving along the health continuum.

The aesthetic, the art, is more difficult to describe and, Carper suggests, has been given less attention, as this type of knowing is associated with the (now-deprecated) apprenticeship system of learning in which (under the best circumstances) the student gained knowledge about the less tangible aspects of care from observation and interaction with skilled practitioners. Aesthetics is the appreciation of beauty and, as Titchen and Hardy (2009: 68) comment: '... aesthetics enables the giving of care that is not only effective but also pleasing to give and receive and which potentially enhances human flourishing for the giver and receiver.'

Rhodes argues strongly for the recognition of the aesthetic component of nurse-midwifery practice and for the study of the philosophy of aesthetics. She comments:

> Through aesthetics we can come to understand the various meanings of 'art' and begin to apply these concepts to scholarly and clinical work. It is the art of nurse-midwifery that will distinguish us from other obstetrical/gynecologic practitioners and philosophically make our research nurse-midwifery research. We must begin to explicate in scholarly works the value and relationship of aesthetics to the discipline of nurse-midwifery and nurse-midwifery practice. (Rhodes, 1988: 284)

The third type of knowledge that Carper (1992) describes is personal knowledge. This is considered the most difficult to articulate but is concerned with the individual nurse's or midwife's knowledge of themselves: 'Personal knowledge is concerned with the knowing, encountering and actualizing of the concrete, individual self. One does not know about the self; one strives simply to know the self' (Carper, 1992: 220). This personal knowledge is vital if nurses and midwives are going to be able to avoid objectifying people and to use themselves in the therapeutic relationship (Carper 1992). Midwives whose personal philosophy of themselves is that they should be open and intuitive with women for whom they are caring will clearly provide different care from midwives whose view is that a more detached attitude should be taken (for example, see Chapter 8).

The final type of knowledge that Carper (1992) describes is ethical knowledge, which is concerned with moral codes and provides the basis for ethical decision-making in practice. Combined, these four types of knowing (midwifery science; the art of midwifery; the personal knowledge of the midwife; and the ethical, moral component) describe and demonstrate the values, beliefs and philosophy of care held by the individual midwife.

Clarification of these four patterns of knowing may assist midwives in articulating their philosophies of midwifery care and of life. This is an essential first step in describing practice theories, which will be fundamentally affected by personal philosophies; in choosing between pre-existing conceptual models, some of which will be closer to one's own personal philosophy than others; and in developing models for midwifery care.

Conceptual models

Conceptual models provide an abstract representation of the ideas upon which a discipline is based. Conceptual models or conceptual frameworks of nursing are: 'abstract models of what nursing is, or should be' (Aggleton and Chalmers, 1986: 4). Conceptual models are constructed in various ways but may bring together information and insights from a variety of disciplines, from personal and general philosophies, from observation of practice and from research, to help provide a framework within which practice, education and research in a discipline can be better understood and around which these three activities can be organized.

Fawcett (2005: 16) defines a conceptual model as: 'a set of relatively abstract and general concepts that address the phenomena of central interest to a discipline, the propositions that broadly describe those concepts, and the propositions that state relatively abstract and general relations between two or more of the concepts'. Fawcett comments (2006: 500) that different conceptual models provide different ways of looking at nursing practice and: 'Each conceptual model of nursing, then, provides an alternative guide to the way that nurses work with patients.' Similarly, the conceptual models discussed later in this book provide alternative guides to the way that midwives might interact and provide care with and for women and their families.

Models provide a framework for understanding and developing practice, for guiding actions, for organizing education and for identifying research questions to be asked. They may be represented in various ways: as mental, physical or symbolic models (Lancaster and Lancaster, 1992). A mental model is described in language that identifies the relationships between concepts. A physical model may be a representation of reality; for example, an architect's model of a birth centre, which demonstrates in physical terms the ways in which the model facilitates choice (alternative facilities), privacy, continuity, relationship to nature and other important concepts. A symbolic model may be in the form of a diagram, mathematical formulation or other representation. Robinson (1992) argues with the comparison that is sometimes made between nursing models and these models, and suggests that, while nurses and midwives use such models in their practice (including, for example, diagrams illustrating the onset of labour) conceptual models cannot be represented in this concrete way. Pearson and Vaughan (1986) consider that conceptual models are, in essence, the same as the more physical models described above but that they may be described as descriptive pictures that represent practice: 'pictures composed of ideas and values and written down in a clear way' (Pearson and Vaughan, 1986: 2).

Four ideas, or concepts, are central to all nursing/midwifery models:

- person
- health
- environment
- nursing/midwifery.

All models can be analyzed in terms of the emphasis given within each model to these elements or concepts (see, for example, Fawcett, 1984; Kershaw and Salvage, 1986; Fitzpatrick and Whall, 1989; Moody, 1990; Marriner-Tomey and Alligood, 2006; Carter, 2010). Each model gives greater or less weight to different elements. For example, the models of Florence Nightingale and Neuman emphasize the effects of the environment or society on health; for Rogers and Parse the person or individual is the central focus of their models (Marriner-Tomey and Alligood, 2006). In addition to reflecting the views of individual theorists, concern with the different elements reflects changes in society and nursing practice (Fitzpatrick and Whall, 1989).

Each of these models is concerned with the person, the individual – what are the characteristics of the person and how does the person interrelate with the world? For example, King describes the person as follows: 'Human beings are viewed as open systems interacting with the environment, each exhibiting permeable boundaries permitting an exchange of matter, energy and information' (Gonot, 1989: 273; Sieloff, 2006). Orem's view of the person is described by Johnston (1989) as follows: 'In discussing the nature of the person, she considers the person as self-reliant and responsible for self-care and the well-being of dependents. Self-care is a requirement for persons. It is the capacity to reflect upon personal experience of self and environment' (Johnston, 1989: 170; Taylor, 2006).

Similarly, each model defines and elaborates a view of the concepts of environment (society), health and nursing practice. The particular philosophical orientation of the theorist, whether nurse or midwife, will determine the way in which they define person, health, environment and their sphere of practice. Pearson and Vaughan (1986) and Carveth (1987) summarize the main traditions on which models are based and which provide a means of classification. Systems models are based on systems theory in which closed and open systems are described. These models describe the process by which the individual seeks to maintain and adapt to or cope with changes in their external and internal environments. The models developed by Roy, Neuman and King are examples of systems models (Marriner-Tomey and Alligood, 2006).

Another group of models is based on developmental theory. These models – for example, the Self-Care Deficit Theory developed by Orem – are centrally concerned with growth and change, and the function of the nurse or midwife in facilitating this process. The inclusion in the activities of living model developed by Roper *et al.* (1985) of the concept of the life span is an example of the inclusion of developmental theory in a nursing model. A number of the models developed in relation to the care of the childbearing woman that are discussed in Chapter 3 are concerned with the developmental process involved in becoming a mother and can, therefore, be classified as developmental models (Rubin, 1984; Mercer, 1986).

The models developed by Rubin (1984) and Mercer (1986) are also based on symbolic interaction theory, which is the theory that underpins the third group of nursing models. Symbolic interaction theory is concerned with the interaction between the individual and the environment, and the interpretation that the individual puts on that interaction. Individuals construct their own roles (or ways of behaving) through the process of interaction with the environment, composed of other people, their expectations and the expectations implicit in the roles held by those individuals. 'The symbolic interactionists operate on three premises: that the human being has a self; that human action is constructed by that self; that human action occurs within a social setting' (Field, 1983: 4).

These models put emphasis on understanding, empathizing with the individual's view of their world. If the process of childbearing is viewed as a process in which the woman adopts and develops new understandings of herself, her relationships and her roles (for example, as a daughter, friend and new mother), then it is clear why symbolic interaction is the basis of models concerned with attainment of the maternal role or becoming a mother (Rubin, 1984; Mercer, 1986; Meighan, 2006).

Paradigms

In much of the literature on models and theory building, the four concepts identified (person, health, environment and nursing) are described as 'metaparadigm' concepts (Fawcett, 1984; Carveth, 1987; Moody, 1990; Alligood, 2006). A paradigm is described as the world view of a discipline: 'different disciplines often use different approaches to enquiry, according to the particular world-view, and hence paradigm they pursue' (Vaughan, 1992: 10). Robinson (1992) discusses the use of the term 'paradigm' by the physicist Kuhn (1970 [1962]), who used the term to describe a world view held by a discipline; for example, physicists once held the world view that the world was flat. Changes in the paradigm that the world was flat led to a huge shift, or paradigm shift, in the science of physics. Meleis (2007) notes that Kuhn defined 'paradigm' in a number of different and conflicting ways, which provides one example of the difficulties inherent in defining the terms commonly used in theory development work.

Vaughan (1992) describes three world views: that of the natural sciences, that of naturalism and that of critical social theory. The first paradigm is that found in the basic sciences, and knowledge is developed in this paradigm through positivism and experimentation. In the naturalism paradigm, knowledge is developed through observation of the natural world and attempts to explain the world through the experience of those in it. In the third paradigm, critical social theory, the individual is placed centrally in the development of theory, which is developed by the reflection of the individual on his or her own world or their own practice. Other authors categorize paradigms in different ways. For example, McKenna and Slevin (2008) describe four paradigms: systems paradigm theories, concerned with inter-relationships in systems; interactional paradigm theories, based on symbolic interaction; the development paradigm, involving continual development and growth, and the behavioural paradigm, concerned with how people meet their needs.

The term 'paradigm' is also used by some authors (for example, Moody, 1990) to describe a conceptual model. Robinson (1992) argues that the models that have been developed in nursing do not constitute such paradigms, or world views of nursing that are held in common by many nurses, and the description of paradigms given by Vaughan (1992), would support this analysis. Philosophies and conceptual models may be considered to be derived from paradigms so that a range of conceptual models may be derived from one paradigm, as illustrated in relation to natural sciences in Table 2.1. For example, developmental models and systems models may all be described as emanating from the natural sciences world view or paradigm, while symbolic interactionist models may be seen to be based on the naturalism world view or paradigm (according to one classification approach). These conceptual models are based on and give rise to a range of theories about practice. The theories comprise a number of concepts that, when they are described in measurable terms, may be examined in practice and through research (Proctor and

Table 2.1   The relationship between paradigms, philosophies, models, theories and concepts

Natural science paradigm *Philosophies* *Conceptual models*	
Developmental models, e.g.	Systems models, e.g.

– Orem
– Roper, Logan and Tierney
  |
	– Roy
	– Neuman
	  |

A range of theories derived from each model
  |
	A range of theories derived from each model
	  |

A range of concepts that are related together in theories
  |
	A range of concepts that are related together in theories
	  |

Indicators of those concepts in practice	Indicators of those concepts in practice

Source: Bryar (1995).

Renfrew, 2000). This examination, in turn, either strengthens or challenges the theory, the model, the philosophy and the paradigm.

The four concepts of person, health, environment and nursing/midwifery are metaparadigm concepts, in the sense that they appear to be the central concepts underpinning practice. (It could be suggested that the apparently universal acceptance of these metaparadigm concepts may limit imagination and thinking about other concepts that might be important.) Any paradigm on which midwifery/nursing is based should therefore contain an understanding of these concepts. In the following, these metaparadigm concepts are referred to as 'concepts', as they are considered in the context of conceptual models and theories rather than in the context of paradigms.

Concepts

From the description of conceptual models, it is clear that the basic elements of a model are the concepts. But what is a concept? One definition of 'concept' with which midwives will be familiar is the use of the word to mean: 'to conceive in the womb' (Simpson and Wiener, 1989: 653). However, this is not the meaning that is generally ascribed to the noun 'concept', used in the context of theory building. The phenomena that are brought together in a model are labelled 'concepts': 'These phenomena are classified into concepts, which are words bringing forth mental images of the properties of things. Concepts may be abstract ideas, such as adaptation and equilibrium, or concrete ones, such as table and chair' (Fawcett, 1992: 425).

McKenna and Slevin (2008: 4–5) provide the helpful image of a wall: the concepts are the bricks, which may be of different shapes, connected together by propositions, the mortar, to form a theory – the wall. The term 'concept' is the label given to classes of ideas and things in the world, and part of the process of learning involves the development of the understanding of concepts: 'Our world is filled with sets of objects, events and ideas that share some common quality while differing in other characteristics. An organism that learns to respond to the common quality of a given set has learned a concept' (Sills, 1972: 206).

This description indicates that a concept can be applied to an idea, an event or a group of objects. While the idea (concept) that other 'organisms' may recognize concepts as concepts may be questioned, this description shows that the individual's understanding of concepts develops through learning and observation. For example, a child learns through observation to identify the colour blue from the other properties of an object such as its weight or size (Sills, 1972; Chapman, 1985). Through observation and experience, the individual develops a concept or idea of body-weight and the normal range of body-weight. The individual's mental picture, idea or concept of ideal body-weight will be influenced by the society within which they live, the social prestige given to those who are very heavy or very slim, access to food and health messages related to weight. Weight is a concrete concept. Other concepts are more abstract; for example, anxiety. Through experience and observation, an idea of the physical and psychological factors that combine together to produce the concept anxiety is developed. Concepts enable us to make sense of our world:

> Concepts are linguistic labels that selectively categorise elements of reality. Concepts are mental images that help organise the facts in our world, thus enabling us to go about our daily activities in a more orderly fashion. Concepts are not real but invented to represent reality. (Moody, 1990: 148)

Concepts are labels, not the things themselves. To observe or develop some aspect of a concept, it has to be described or defined in more explicit, observable or measurable terms. Once this has been done, the concept can be examined and tested through research. Thompson *et al.* (1989), in a discussion of the process of theory building in nurse-midwifery, provide an example of this process. These authors identify six concepts that are: 'intended to promote the optimal health and wellbeing of women' (Thompson *et al.*, 1989: 124). These concepts are: safe; satisfying; respecting human dignity and self-determination; respecting cultural and ethnic diversity; family-centred; and health-promoting. Each of these concepts is defined and the components of the concept specified as shown in Box 2.1.

Each of the components is then described in terms of an indicator of that component in practice (see Box 2.2).

This process of identification of concepts, definition and development of indicators demonstrates the process by which model building – which involves the statement of the underlying philosophy of the midwife, the naming of concepts and the description of relationships between concepts, the proposition of theories and measurement of the concepts in practice – relates to the actual provision of care. A model that includes the concept of 'satisfying' as an aspect of midwifery care will result in a different experience of care (if that model is put into practice) than a model that does not include this concept. This process is examined further in Part II; see, for example, Chapters 11 and 13.

Box 2.1   Definition and components of the concept: satisfying

Definition: actions that maximize congruence of woman's/family's preferences for care and expectations of outcomes with realities and actual health outcomes.

Components:
1 Identifies client preferences for pregnancy care;
2 Helps mobilize resources throughout pregnancy to meet client preferences;
3 Meets birth expectations of client and family, when possible;
4 Minimizes the negative aspects of health systems that affect the client;
5 Applies current theory and research in order to provide the highest quality nurse midwifery care.

Source: Thompson *et al.* (1989: 125).

Box 2.2   Indicators used to measure one component of the concept: satisfying

Components and indicators:
- Identifies client preferences for pregnancy or gynecologic care;
- Elicits and listens for client identification of preferences;
- Tailors schedule of prenatal or gyn visits to needs and preferences of client;
- Initiates information-seeking process about supplementary care that can be adapted to client preferences;
- Identifies care options, including CNM or MD as the provider or co-manager;
- Provides continuity of care; including 24-hour access.

Source: Thompson *et al.* (1989: 127).

Theory

Conceptual models provide the broad framework of ideas about midwifery care. These models are comprised of concepts. Theories may be derived from conceptual models (through a process of deductive theorizing) or may be derived from observation (through a process of inductive theorizing). Theories contribute to the construction and testing of conceptual models and are more limited in scope than models. Theories may (if they are predictive theories) suggest relationships between concepts in the form: 'if ... then ...' (Agyris and Schön, 1974: 5). Using the example above, a theory could be that: if the midwife listens to and identifies the woman's preferences, then the woman will experience greater satisfaction in the care that is provided.

Theory is essentially about providing explanations of events, actions and phenomena. These explanations may arise through a process of thinking, through observation or through a combination of thinking (incorporating prior knowledge) with observation. Once an explanation or theory has been expressed, it can then be tested in practice and through research. Theory that is predictive of practice is developed through a process that moves through descriptive or factor-isolating theory, explanatory theory and predictive theory finally arriving at theory that is prescriptive (Dickoff and James, 1992, see this chapter: pp. 40–2; Alligood, 2006).

The dictionary provides two definitions of the word 'theory':

a conception or mental scheme of something to be done, or of the method of doing it; a systematic statement of rules or principles to be followed;

a scheme or system of ideas or statements held as an explanation or account of a group of facts or phenomena; a hypothesis that has been confirmed or established by observation or experiment, and is propounded or accepted as accounting for the known facts; a statement of what are held to be the general laws, principles, or causes of something known or observed. (Simpson and Weiner, 1989: 902)

A theory is a mental construct that seeks to clarify the relationships between facts and phenomena (between concepts). Moody (1990) cites Silva's (1981) definition of the term 'theory', which demonstrates the relationship between philosophy and theory: 'The term theory refers to a set of logically inter-related statements of significance (concepts, propositions, definitions) that have been derived from philosophic beliefs or scientific data and from which questions or hypotheses can be deduced, tested and verified' (Silva, 1981, cited by Moody, 1990: 23).

Moody (1990) goes on to discuss the value and utility of theories in practice and research: 'Theories are invented to assist us in describing, explaining, predicting and understanding phenomena of concern. In relation to research, theory helps us to interpret scientific findings in a meaningful and generalis-able way' (Moody, 1990: 23). In conclusion, Moody (1990) provides this succinct summary of the term: 'A theory is a set of concepts or inter-related statements that may be tested empirically and serve to explain, describe or predict phenomena of interest to the discipline' (Moody, 1990: 57).

Concepts are described as the building blocks of theory (Chapman, 1985). Concepts brought together in theory provide an explanation of reality or hypothesis which may then be tested through observation in practice or through research (Bick, 2000). For example, in the 1920s the obstetrician Grantly Dick-Read brought together the concepts of fear and tension in a model to explain the pain that he had observed in women he was caring for in labour. The three concepts of fear, tension and pain were described by Grantly Dick-Read as follows:

> Fear is a natural protective emotion without which few of us would survive. When through association or indoctrination there is fear of childbirth, resistant actions and reactions are brought to the mechanism of the organs of reproduction. This discord disturbs the harmony or polarity of muscle action, causing tension, which in turn gives rise to nervous impulses inter-preted in the brain as pain. (Dick-Read, Wessel and Ellis, 1987: 196)

This feedback relationship can be illustrated, as shown in Figure 2.1. This theory – of the relationship between fear, tension and pain – was then addressed by Dick-Read through the provision of information on the process of labour in childbirth preparation classes, books and other means.

The relationship between uncertainty, anxiety and pain (Figure 2.1) has also been extensively explored in the field of surgical nursing. Hayward (1975) provides detailed definitions of these three concepts, describing the knowledge base from which these concepts were drawn. In a description of an experimental study of this theory, information is provided of the ways in which these concepts were measured, including using a pain measure and

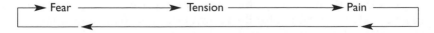

Figure 2.1   The feedback relationship between fear, tension and pain

recording administration of analgesia. This study found that people who had information about their surgery and what they should expect after the operation experienced less pain than people who did not have this information. In a study of information given to women in labour, Kirkham (1989) has shown that, while women wanted information, there was no consistency in the information they were given and the midwives were constrained, in a number of ways, from giving information. Kirkham (1989) refers to Hayward's (1975) study and comments on the lack of application of these findings in care of the childbearing woman. Reference could also be made to the earlier work by Grantly Dick-Read on this theory, which suggests an if ... then ... relationship between information and pain.

Where does theory come from?

Having established some understanding of the terms 'theory', 'model' and 'concept', this section will consider how theory is developed, and how knowledge is developed. Morse (1992) indicates that theory is developed from available information. This information may be available in the form of knowledge in a range of disciplines such as sociology, physiology or history, or in the form of data or evidence from practice (empirical information). In the first case, theory is developed by deductive reasoning from the knowledge base that is already available; in the second case, theory is developed inductively from the evidence. In both cases, the theory can then be further tested, the theory developed and the knowledge base extended.

Deductive theory

The identification of concepts and theories using the deductive approach involves examination of pre-existing knowledge or theory, which is then applied to the practice of midwifery. This knowledge and theory may be part of the knowledge base of other disciplines, such as psychology; it may be found in models or theories of nursing; or it may be found in the literature about and on midwifery.

Use of theory from other disciplines
Midwifery practice draws on a wide range of theory from many disciplines. As Price and Price (1993) comment: 'We, like the medical profession, should be comfortable in drawing on theory from other domains, such as physiology, pharmacology, psychology or sociology. Such theory helps us to anticipate, interpret and react to the changes in a woman's health status during pregnancy and beyond' (Price and Price, 1993: 235).

One example of the utilization of theory from other disciplines in midwifery is provided by the range of theories about social deprivation and health that are derived from sociological theory (Stringer, 2007). There is a great deal of evidence in the form of mortality and morbidity statistics that people in areas of deprivation experience poorer health than people who live in less deprived areas: this experience is part of the North–South divide in Britain and the North–South divide throughout the world. Theories have been propounded from many fields in relation to deprivation and health. In sociology, for example, the following theories have been deduced from the knowledge base of sociology to provide an explanation of the relationship between ill health and poverty:

- artefact theory – that the relationships are spurious and due to artefacts in data collection
- social selection theory – that those in poor health cannot work and therefore move down into lower social classes
- materialist theory – that material circumstances such as income and housing are the most important factors
- cultural/behavioural theories – that class differences in health beliefs and behaviour have the most profound effects on health. (Jewson, 1993)

Each of these theories can be examined in relation to data to assess the extent to which the theory provides a true explanation of reality. In the example above, theory is derived from one discipline. Theory may also be deduced or derived from a combination of disciplines; for example, sociology and psychology in the combination of the social determinants of health model with theories of motivation and behaviour change to explore public health strategies (Edwards and Byrom, 2007). Other examples of the use of theory are presented in Chapters 4 and 5, which provide a detailed discussion of the use of one theory – motivation theory – drawn from psychology in care of breast-feeding women while, in Chapter 14, social political theory is explored in relation to the model of partnership in midwifery practice.

The process, of concept clarification in these underlying disciplines, is found, for example, in textbooks on midwifery (Bennett and Brown, 1993; Silverton, 1993). Taking the example of labour, Silverton (1993) describes the need to understand the anatomy of the pelvis, the mechanism of muscle contraction and the physiology of uterine contractions, the mechanisms of labour (which include an understanding of the anatomy of the foetal skull), and the physiology of the separation of the placenta. An understanding of these concepts and the interrelationships between the concepts (theories about the concepts) contributes to understanding the process and mechanisms of labour.

This knowledge and theory appears quite straightforward and un-problematic, but the way this knowledge is put into practice is where the personal concepts, theories and models of the midwife come into operation, and where midwives may find conflict between their own models and those of the organization or those of other health care practitioners (Field, 1983, see ch. 3). Planning of labour care may involve establishing an atmosphere of mutual trust using a birth plan, but it also must take account of the local facilities (Silverton, 1993), hospital policies (which form the interpretation of theory) and the model of care supported by the organization. Concepts and theory, in this sense, are not value-free. While the physiology of labour may be complex, it can be understood by the research scientist, the child-bearing woman and the new student midwife on different levels. However, the interpretation of that physiological process will vary from place to place. Interpretations may emphasize the waiting and watching approach, epitomized in the pregnancy as a normal life-event; or a more active, interventionist approach may be taken to the physiology of childbirth (Rothman, 1983, see, for example, Chapters 8 and 9).

In Chapter 3, examples are given of theories for midwifery practice that show that, to a greater or lesser extent, these theorists have all based their work on pre-existing theory in other disciplines. In their discussion of Mercer's work, Bee and Oetting (1989) and Meighan (2006) refer to her use of theory from the fields of social interactionism and psychology, and to her constant exploration of available theory:

> Early in Mercer's research, she drew from Mead's interactionist theory of self and Von Bertalanffy's general systems theory. As her research developed into attainment of the maternal role, she also combined the work of Werner and Erikson with Burr and associates' theory to develop a theoretical framework of role theory from an interactionist approach. (Bee and Oetting, 1989: 293)

> Although much of her work involved testing and extending Rubin's theories, she has consistently looked to the research of others in the development and expansion of her theory. (Meighan, 2006: 607)

Mercer (1986) describes in detail the theoretical sources for the variables that she examines in her work on attainment of the maternal role – becoming a mother. These sources range across a large number of disciplines, including psychology, sociology, anthropology, medicine and others, and include reference to different schools of thought within these disciplines. Having identified these concepts in the literature of a range of disciplines, Mercer then went on to test the importance of each of these concepts, in particular that of age, in attainment of the maternal role – becoming a mother (Mercer, 1986; Meighan, 2006).

Use of theory in the form of nursing models

A number of midwives have adapted and applied nursing models to midwifery practice. For example, Methven (1986) demonstrated the utility of Orem's model of self-care in the antenatal care of the childbearing woman. She argued that the underlying self-care philosophy of this model, which is based on respect for the individual, fitted very well with midwifery practice. The type of relationship that the model describes between the nurse (or midwife) and the patient (or childbearing woman), is one of partnership, in which the nurse (or midwife) acts to compensate for those activities that the individual is unable (for whatever reason) to perform:

> The analysis of the nurse's role, delineated by Orem, would appear to be wholly consistent with the concept of the midwife being 'with the mother' in order to 'help' her during a normal pregnancy, delivery and puerperium.

In this way the status of the mother is not reduced to that of 'patient' and the ideal of 'partnership of care' remains possible. (Methven, 1986: 15)

This model also has as a central feature the promotion of health, which is a key concept in midwifery practice. Other nursing models have been used by other midwives. In all cases, questions need to be asked about the extent to which the philosophy and theory that inform the model and the four concepts of person, health, environment and practice are applicable to midwifery.

Spires (1991), for example, argued that the Neuman Systems Model was applicable to midwifery care because it is concerned with health and the ability of the individual to cope with changes in health status, such as those that occur in pregnancy which, while it may be a state of health, involves changes in bodily function as well as in social and psychological functions. This model also places the individual firmly within their social context and requires a detailed assessment of the environment within which the person lives. Ball (1987) has demonstrated the importance of the social context of the woman's life on her adaptation to motherhood, which provides support for the value of the Neuman model to care of the childbearing woman.

Literature on or about midwifery
The third strand to the deductive identification of concepts, theories and models involves the examination of literature specifically on midwifery. Such an examination aims to identify within that literature the values and concepts held by midwives that may then be tested and related together in the process of theory building. Several of the authors of chapters in Part II take this approach to identify the concepts that are central to midwifery (see, for example, Chapters 12 and 13). In illustration, Lehrman describes the process that she adopted to identify the concepts that she then examined in a study of antenatal care:

> Some categories were developed following a review of articles from professional journals written by nurse-midwives during the past 25 years. These articles contained a consistent reoccurrence of concepts considered to be aspects of nurse-midwifery practice. These were extracted from the literature and grouped, resulting in eight aspects of nurse-midwifery practice. (Lehrman, 1981: 29)

The concepts that Lehrman (1981) identified in this painstaking way are shown in Box 2.3. Lehrman (1988) provides further evidence of the utility of this approach to identification of shared concepts in a study of care in labour based on the Nurse-Midwifery Practice Model. She describes the development of this model as being partly based on the identification of the concepts that are included in the philosophy of the American College of Nurse-Midwives. Thompson *et al.* (1989) have described the process of identifying concepts, again, based initially on the American College philosophy. From the philosophy, these authors identified seven concepts of nurse-midwifery practice, shown in Box 2.3

Box 2.3   Concepts identified from the literature by Lehrman and Thompson et al.

Non-interventionist care	'nurse-midwifery is safe
Flexibility in care	is satisfying
Participative care	respects human dignity
Consumer advocacy	respects cultural and ethnic diversity
Time	promotes self-determination
Continuity of care	is family centred
Family-centred care	promotes health'
Education and counselling as part of care	

Source: Lehrman (1981).   *Source*: Thompson et al. (1989: 122).

Box 2.3 immediately identifies the differences between the concepts identified in the philosophy (Thompson *et al.* 1989) and those identified by Lehrman (1981) from the literature. This difference may reflect changes in thinking between 1981 and 1989, or it may reflect differences between those who draft philosophies and the broader cross-section of nurse-midwives who may write articles.

Thompson *et al.* (1989) go on to describe the process they went through to refine, define and develop indicators for these concepts. This involved making video-tapes of antenatal visits, which were then reviewed by a panel of nurse-midwives and a researcher, who was not a nurse-midwife. They identified indicators of each of the concepts. A number of nurse-midwives then completed a questionnaire about what they thought was special about nurse-midwifery care. The indicators identified by the panel were combined with the results from the questionnaires and the results of a literature search regarding client views of nurse-midwifery practice. The concepts and indicators were then reviewed by several different groups of nurse-midwives and finally, 'the group indicated that the concepts were sufficiently comprehensive to delineate the nurse-midwifery care process, that the definitions were essentially accurate, and that the concept components were adequate' (Thompson *et al.*, 1989: 122). During this process, it was decided that the concepts of 'respects human dignity' and 'promotes self-determination' were so similar that they were merged and formed one concept: respecting human dignity and self-determination (see p. 26). The delineation of these concepts and identification of the indicators of these concepts in practice can now be used to assess whether these six concepts do, in fact, describe nurse-midwifery practice or not.

Inductive theory

Theory may also be developed inductively through the collection of evidence from practice. There are various approaches to this type of theory development, including reflection-in-action, qualitative research and critical social theory. Schön describes reflection-in-action as follows:

> When someone reflects-in-action, he becomes a researcher in the practice context. He is not dependent on the categories of established theory and technique, but develops a new theory of the unique case. His inquiry is not limited to a deliberation about means which depends on a prior agreement about ends. (Schön, 1983: 68)

Qualitative research is aimed at understanding the views, feelings, attitudes and lives of a group of people through the collection of data about their experiences and lives through interviews, observation or other methods (Hakim, 1987). The information collected is then analyzed, and concepts in the data are identified and relationships between these concepts suggested. This process is illustrated in Kirkham's (1989) study in which she observed women in labour and identified, among other concepts, those of labelling, ward order and verbal asepsis in the data collected. This type of research then provides the basis for further deductive studies testing the relationships between the concepts, which might then be related in a model of midwifery care and information-giving in labour.

In recent years, the inductive approach to theory development based on reflection-in-action has received a great deal of attention in nursing due to the work of Benner and Wrubel (1989), and the use of reflection in the educational preparation of midwives and in midwifery practice (Hannigan 2001; Collington and Hunt, 2006) Benner has pioneered the use of narrative descriptions of actual clinical practice as a means of describing and identifying the factors that constitute expert nursing practice. Alexander (1989) contrasts the approach taken by Benner and Wrubel (1989) (and others, including Agyris and Schön, 1974) with the deductive (positivistic) approach to theory development:

> Utilising the scientific approach, one would look for lawlike relational statements to predict practice. Nevertheless, employing the qualitative methods in an interpretative approach, Benner describes expert nursing practice in many exemplars. Positivistic science takes an alternative approach by seeking formulas and models to apply. Her work seems to be hypotheses generating rather than hypotheses testing. Benner provides no universal 'how to' for nursing practice, but rather provides a methodology for uncovering and entering into the situated meaning of expert nursing care. (Alexander, 1989: 196)

Using this method, midwives describe clinical practice events and use these as the starting point for ideas (theories) about clinical interventions that may be more or less helpful. These theories can then be tried out in subsequent clinical situations. The basis of this approach is an attempt to elucidate the theories-in-use that are used by the skilled nurse or midwife, based on the view that formal (deductive) theory cannot provide the total explanation for an event in clinical practice. Expert clinical practice is an amalgam of deductive theory with observation, interpretation and experimentation by the practitioner in the field of practice (Gibbs, 1988). Agyris and Schön (1974) illustrate this with the example of grammar and speech. Few people can describe the theories of grammar but everyone demonstrates their own interpretation of these theories in their use of grammar, their theory-in-use of grammar. Alexander describes this process in Benner's work:

> Benner stated that theory is crucial in order to form the right questions to ask in a clinical situation; theory directs the practitioner in looking for problems and anticipating care needs. There is always more to any situation than theory predicts. The skilled practice of nursing exceeds the bounds of formal theory. Concrete experience provides the learning about the exceptions and shades of meaning in a situation. The knowledge embedded in practice discovers and interprets theory, precedes or extends theory, and synthesises and adapts theory in caring nursing practice. (Alexander, 1989: 193)

Midwives may have sympathy with this description of the inductive development of theory. Benner and Wrubel (1989) provide a challenge to all clinical practitioners, including midwives, to describe and tease out from descriptions of clinical care those factors that are significant in that care. Descriptions of these factors and the relationships between the factors (hypotheses) can then be tested in other clinical situations and practice theory developed. However, exploration of this type of theory is not easy and midwives, in common with other clinical practitioners, may prefer to keep away from the exploration and misunderstandings of the 'swampy lowlands': 'In the varied topography of professional practice, there is a high hard ground where practitioners can make effective use of research-based theory and technique, and there is a swampy lowland where situations are confusing "messes" incapable of technical solution' (Schön, 1983: 42).

One danger that needs to be guarded against in the exploration of the 'swampy lowlands' is that creative practice may be assumed to rest on experience alone, rather than being an expression of the interpretation of knowledge and deductive theory from a range of disciplines that is transformed by the skilled practitioner in their theory-in-use, as Benner and Wrubel (1989) acknowledge. Powell (1989) expressed concern about nursing care when she observed that: 'The nurse would try various methods of assisting the patient, often producing helpful results but in a time consuming and essentially unthinking way' (Powell, 1989: 829). This author argues for the careful combination of theory (deductive theory) with theorizing from practice (inductive theory):

> The need is, therefore, for theories of practice, based on sound theories-in-use, where an essential ingredient would appear to be an in-depth knowledge base in both nursing theory and contributing disciplines. Should this be of poor quality, the theories of practice will be ineffective in terms of patient care and use of resources, human and material. (Powell, 1989: 830)

The identification of concepts, theories and models using an inductive approach starts from the practice of midwifery, rather than from the disciplines or literature that are used in that care. Three inductive approaches may be identified: those associated with qualitative research; those that involve efforts to expose shared meanings; and those that focus on the exposure of practice theory.

Qualitative research
The main aim of qualitative research is to describe the world from the perspective of the participants in that world. Qualitative researchers try to understand the meaning individuals ascribe to their life experience and, in this case, their experience of birth, life after birth and the role of the midwife in their life-world (Sinclair 2004). The person who is collecting information, or undertaking research and collecting data, uses methods that enable the individuals, who are being observed in various ways, to demonstrate or report their feelings, attitudes, beliefs and views about their world (Field and Morse, 1985). This approach contrasts with the deductive method, in which the researcher determines from the literature and available theory the concepts that are important in relation to that aspect of care. In deductive research, a questionnaire or some other measurement tool would then be developed that would be used to measure the existence of the concepts in practice (Proctor and Renfrew, 2000).

In inductive research, data are collected about an area of interest by observation, open or semi-structured interviews and other means. The aim is to provide the subjects with the opportunity to express their own views, rather than being limited – for example, by a questionnaire – to the issues that the researcher has decided are important. The informants have the opportunity to identify issues and aspects of their lives or their midwifery care that the researcher using a deductive approach might never have identified if they did not form part of the deductive theory on which their study was built. Qualitative research has the potential to uncover people's real feelings about their lives, their midwifery care or, for midwives, to describe the reality of being a midwife.

Through the systematic collection and analysis of data, categories are identified that are further refined and identified as concepts that form part of the world view of that group of people. Once these concepts have been described, it is then possible to go on to test their validity and meaning for other groups of people through deductive research (research that is developed, or deduced, from the concepts identified in the qualitative research). This description indicates that qualitative research can be described, using Dickoff and James's (1992) classification (see pp. 41–2), as factor-isolating theory, as it is aimed at uncovering the factors or concepts that make up individuals' theories and models of their world (see, for example, Chapter 7).

In midwifery, there are a number of studies that have used this approach to concept identification. Kirkham (1989) undertook a study of the flow of information between midwives and women during labour in which she observed 113 labours and collected information by taking notes: 'I wanted to know what actually happens in labour and therefore chose observation as my principal research method. I undertook continuous observations of labour during which I took written notes' (Kirkham, 1989: 117). In addition, Kirkham

(1989) undertook interviews with women who were pregnant, the women whose labours had been observed and midwives. Analysis involved categorization of the observations. As this study started from a question about information in labour, the categories developed reflect this. The categories identified include: social class, labelling of patients, and the order of the ward; the inhibiting effect of senior staff (on information-giving) and verbal asepsis. This last concept, Kirkham describes as a means that the midwives used so that they did not have to engage with the worries or concerns expressed by the women. For example:

Woman: Is there only one sort of injection?
Sister: Don't be thinking six hours ahead or four hours ahead. See how it goes. I say see how it goes. [Changes subject]. (Kirkham, 1989: 125)

The identification of the concept of verbal asepsis by Kirkham (1989) could probably not have occurred from a consideration of pre-existing theory. Examination of the literature on midwifery (see, for example, Box 2.3) would suggest that this is a concept that is very foreign to midwives, who emphasize participation and sharing of information in the rhetoric about midwifery care. The identification of this concept opens up the possibility that further data may be collected about care in labour, to discover if this concept is found in settings other than those investigated by Kirkham (1989). This data may be collected in formal research studies, but it may also be collected by all midwives who are involved in the care of women during childbirth. For example, what language is used in the labour ward where you are working, and does this language encourage the woman to be a partner in her care? This study provides one example of the value of qualitative studies in the identification of concepts. These concepts, and the factors that support or reduce the impact of a concept, should then be explored through further research, which would lead to the development of tested practice-derived theory.

Identifying shared meanings
Implicit in much of the discussion in this book is the need for midwives to make explicit to themselves, and others, the concepts that form their pictures of midwifery care. It is suggested that this process will enable discussion about concepts that are shared and those that are not held in common. Most midwifery care is provided within the context of organizations, hospitals or teams. There are few midwives who work in isolated practice, although, like many primary health care practitioners, many community midwives may not be working in teams that have much face-to-face interaction. Midwifery practice involves teamwork to a greater or lesser extent, and teamwork will be facilitated for those teams or other work groups if they understand each other's approaches to care and come to some understanding of their shared or different approaches.

A number of authors provide evidence of ways in which shared meanings may be identified and developed. Henderson (1990) describes a process that occurred over a period of four years in a maternity unit. This process began with the introduction of birth plans and individualized care. This was followed by discussion of the philosophy of care, 'with discussions of the beliefs and values of mothers and midwives being important considerations' (Henderson, 1990: 64). Following an examination and rejection of current models, it was decided that the midwives would develop their own model based on their own care practices. Working groups were set up in which staff identified the 'elements of care' (Henderson, 1990: 66) and decided that they wanted to base the model on Maslow's hierarchy of needs. With reference to the literature, the Human Needs Model of Midwifery was devised and used in practice. At the same time, 'the midwives highlighted the need to review existing documenta-tion' (Henderson, 1990: 65) and developed new documentation to facilitate the use of the model. Henderson concludes that the model: 'affords midwives the opportunity to discuss their values and beliefs, thus allowing them to control the care they give. The model presented here reflects the views, philosophies and assumptions of one group of midwives. It is a framework serving to guide practice, a structured way to plan, implement and evaluate care' (Henderson, 1990: 66–7).

This description of the process of developing shared meanings from the meanings of individual midwives, which took four years, illustrates the time that is needed to work through this process of change. Walsh, in Chapter 8, illustrates the impact on care of shared meanings in a midwifery-led unit, while Gillen and colleagues in Chapter 13 demonstrate the value of uncover-ing shared meanings in relation to bullying in midwifery.

Practice theory
Qualitative research methods and the process of identifying shared meanings can both be described as approaches to theory development that are within the naturalism paradigm (Vaughan, 1992). The process of exploring practice through description and identification of the elements in that practice may be described as occurring within the paradigm of critical social theory, or it may simply be considered as the best starting place for identifying the concepts that midwives demonstrate in their practice.

The important point here is the demonstration or description of the concepts in practice. Rather than midwives describing what they think they should do, the emphasis here is on the midwives describing or demonstrating what they actually do in practice. These descriptions aim to identify the midwives' theories-in-use rather than their espoused theories-in-action (Agyris and Schön, 1974). Such espoused theories are formed of the past learning of the individual and are the sort of theories that people will describe if asked how they would behave in certain circumstances. It might be argued that it is espoused theories that are found in philosophies and in other writings. What is more important, however, is the way that midwives and others act in prac-tice which, Agyris and Schön (1974) argue, demonstrates their theories-in-use. As discussed in Chapter 3, there may be organizational reasons (in addition to educational or other reasons) for any disparity between espoused theories and theories-in-use. For example, midwives were found in one study to hold the theory (espoused theory) that individualized care of the childbearing woman was very important. In practice, their care was constrained by organizational policies and other demands, so that there was a gap between this espoused theory and the theory-in-use that the midwives demonstrated in their practice (Bryar, 1985). Chapters 7 and 11 explore these differences in more detail.

Agyris and Schön (1974) describe a process that helps individuals to identify their theories-in-use (or practice theories). Individuals are asked to write about 'a challenging intervention or interaction with one or more individuals that (1) you have already experienced or (2) you might expect to experience in the near future' (Agyris and Schön, 1974: 41). The description identifies on one half of the paper what was going on in the writer's mind during the incident, and the other half describes, as closely as possible, the content of the intervention/interaction. The description of the incident is then discussed in a group setting. Reflection by the individual and discussion with the group helps in the identification of the underlying attitudes and concepts held by the writer. Awareness of these attitudes and concepts, and the behaviours or actions that are associated with these concepts, can then lead to change, modification or conscious testing of the concepts and theories in practice. Agyris and Schön are concerned with achieving change rather than undertaking this activity as an aid to theory building but many midwives, seeking to provide a new form of midwifery care, would probably agree with these authors' aim for this process:

> Understanding how we diagnose and construct our experience, take action, and monitor our behaviour while simultaneously achieving our goals is crucial to understanding and enhancing effectiveness. If we learn to behave differently and to make these new behaviours stick, we will begin to create a new world. (Agyris and Schön, 1974: xi)

Exposure of practice theory through description and teasing-out the concepts implicit in the actions described appears to have the potential to assist midwives in speaking about midwifery practice. Sharing these descriptions may help to identify shared concepts, as well as differences in thinking. These concepts can then be explored through further story-telling, observation of practice and research.

Combining deductive and inductive theory

There is an argument within the nursing literature that more weight has been given in the past to models, theory and knowledge derived from disciplines outside nursing than to theory that has now been developed from practice. The same arguments could possibly apply in midwifery. To make the point more strongly for the value of practice theory, advocates of experiential learning have decried the value of knowledge from sources other than the experiential, practice base, as discussed. Boud *et al.* (1985: 43) epitomize this approach in their description of experiential learning as freeing people: 'from the drudgery of organising complicated bodies of knowledge'. This leads to the danger that practitioners may have inadequate knowledge, for example, of physiology or psychology, which limits their ability to be creative in practice situations in the way envisaged in Benner's (1984) model of the expert practitioner.

Myths and other messages about learning support this denial. For example, a poster depicts Einstein with the quotation: 'Imagination is more important than knowledge', implying that we, who have little or no knowledge, can achieve as much as Einstein through the use of our imaginations! Newton provides the most ironic example of this type of myth. Newton was an architect of the deductive, scientific method but has been portrayed as one of the chief exponents of experiential learning – through the experience of an apple falling on his head, he discovered gravity! The reality of this discovery is, in fact, very different. Newton spent many years studying prior to developing his theory about gravity. In 1661, when he was 19, he went to university, where he studied the official curriculum of Greek philosophy and his own unofficial curriculum of seventeenth-century philosophers, scientists and mathematicians. This knowledge provided the foundation for his discoveries and theories in mathematics, dynamics, optics and many other fields (Fauvel et al., 1989).

The amount of work involved in studying in the way that Newton studied is enormous. Is it for this reason that the myth of the apple is so strong? It is much more comfortable to think that we might one day sit under an apple tree (or care for a woman during the childbearing process) and discover one of the secrets of the universe than that we might have to spend many years absorbing the accumulated knowledge of our forebears and then examine our own experience in the light of that knowledge. However, subject areas are called 'disciplines' for a reason.

Creative midwifery practice, it is suggested, must be dependent on the utilization of theory derived from a range of disciplines in combination with practice theories.

Levels of theory

In the preceding discussion, the basic form of a theory has been described as a means of stating relationships between concepts. Theories may be described according to their scope. Although different terms are used by different authors, the following are commonly described: microtheories, middle-range theories and grand theory, paradigms and meta-theory. In addition, Moody (1990) identifies practice theory as a separate category. Practice theory, as discussed, is derived from direct observation and reflection on practice, using an inductive process. Both microtheories and middle-range theories may be derived, at least in part, from such a process. Thus, it may be more useful to consider practice theory as one type of microtheory, other types of microtheory being derived from deductive reasoning.

Microtheories are described by Keck (1989) as: 'the least complex [theories]. They contain the least complex concepts and refer to scientific, easily defined phenomena. They are narrow in scope because they attempt to explain a small aspect of reality. They are primarily composed of enumerative or associative concepts' (Keck, 1989: 21–2).

Middle-range theories are theories at the next level of complexity (Marriner-Tomey, 1989). Moody (1990) cites Merton's (1968) definition of middle-range theories as: 'those that examine a portion of reality and identify a few key variables: Propositions are clearly formulated and testable hypotheses can be derived' (Moody, 1990: 55).

Moody (1990) comments that middle-range theories are often developed by qualitative or ethnographic studies in which data are collected about an area of practice or experience. Variables or concepts are identified in the data, and suggestions (propositions or hypotheses) are then made about the relationship between the different variables. These relationships can then be tested by further research. Lehrman (1989) describes the model she has developed, the Nurse-Midwifery Practice Model, as a middle-range theory, and describes research aimed at testing relationships between concepts in the part of the model that is concerned with care in labour (Lehrman, 1988). As Alligood (2006: 8) comments: 'Middle range theories are more precise and focus on answering specific nursing practice questions.'

Grand theories are 'the most complex and broadest in scope. They attempt to explain areas in a discipline. They are composed of summative concepts and incorporate numerous narrow range theories' (Keck, 1989: 22).

The final level of theory is meta-theory, which is 'the analysis of theory or theorising about theory in a discipline' (Moody, 1990: 55). Meta-analysis is a method made familiar in midwifery practice through the work of Enkin *et al.* (1991) who, with their colleagues, synthesized research in areas of pregnancy and childbirth, work continued by the Cochrane Collaboration. This research has been combined and analyzed to produce information about the most effective methods of care. In the same way, theories may be analyzed and considered in relation to the concepts included in the theories, the relevance of the theories to the discipline, the strength of relationships between concepts, and so on.

Types of theory

Four types of theory have been described by Dickoff and James (1992) – two philosophers who have worked closely with nurses and nurse-midwives (see p. 60) for many years – in their classic paper 'A Theory of Theories: A Position Paper', written in 1968. Theories may describe, explain, predict, produce or shape reality. Moody (1990) summarizes these four levels of theory:

(1)   factor-isolating theories: observing, describing and naming concepts
(2)   factor-relating theories: relating named concepts to one another
(3)   situation-relating theories: inter-relationships among concepts or propositions
(4)   situation-producing theories: prescribing activities necessary to reach defined goals (also known as prescriptive theories). (Moody, 1990: 54)

The first level of theory identifies and describes or names concepts. Dickoff *et al.* (1992a) describe this as 'naming theory' and point out that, if concepts have not been named, further levels of theory development are impossible. Much of midwifery research is descriptive and aimed at this first level of theory: naming the concepts in midwifery (see, for example, Chapters 11 and 12).

Factor-relating theories suggest inter-relationships between concepts. Such theories are often the outcome of qualitative research in which factors have been named and then relationships between them suggested (see, for example, Chapter 9). Situation-relating theories are the third level of theory and are predictive theories. Such theories predict that, if one factor or variable is altered, there will be a change in one or more other variables.

The fourth level of theory is described as situation-producing theory and is aimed at bringing about change: 'predictive theory says if A happens then B happens; prescriptive or situation-producing theory says B is among the things conceived as appropriate to bring into being and so here is how to bring about A, or here is how to facilitate A's production of B, and so on' (Dickoff *et al.*, 1992a: 477–8).

Dickoff *et al.* (1992b) concluded in 1968 that none of the existing theories of nursing met their criteria for a fourth level situation-producing theory. There are, however, multiple theories of the first, second and third types. In fact, there are so many theories and models of and for nursing that Whall (1989) has argued that, rather than develop new theories, nurses should be developing and refining those already available. This is a point that midwives may need to consider as theoretical development proceeds: are there ways of networking and sharing ideas about theory development that may be more useful for care of the childbearing woman than the development of multiple theories? The argument in opposition to this is that each human being, and their circumstance, is unique and therefore multiple theories are needed. Might there be, however, concepts that would be inherent in any model of midwifery practice?

Concepts basic to midwifery

Earlier, the four concepts that are described as being basic to all models of nursing were described: the person, health, the environment and nursing. For midwifery, these elements could be:

- person (the woman, child, partner and others)
- health
- environment
- midwifery.

Theories or models of or for midwifery practice would therefore contain these concepts. In Part II, a number of theories of midwifery practice are presented, and questions can be asked to the extent to which they contain these four

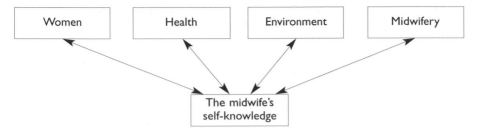

Figure 2.2   Concepts central to midwifery care

elements. But, prior to examining these theories, it may be worth considering the following questions relating to these concepts:

- How do I think about people: the women and families I care for?
- How do I think about health?
- How do I think about the environment and society?
- How do I think about midwifery practice?

Thinking about these areas brings together knowledge from other disciplines such as psychology, our own experiences as women (or men), and our values and attitudes, developed throughout our lives. And it is this element, it is suggested, that is missing from the characterization of models as being concerned with the concepts of person, health, environment and midwifery. A fifth element is the personal or self-knowledge discussed earlier (Carper, 1992). It may be suggested that any model of midwifery should also include the concept of personal knowledge that underpins the other concepts as shown in Figure 2.2.

A conceptual model of midwifery would provide a picture of midwifery practice and care, and help provide answers to questions about what constitutes midwifery practice. Two models have a significant impact on midwifery practice: the medical model, and the model of pregnancy as a normal life-event.

The medical model

The medical model is of great importance to midwifery care, as the influence of this model pervades society, health care organizations and the educational preparation of many health care practitioners. When alternative models of practice are being discussed, it is necessary to have a thorough understanding of this important model used by doctors to support their practice:

> A practising physician is an actor, not a scholar or philosopher. He needs a conceptual model but one that reduces the reality with which he deals to the bare essentials. If this model is useful in the sense of providing him with serviceable tools, he does not care too much about its over simplicity and poor correspondence with the external reality. The medical model has served him admirably in this respect. (Vouri and Rimpela, 1981: 227)

health, and contrasts this with evidence of the improvements in health achieved through improvements in nutrition, sanitation and the control of other environmental factors. In relation to the health of childbearing women, the traditional medical model argument of effectiveness is illustrated by inflexible systems of antenatal care that are based on the proposition that attendance by individual women for a set number of antenatal examinations will reduce perinatal mortality. The social health model that McKeown (1989) and others (see, for example, Marmot, 2005; WHO, 2008) describe attributes' improvements in perinatal outcome to improvements in diet, education and other factors, as well as medical interventions.

The third element in the medical model is the understanding of the nature of diseases. Stacey (1988) provides a description of the systems of belief about disease causation in Britain in the Middle Ages and the importance of beliefs in good and evil powers, in the power of healing, and in the Galenic tradition of the four humours and efforts to restore balance in the humours when someone was ill. Paracelsus, working in the sixteenth century, is identified as the person who changed the focus of attention from the cause of the disease (for example, an outside spiritual influence) to the disease itself, thus helping to change the focus of medical attention from the patient to the disease – the disease process being seen as independent of the patient (Stacey, 1988). Scientific discoveries – in particular, the discovery and understanding of cell structure – increased knowledge of the process of disease. This understanding continues to grow today with the increasing knowledge, for example, of the effects of genetic factors on disease. Cell theory – that: 'the essence of disease was to be found in the altered functioning of cells' (Vuori and Rimpela, 1981: 222) – had consequences for the practice of medicine and the relationship of the medical practitioner and the person who was unwell as the focus became narrowed on the organ, the cell, the DNA, which Vuori and Rimpela (1981) argue reduced the holistic approach.

This compartmentalization has significant effects on medical practice and on the practice of other health care practitioners who hold this model. The narrow focus is in opposition to holistic care, and the focus on the disease and the part that is diseased has the consequence of helping medicine to be largely reactive in its practice, rather than proactive and preventive. The medical practitioner is there to react and treat when something has gone wrong, the 'fire brigade approach' (Macdonald, 1993: 34): 'The emphasis is on waiting for something to go wrong; the sufferer then approaches the medical professional, the problem is diagnosed and dealt with' (Macdonald, 1993: 34).

The three main elements of the medical model are summarized by Vouri and Rimpela (1981) as the control of nature by human beings; a mechanistic view of human beings; and an understanding of disease that separates human beings from the environment and social context in which they live. These elements are illustrated in Figure 2.3, which also shows some of the consequences of this model for the practice of medicine and for the practice of other disciplines that work closely with medicine; for example, midwifery.

The medical model clearly has utility in the diagnosis and treatment of ill health, but it also has negative consequences. In its extreme form, the model

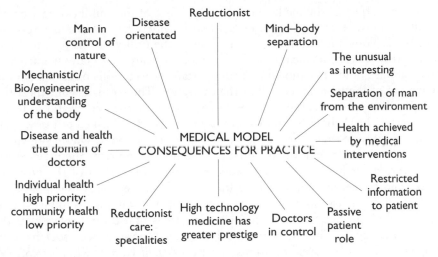

Figure 2.3   The medical model: consequences for practice

Source: Bryar (1995).

fragments and objectifies the individual, who experiences care from detached professionals who tend to make all the decisions about care.

Organizations that hold the medical model will be organized in ways that enable the treatment of individual parts of the body, in departments and specialities. Health professionals who hold the medical model will provide care that focuses on a particular organ or aspect of the person.

Care by midwives who hold the medical model will also demonstrate the features described above. Women will be viewed in terms of their pregnancy, rather than as individuals with unique personal and family concerns. Care will be organized around the ability to control the process of childbirth, to reduce professional uncertainty, and women will experience little or no control or choice in their care (see Chapters 7 and 11).

McKeown summarizes the elements of medical practice as follows:

> In the broadest sense, the medical role is in the three areas: prevention of disease by personal and non-personal measures; care of patients who require investigation and treatment; and care of the sick who are not thought to need active intervention. Medical interest and resources are focused on the second area and, to a lesser extent, on personal prevention by immunization; the other responsibilities are relatively neglected. (McKeown, 1989: 197)

Midwifery care can be summarized as the support of women and families who are well; promoting health and preventative measures and helping in role development; and, in some instances, caring for women who are ill and in need of investigation, treatment and care. Comparison of the purposes of medicine and midwifery indicates that the medical model may not be the most suitable model on which to base midwifery care.

Another effect of the medical model in the care of the childbearing woman results from the fact that it is a model that is widely held and understood in society. As Vouri and Rimpela (1981) discuss, the utility of this model is one of its strengths. The medical model is the model of care that many women and their families hold. The model indicates certain expectations of care from the viewpoint of the woman as well as the care-giver. The woman will expect the obstetrician, the medical man, to be in control, to be the expert and to make decisions on her behalf. She may therefore feel resentful if asked to make decisions, or if she receives care from other health professionals whom she views as being less expert than the doctors; for example, midwives. She may expect those caring for her to be mainly concerned with the health of the growing foetus and concerned about her health as it affects the foetus. She may then find it difficult to understand why carers (for example, midwives) are concerned about her feelings, behaviours or needs that do not relate directly to the pregnancy. The medical model thus has consequences for the way women view care, their expectations of care and their view of what is expected of them. Alternative models of care need to be considered in relation to the models held by childbearing women, as well as professional groups.

Pregnancy as a normal life-event versus the medical/obstetric model of pregnancy

The continuum between these models and the main beliefs and consequences for action associated with these models are illustrated in Figure 2.4.

The medical/obstetric model of pregnancy defines pregnancy as a potentially pathological condition requiring medical intervention. This model stresses physical care, rather than care of the whole person (Weitz and Sullivan, 1985). Pregnancy is treated as an illness, and women are encouraged to view themselves as patients (Comaroff, 1977). The outcomes of care within

Medical model of pregnancy ◄──────► Pregnancy as a normal life-event

Perspectives	Perspectives
1 Normal in retrospect	1 Normal in anticipation
2 The unusual case as interesting	2 Each pregnancy a unique event
3 Prevention of physical complications	3 Development of the individual through experience of pregnancy
4 Doctor in charge	4 Woman and family major decision-makers
5 Information restricted	5 Information shared

Outcomes	Outcomes
1 Live, healthy mother and baby	1 Live, healthy mother and baby and satisfaction of individual needs

Figure 2.4   Continuum contrasting the medical model of pregnancy and the model of pregnancy as a normal life-event

Source: Reproduced from Bryar (1985, diagram 5.3: 61).

this model are measured by physical and physiological criteria (Oakley, 1980). As Chalmers *et al.* (1980) comment: 'Clinicians see reproduction as a medical and potentially pathological process, the success of which is to be measured in terms of perinatal mortality rates and guaranteed by the surveillance of professional experts' (Chalmers *et al.*, 1980: 844).

Oakley (1979; 1980) has described the medical/obstetric model as consisting of the following features:

- the definition of pregnancy as a medical, and therefore pathological, process about which doctors are the sole experts
- the limited definition of the criteria of reproductive success – perinatal and maternal mortality rates
- the divorce of reproduction, as an illness, from its social context and the typification of women as, by nature, maternal.

The alternative model of pregnancy emphasizes pregnancy as a normal life-event:

> The medical definition of pregnancy is opposed, both within the health services and in wider society, by a cogent view which asserts that pregnancy and childbirth are natural processes; as such they are best managed by the woman herself, with assistance from, rather than control by professional agents. (Comaroff, 1977: 115)

Within this model, pregnancy is viewed as a natural process and a period of growth (Breen, 1975; Weitz and Sullivan, 1985) in which decision-making is restored to women, preventing the potentially serious consequences of the passive role assigned to them within the medical model (Gaskin, 1977 [2002]; National Childbirth Trust, 1981; Brackbill *et al.*, 1984). This model of pregnancy puts the woman at the centre, rather than the obstetrician or the midwife. She is the person who is able to make choices and reach decisions about the type of care she would prefer and where she would prefer her baby to be born based on information from, among others, the midwives, doctors and obstetricians who may be involved in her care.

Opoku (1992) identifies two uses of the term 'normal' in the literature. The first uses the word to mean common and: 'includes common procedures such as episiotomy, artificial rupture of membranes, intravenous infusions and electronic foetal monitoring' (Opoku, 1992: 121). The second use of the term 'normal' is in the sense of natural, birth without intervention. In the continuum above, the model of pregnancy as a normal life-event, however, encompasses something more than these essentially medical definitions: the growth and development of the individual woman.

Currell (1990) considers that there is a need to put the focus on the woman (rather than the health professional). Childbirth is, then, seen as a process that is a part of the wider life processes experienced by the woman: a time of great opportunity for growth but, equally, a time of great potential harm and restrictions on growth. Midwives and obstetricians are therefore in a crucial position either to assist or to inhibit the woman, and potentially her child, to grow. Nurse-midwives in the USA have identified this change in roles and personal growth as the focus of their models of attainment of the maternal role (see Chapter 3; Rubin, 1984; Mercer, 1986).

The medical/obstetric and pregnancy as normal life-event models have been presented at the opposite ends of a continuum. The question then is: What is the model that midwives hold or, what are the models that midwives hold? Opoku (1992) describes the use of the 'normal' pregnancy model by midwives in their efforts to resist medical interventions and to take charge of twin or breech births. This use of the model, as a tool to oppose the power of another profession, is similar to the use of bonding to achieve change in the care of mothers and babies in hospital. However, in the 1970s and early 1980s studies showed that midwives aligned themselves with an obstetric model of pregnancy. The majority of midwives work in hospitals in which the care of women as patients has been described (Thomson, 1980; Kirkham, 1983; 1989). Comaroff observed that midwives demonstrated in their practice adherence to an obstetric model:

> This paradigm was expressed at a number of levels: in explicit reference to the management of women as 'patients'; in the exclusion of non-medical aspects of childbirth from communications with them, in their encouragement of reliance upon medical control over labour; in a reluctance to demystify technical knowledge for the women with whom they dealt. (Comaroff, 1977: 126)

Midwives were observed by Kirkham (1983) to give limited information to women, thus limiting their potential for making decisions. Laryea (1980) found that women postnatally emphasized their need for emotional support and teaching, while the midwives emphasized physical care, utilizing a medical model of pregnancy. The women were reluctant to express their views to midwives, whom they considered did not understand how they felt.

The flexibility of the term 'normal' highlighted by Opoku (1992) means that this term can be used to cover a type of care that includes a great deal of professional control: 'The "normal" model is not against home births supported by adequate backup for emergencies and it favours "low-tech" births in consultant or GP units' (Opoku, 1992: 121). Arney (1982) argues that the type of control described by Opoku (a midwife) is a feature of the hidden control built into alternative forms of care. The great fear for obstetricians, Arney (1982) suggests, is not the case that has been mishandled and ends in tragedy but, rather, the woman who has her baby outside of and unknown by the system of obstetrical care. He describes the alternative birth centres and places such as the Farm in Tennessee (Gaskin, 1977 [2002]) as providing alternative care but within obstetric control. These alternatives have been developed within the obstetric rule (medical model), which maintains safety as the most important factor. Through provision of such alternatives, Arney argues that the woman becomes responsible for her safety (for maintenance of the obstetric rule), making it even harder for her to opt out of the care system:

> Alternatives to birth have arisen not in opposition to the rule that birth should occur within a flexible system of obstetrical alternatives in which a woman's experience can gain prominence against a background of obstetrical expertise and safety; alternatives have arisen within this rule. The rule informs and facilitates alternatives, and the rule, in turn, is strengthened by their existence as they push the apparent limitations imposed by the rule further and further outward. The rule comes to resemble a liberating rather than constraining force ... The world of imagined possibilities comes to be defined in terms of the options available under the rule. The 'flexible systems' rule constrains imagination and becomes the force that holds together the panoptic machine that controls birth. (Arney, 1982: 240)

DeVries (1993) argued that midwives have lost power and are in danger as a profession, as they have defined their area of practice as the normal, as low-risk. He argues that professional power is associated with emphasizing risk. However, Welford (1993), in a discussion of birthing rooms, suggests that this definition of low risk may, in fact, increase midwifery power. Through the definition of low-risk, obstetricians are excluded from care but that care, such as that provided in birthing rooms by midwives, takes place within the confines of the hospital, reducing obstetric concern (Arney, 1982). Welford (1993) suggests that the establishment of birthing rooms may, in fact, reduce women's choice and prevent the establishment of truly radical services: 'I would argue that the birthing room as we know it is actually a compromise between truly radical changes that might allow the birthplace to empower women and midwives and what more traditional colleagues feel comfortable with' (Welford, 1993: 35). The analyses by Arney (1982) and Welford (1993) may be painful for midwives, but they need to be considered as efforts are made to identify midwifery models of care. These authors indicate the need to examine each value carefully and thoroughly for its true meaning and the consequences it has for practice.

The midwife, according to some authors, frequently appears to hold a medical/obstetric model of pregnancy and this model may, in some cases, be reinforced by the setting within which they work (see Chapter 3 and Chapter 7). The adoption of the medical model may have benefits for the midwife at the individual and professional levels. The presentation by the midwife of a stereotyped image may prevent 'patients' discussing threatening topics with the midwife (Jourard, 1971; Comaroff, 1977). The alternative model may lead to the discussion of such topics as the woman's emotional needs, or psycho-social aspects of pregnancy that the midwife may not feel prepared (either emotionally or professionally) to discuss (Breen, 1975; Laryea, 1980). Examination of our personal models helps to identify our own model of practice, and enables discussion in the midwifery team of the similarities and differences in the models held by different members of the team.

Conclusion

In summary, conceptual models provide an abstract picture of the thinking of one or more people about some aspect of the world; in the case of midwifery, midwifery care. Theories are formulated from an understanding of the relationships between concepts, and may be tested through observation and other forms of research. Models and theories are mental constructs and this must always be remembered. They are mental constructs or images developed to provide greater understanding of events in the physical, psychological or social worlds. Models and theories are not concrete objects and are intended to be tested, modified or abandoned in the light of new evidence. For example, the theory that the world was flat was abandoned (by most people) when new evidence was discovered. As an advertisement for beer that shows a picture of a flat earth puts it, 'When you know what's what and what's not.' Morse has cautioned against the danger of 'believing in theories':

> Theories, theoretical frameworks, and models have been taught to students as facts, as correct and as dogma. Students have been examined on the material, graded and instructed to somehow use these theories in practice. What they have not been taught is that theories are only tools; that theories are means for organising data, for making sense of and explaining reality, so that confusion is rendered comprehensible and predictable. Students have not been taught that theories are merely someone's best guess about the nature of reality – given the available information – and as such, they must be tested, modified, and tested again. (Morse, 1992: 259)

In this chapter, the aim has been to present and define terms used in theory building, and to consider ways that theory may be built. Two broad approaches to theory building have been described here: deductive approaches and inductive approaches. Additional approaches to concept identification – and, thus, theory building – are described in Part II (see, for example, Chapters 11 and 13). Deductive approaches include: use of theory from other disciplines; the use of theory in the form of nursing models; and the use of literature on and about midwifery. Inductive approaches include: qualitative research; identification of shared meanings; and practice theory. Different approaches will be suitable for different situations and for different people. Deductive and inductive approaches and combination of these approaches provide enormous possibilities for the further development of theory of and for midwifery practice. This future development will help further to answer the questions with which this book commenced: How do I care? How do you care?

ACTIVITIES

Undergraduate

The judicious and best use of evidence to inform practice is a major aspect of your role. Reflect on one clinical case in which the decision-making was based on collating multiple data, including that valued by proponents of the medical model and the social model of midwifery. Consider the value of different ways of seeing and knowing in practice.

Postgraduate

Schön describes reflection-in-action as follows:

> When someone reflects-in-action, he becomes a researcher in the practice context. He is not dependent on the categories of established theory and technique, but develops a new theory of the unique case. His inquiry is not limited to a deliberation about means which depends on a prior agreement about ends. (Schön, 1983: 68)

Using examples from the literature and practice, deliberate on the meaning of this statement, and analyze the tensions that could arise when it is applied to practice.

References

Aggleton, P. and Chalmers, H. (1986) *Nursing Models and the Nursing Process.* London: Macmillan.

Agyris, C. and Schön, D.A. (1974) *Theory in Practice. Increasing Professional Effectiveness.* San Francisco, CA: Jossey-Bass.

Alexander, J.E. (1989) 'From Novice to Expert: Excellence and Power in Clinical Nursing Practice', in A. Marriner-Tomey (ed.), *Nursing Theorists and Their Work,* 2nd edn. St Louis, MO: C.V. Mosby, ch. 16: 187–99.

Alligood, M.R. (2006) 'Introduction to Nursing Theory: Its History, Significance, and Analysis', in M.R. Marriner-Tomey and A. Alligood, *Nursing Theory, Utilization & Application,* 3rd edn. St Louis, MO: Elsevier Mosby, ch. 1: 3–15.

Alligood, M.R. and Marriner-Tomey, A. (2006) *Nursing Theory, Utilization & Application,* 3rd edn. St Louis, MO: Elsevier Mosby.

Arney, W.R. (1982) *Power and the Profession of Obstetrics.* Chicago, IL: University of Chicago Press.

Ball, J.A. (1987) *Reactions to Motherhood. The Role of Postnatal Care.* Cambridge: Cambridge University Press.

Bee, A.M. and Oetting, S. (1989) 'Ramona T. Mercer: Maternal role attainment', in A. Marriner-Tomey (ed.), *Nursing Theorists and Their Work,* 2nd edn. St Louis, MO: C.V. Mosby, ch. 24: 292–306.

Benner, P. (1984) *From Novice to Expert. Excellence and Power in Clinical Nursing Practice.* Menlo Park, CA: Addison-Wesley.

Benner, P. and Wrubel, J. (1989) *The Primacy of Caring. Stress and Coping in Health and Illness.* Menlo Park, CA: Addison-Wesley.

Bennett, V.R. and Brown, L.K. (eds) (1993) *Myles Textbook for Midwives,* 12th edn. Edinburgh: Churchill Livingstone.

Bick, D. (2000) 'Asking Questions about Practice and Using Appropriate Research Methods', in S. Proctor and M. Renfrew (eds), Linking *Research and Practice in Midwifery. A Guide to Evidence-Based Practice*. Edinburgh: Balliere Tindall, ch. 7: 125–38.

Boud, D., Keogh, R. and Walker, D. (1985) Reflection: Turning Experience into Learning. London: Kogan Page.

Brackbill, Y., Rice, J. and Young, D. (1984) *Birth Trap. The Legal Low-Down on High-Tech Obstetrics*. St Louis, MO: C.V. Mosby.

Breen, D. (1975) *The Birth of a First Child: Towards an Understanding of Femininity*. London: Tavistock Publications.

Bryar, R. (1985) 'A Study of the Introduction of the Nursing Process in a Maternity Unit', Unpublished MPhil thesis. London: Southbank Polytechnic.

Bryar, R. (1995) *Theory for Midwifery Practice*, 1st edn. London: Macmillan.

Comaroff, J. (1977) 'Conflicting Paradigms of Pregnancy: Managing Ambiguity in Ante-natal Encounters', in A. Davis and G. Horobin (eds), *Medical Encounters: The Experience of Illness and Treatment*. London: Croom Helm, ch. 8: 115–34.

Carper, B.A. (1992) 'Fundamental Patterns of Knowing in Nursing', in L.H. Nicholl (ed), *Perspectives on Nursing Theory*, 2nd edn. Philadelphia, PA: J.B. Lippincott, ch. 19: 216–24.

Carter, S.K. (2010) 'Beyond Control: Body and Self in Women's Childbearing Narratives', *Sociology of Health and Illness E Article*, first published online 23 July 2010, no. doi: 10.1111/j.1467-9566.2010.01261.x (accessed 15 August 2010).

Carveth, J.A. (1987) 'Conceptual Models in Nurse-Midwifery', *Journal of Nurse-Midwifery*, 32(1): 20–5.

Chalmers, I., Oakley, A. and MacFarlane, A. (1980) 'Perinatal Health Services: An Immodest Proposal', *British Medical Journal*, 280(6,217): 842–5.

Chapman, C.M. (1985) *Theory of Nursing: Practical Application*. London: Harper & Row.

Chinn, P.L. and Kramer, M.K. (1991) *Theory and Nursing: A Systematic Approach. Mosby Year Book*. St Louis, MO: Mosby.

Chinn, P.L., and Kramer, M.K. (2008) *Integrated Theory and Knowledge Development in Nursing*, 7th edn. St Louis, MO: Mosby Elsevier.

Collington, V. and Hunt, S.C. (2006) 'Reflection in Midwifery Education and Practice: An Exploratory Analysis', *Evidence Based Midwifery*, 4(3): 76–82.

Comaroff, J. (1977) 'Conflicting Paradigms of Pregnancy: Managing ambiguity in ante-natal encounters', in A. Davis and G. Horobin (eds), *Medical Encounters: The Experience of Illness and Treatment*. London: Croom Helm, ch. 8: 115–34.

Cronin, P. and Rawlings-Anderson, K. (2004) *Knowledge for Contemporary Nursing Practice*. Edinburgh: Mosby.

Currell, R. (1990) 'The Organisation of Midwifery Care', in J. Alexander, V. Levy and S. Roch (eds), *Midwifery Care. Antenatal Care. A Research-Based Approach*. London: Macmillan, ch. 2: 20–41.

DeVries, R.G. (1993) 'A Cross-National View of the Status of Midwives', in E. Riska, and K. Wegar (eds), *Gender, Work and Medicine: Women and the Medical Division of Labour*. London: Sage.

Dick-Read, G., Wessel, H. and Ellis, H.F. (1987) *Childbirth without Fear: The Original Approach to Natural Childbirth*, 5th edn. New York, NY: Harper & Row.

Dickoff, J. and James, P. (1992) 'A Theory of Theories: A Position Paper', in L.H. Nicholl (ed.), *Perspectives on Nursing Theory*, 2nd edn. Philadelphia, PA: J.B. Lippincott, ch. 8: 99–111.

Dickoff, J., James, P. and Wiedenbach, E. (1992a) 'Theory in a Practice Discipline, Part I: Practice Oriented Theory', in L.H. Nicholl (ed.), *Perspectives on Nursing Theory*, 2nd edn. Philadelphia, PA: J.B. Lippincott, ch. 46: 468–500.

Dickoff, J., James, P. and Wiedenbach, E. (1992b) 'Theory in a Practice Discipline, Part II: Practice Oriented Research', in L.H. Nicholl (ed.), *Perspectives on Nursing Theory*, 2nd edn. Philadelphia, PA: J.B. Lippincott, ch. 53: 585–98.

Downe, S. (1991). 'The Midwife as Practitioner: Midwifery Standards – Uniformity or Quality?', *Midwives Chronicle and Nursing Notes*, 104(1,236): 3–4.

Dubos, R. (1960) *Mirage of Health*. London: George Allen & Unwin. Cited by McKeown, T. (1989) *The Role of Medicine: Dream, Mirage or Nemesis?* Oxford: Basil Blackwell.

Edwards, G. and Byrom, S. (eds) (2007) *Essential Midwifery Practice: Public Health*. Chichester: Wiley-Blackwell.

Enkin, M., Keirse, M.J.N.C. and Chalmers, I. (1991). *A Guide to Effective Care in Pregnancy and Childbirth*. Oxford: Oxford University Press.

Fauvel, J., Flood, R., Shortland, M. and Wilson, R. (1989) *Let Newton Be!* Oxford: Oxford University Press.

Fawcett, J. (1984) *Analysis and Evaluation of Conceptual Models of Nursing*. Philadelphia, PA: F.A. Davis.

Fawcett, J. (1992) 'A Framework for Analysis and Evaluation of Conceptual Models of Nursing', in L.H. Nicholl (ed.), *Perspectives on Nursing Theory*, 2nd edn. Philadelphia, PA: J.B. Lippincott, ch. 41: 424–41.

Fawcett J. (2005) *Contemporary Nursing Knowledge: Analysis and Evaluation of Nursing Models and Theories*. Philadelphia, PA: F.A. Davies.

Fawcett J. (2006) 'Nursing Philosophies, Models, and Theories: A Focus on the Future', in Marriner-Tomey, A. and Alligood, M.R. (2006) *Nursing Theorists and Their Work*, 6th edn. St Louis, MO: Elsevier Mosby, ch. 22: 495–516.

Field, P.A. (1983) 'An Ethnography: Four Public Health Nurses' Perspectives of Nursing', *Journal of Advanced Nursing*, 8(1): 3–12.

Field, P.A. and Morse, J.M. (1985) *Nursing Research: The Application of Qualitative Approaches*. London: Croom Helm.

Fitzpatrick, J.J. and Whall, A.L. (1989) *Conceptual Models of Nursing: Analysis and Application*, 2nd edn. Norwalk, CT: Appleton & Lange.

Gaskin, I.M. (2002) *Spiritual Midwifery*. 4th edn. Summertown: Book Publishing Co.

Gibbs, G. (1988) *Learning by Doing: A Guide to Teaching and Learning Methods*. Oxford: Oxford Further Education Unit, Oxford Polytechnic.

Gonot, P.J. (1989) 'Imogene M. King's Conceptual Framework for Nursing', in J.J. Fitzpatrick and A.L. Whall (eds), *Conceptual Models of Nursing. Analysis and Application*, 2nd edn. Norwalk, CT: Appleton & Lange, ch. 18: 271–83.

Hakim, C. (1987) *Research Design. Strategies and Choices in the Design of Social Research*. London: Unwin Hyman.

Hannigan, B. (2001) 'A Discussion of the Strengths and Weaknesses of "Reflection", in Nursing Practice and Education', *Journal of Clinical Nursing*, 10(2), 278–83.

Hardy, S., Titchen, A., McCormack, B. and Manley, K. (eds) (2009) *Revealing Nursing Expertise Through Practitioner Inquiry*. Chichester: Wiley-Blackwell.

Hayward, J. (1975) *Information – A Prescription Against Pain*. London: Royal College of Nursing.

Henderson, C. (1990) 'Models and Midwifery', in B. Kershaw and J. Salvage (eds), *Models for Nursing 2*. London: Scutari Press, ch. 7: 57–67.

Jewson, N. (1993) 'Inequalities and Differences in Health', in S. Taylor and D. Field (eds), *Sociology of Health and Health Care: An Introduction for Nurses*. Oxford: Blackwell Scientific Publications, ch. 4: 57–93.

Johnston, R.L. (1989). 'Orem's Self Care Model for Nursing', in J.J. Fitzpatrick and A.L. Whall (eds), *Conceptual Models of Nursing*, 2nd edn. Norwalk, CT: Appleton & Lange, ch. 12: 165–84.

Jourard, S.M. (1971) *The Transparent Self*, 2nd edn. New York, NY: Van Nostrand.

Keck, J.F. (1989) 'Terminology of Theory Development', in A. Marriner-Tomey (ed.), *Nursing Theorists and Their Work*, 2nd edn. St Louis, MO: C.V. Mosby. ch. 2: 15–23

Kershaw, B. and Salvage, J. (eds) (1986) *Models for Nursing*. Chichester: John Wiley & Sons.

Kirkham, M. (1983) 'Labouring in the Dark: Limitations on the Giving of Information to Enable Patients to Orientate Themselves to the Likely Events and Timescale of Labour', in J. Wilson-Barnett (ed.), *Nursing Research: Ten Studies in Patient Care. Developments in Nursing Research, Volume 2*. Chichester: John Wiley & Sons, ch. 4: 81–99.

Kirkham, M. (1989) 'Midwives and Information-Giving during Labour', in S. Robinson and A.M. Thomson (eds), *Midwives, Research and Childbirth, Volume I*. London: Chapman & Hall, ch. 6: 117–38.

Kuhn, T. (1970 [1962]) *The Structure of Scientific Revolutions*, 2nd edn. *International Encyclopaedia of United Science*, 2:2. Chicago, IL: Chicago University Press. Cited in J. Robinson (1992) 'Problems with Paradigms in a Caring Profession', *Journal of Advanced Nursing*, 17(5): 632–8.

Lancaster, W. and Lancaster, J. (1992) 'Models and Model Building in Nursing', in L.H. Nicholl (ed.), *Perspectives on Nursing Theory*, 2nd edn. Philadelphia, PA: J.B. Lippincott, ch. 42: 432–41.

Laryea, M.G.G. (1980) 'The Midwives' Role in the Postnatal Care of Primiparae and their Infants in the First 28 Days Following Childbirth', Unpublished MPhil thesis, Newcastle-upon-Tyne Polytechnic, Newcastle-upon-Tyne.

Lehrman, E.-J. (1981) 'Nurse-Midwifery Practice: A Descriptive Study of Prenatal Care', *Journal of Nurse-Midwifery*, 26(3): 27–41.

Lehrman, E.-J. (1988) 'A Theoretical Framework for Nurse-Midwifery Practice', Unpublished PhD thesis, University of Arizona, Arizona.

Lehrman, E.-J. (1989) 'A Theoretical Framework for Nurse-Midwifery Practice', *Dissertation Abstracts International*, 49(12): 5230-B.

Luker, K. (1988) 'Do Models Work?', *Nursing Times*, 84(5): 27–9.

Macdonald, J.J. (1993) *Primary Health Care: Medicine in its Place*. London: Earthscan.

Marriner-Tomey, A. (ed.) (1989) *Nursing Theorists and their Work*, 2nd edn. St Louis, MO: C.V. Mosby.

Marriner-Tomey, A. and Alligood, M.R. (2006) *Nursing Theorists and Their Work*, 6th edn. St Louis, MO: Elsevier Mosby.

Marmot, M. (2005) 'Social Determinants of Health Inequalities', *Lancet*, 365(9464): 1099–104.

McKenna, H.P. and Slevin, O.D. (2008) *Vital Notes for Nurses: Nursing Models, Theories and Practice*. Chichester: Wiley-Blackwell

McKeown, T. (1989) *The Role of Medicine: Dream, Mirage or Nemesis?* Oxford: Basil Blackwell.

Meighan, M. (2006) 'Mercer's Becoming a Mother Theory in Nursing Practice', in M.R. Alligood and A. Marriner-Tomey, *Nursing Theory, Utilization & Application*, 3rd edn. St Louis, MO: Elsevier Mosby, ch. 17: 393–430.

Meleis, A.I. (2007) *Theoretical Nursing. Development & Progress*. Philadelphia, PA: Lippincott Williams & Wilkins.

Mercer, R.T. (1986) *First-Time Motherhood: Experiences from Teens to Forties*. New York, NY: Springer.

Merton, R.K. (1968) *Social Theory and Social Structure*. New York, NY: Free Press. Cited in L.E. Moody (1990), *Advancing Nursing Science through Research, Volume I*. Newbury Park, PA: Sage.

Methven, R.C. (1986) 'Care Plan for a Woman Having Ante-natal Care, Based on Orem's Self-care Model', in C. Webb (cd.), *Women's Health: Midwifery and Gynaecological Nursing*. London: Edward Arnold, ch. 2: 13–41.

Moody, L.E. (1990) *Advancing Nursing Science through Research, Volume I*. Newbury Park, PA: Sage.

Morse, J.M. (1992) 'Editorial: If You Believe in Theories ...', *Qualitative Health Research*, 2(3): 259–61.

National Childbirth Trust (1981) *Change in Antenatal Care*. London: National Childbirth Trust.

Oakley, A. (1979) *Becoming A Mother*. Oxford: Martin Robertson.

Oakley, A. (1980) *Women Confined: Towards a Sociology of Childbirth*. Oxford: Martin Robertson.

Opoku, D.K. (1992) 'Does Inter-Professional Co-operation Matter in the Care of the Birthing Woman?', *Journal of Interprofessional Care*, 6(2): 119–25.

Pearson, A. (1992) 'Knowing Nursing: Emerging Paradigms in Nursing', in K. Robinson and B. Vaughan, *Knowledge for Nursing Practice*. Oxford: Butterworth/Heinemann, ch. 14: 213–26.

Pearson, A. and Vaughan, B. (1986) *Nursing Models for Practice*. London: Heinemann Nursing.

Powell, J.H. (1989) 'The Reflective Practitioner in Nursing', *Journal of Advanced Nursing*, 14(10): 824–32.

Price, A. and Price, B. (1993) 'Midwifery Knowledge: Theory for Action, Theory for Practice', *British Journal of Midwifery*, 1(5): 233–7.

Proctor, S. and Renfrew, M. (eds) (2000) *Linking Research and Practice in Midwifery. A Guide to Evidence-Based Practice*. Edinburgh: Balliere Tindall.

Rhodes, J.M.R. (1988) 'Integrating Philosophy into the Doctoral Preparation for Nurse-Midwives', *Journal of Nurse-Midwifery*, 33(6): 283–4.

Robinson, J.A. (1992) 'Problems with Paradigms in a Caring Profession', *Journal of Advanced Nursing*, 17(5): 632–8.

Rolfe, G. (1996) *Closing the Theory Practice Gap: A New Paradigm for Nursing*. Oxford: Butterworth Heinemann

Roper, N., Logan, W.W. and Tierney, A.J. (1985) *The Elements of Nursing*, 2nd edn. Edinburgh: Churchill Livingstone.

Rothman, B.K. 1983. 'Midwives in Transition: The Structure of a Clinical Revolution', *Social Problems*, 30(3): 262–71.

Rubin, R. (1984) *Maternal Identity and the Maternal Experience*. New York, NY: Springer.

Schein, E.H. (1972) *Professional Education: Some New Directions*. New York, NY: McGraw-Hill.

Schön, D.A. (1983) *The Reflective Practitioner: How Professionals Think in Action*. London: Basic Books, HarperCollins.

Sieloff, C.L. (2006) 'Imogene King: Interacting Systems Framework and Middle Range Theory of Goal Attainment', in A. Marriner-Tomey and M.R. Alligood, *Nursing Theorists and Their Work*, 6th edn. St Louis, MO: Elsevier Mosby, ch. 15: 297–317.

Sills, D.L. (ed.) (1972) *International Encyclopaedia of the Social Sciences, Volumes 3 and 4*. New York, NY: Macmillan/Free Press.

Silva, M. (1981) 'Selection of a Theoretical Framework', in S.D. Krampitz and N. Pavlovich (eds), *Readings for Nursing Research*. St Louis, MO: C.V. Mosby. Cited in L.E. Moody (1990), *Advancing Nursing Science through Research*, Volume 1. Newbury Park, PA: Sage.

Silverton, L. (1993) *The Art and Science of Midwifery*. New York, NY: Prentice Hall.

Simpson, J.A. and Weiner, E.S.C. (eds) (1989) *Oxford English Dictionary*, 2nd edn. Oxford: Clarendon Press.

Sinclair, M. (2004) 'Qualitative Research: A Valuable Contribution to Midwifery Knowledge', *Evidence Based Midwifery*, 2(1): 3.

Smith, A. (1991) 'Newbourne Optimism', *Nursing Times*, 87(16): 56–9.

Spires, L. (1991) 'A Model for Midwifery Practice?', *Modern Midwife*, 1(5): 9–11.

Squire, C. (ed.) (2003) *The Social Context of Birth*. Abingdon: Radcliffe Medical Press.

Stacey, M. (1988) *The Sociology of Health and Healing. A Textbook*. London: Routledge.

Stringer, E. (2007) 'Health and Inequality: What Can Midwives Do?', in G. Edwards and S. Byrom (eds), *Essential Midwifery Practice: Public Health*. Chichester: Wiley-Blackwell, ch. 2: 27–48.

Taylor, S.G. (2006) 'Dorothea E. Orem: Self-care Deficit Theory of Nursing', in A. Mariner Tomey and M.E. Alligood, *Nursing Theorists and Their Work*, 6th edn. St Louis, MO: Elsevier Mosby, ch. 14: 267–96.

Thomson, A.M. (1980) 'Planned or Unplanned? Are Midwives Ready for the 1980s?', *Midwives Chronicle and Nursing Notes*, 93(1,106): 68–72.

Thompson, J.E., Oakley, D., Burke, M., Jay, S. and Conklin, M. (1989) 'Theory Building in Nurse-Midwifery. The Care Process', *Journal of Nurse-Midwifery*, 34(3): 120–30.

Titchen, A. and Hardy, S. (2009) 'A Kaleidoscope of Nursing Expertise: A Literature Review', in S. Hardy, A. Titchen, B. McCormack K. and Manley (eds), *Revealing Nursing Expertise Through Practitioner Inquiry*. Chichester: Wiley-Blackwell, ch. 3: 55–71.

Vaughan, B. (1992) 'The Nature of Nursing Knowledge', in R. Robinson and B. Vaughan, *Knowledge for Nursing Practice*. London: Butterworth/Heinemann, ch. 1: pp. 3–19.

Vouri, H. and Rimpela, M. (1981) 'The Development and Impact of the Medical Model', *Perspectives in Biology and Medicine*, winter: 217–28.

Weitz, R. and Sullivan, D. (1985) 'Licensed Lay Midwifery and the Medical Model of Childbirth', *Sociology of Health and Illness*, 7(1): 36–54.

Welford, H. (1993) 'A Room of One's Own', *Modern Midwife*, 3(5): 34–5.

Whall, A.L. (1989) 'Nursing Theory Issues and Debates', in J.J. Fitzpatrick and A.L. Whall (eds), *Conceptual Models of Nursing. Analysis and Application*, 2nd edn. Norwalk, CT: Appleton & Lange, ch. 2: 15–22.

WHO (2008) *Primary Health Care: Now More than Ever*. WHO: Geneva.

Midwifery Theory Development

Rosamund Bryar and Marlene Sinclair

Key points

- Overview of historical development of midwifery theory
- Provides an outline of the development of theory in midwifery
- Identification of theory to be tested through further research
- Identification of relevance of application of theory to practice.

Introduction

In this chapter, the development of theory in and for midwifery practice is explored. Until the 1990s, it was argued that there had been little or no theory development in midwifery but, in reality, explicit research on the development of midwifery theory has been taking place at least since the 1960s and, as Part II of this book shows, has gained in pace and depth since the 1990s. An overview of the historical development of theory in and for midwifery practice is followed by a description of the theory building work of a number of midwives and nurse-midwives. As Meleis comments, understanding the journey of development of theory in a discipline can inform the work of those taking this work forward:

> By uncovering and understanding a discipline's theoretical journey, members of the discipline learn and build on it. By unfolding the process used in developing the theoretical past, we gain insights that improve our understanding of our current progress, and we are empowered to achieve our disciplinary goals. When we take a critical and reflective stance on the current theoretical discourse, or lack thereof as the case may be, we see

shadows of our past issues and accomplishments as well as visions of the future of our discipline and profession. (Meleis, 2007: 3)

The growth of activity in midwifery theory building owes a great deal to the pioneers of this work, midwives, nurse-midwives and practitioners from other disciplines. The initiation of theory building in midwifery may be attributed to Ernestine Wiedenbach, who qualified in the USA as a nurse in 1925 and worked as a nurse and as a professional writer for the Nursing Information Bureau for 20 years. In 1946, she qualified as a nurse-midwife and worked in clinical practice until she was appointed to Yale in 1952. Nickel *et al.* (1992) comment that during the late 1940s Wiedenbach worked on a project to provide childbirth preparation based on the theories of Dr Grantly Dick-Read.

In discussions of Wiedenbach's contribution to nursing theory, the emphasis is placed on her book *Clinical Nursing: A Helping Art* (1964). However, in 1958 she was the author of *Family-Centred Maternity Nursing*, which she wrote because there were no textbooks that focused on the family. It appears that comments by Dickoff and James on this textbook stimulated her thinking about theory (Nickel *et al.*, 1992). Wiedenbach is considered to have developed her theory inductively from experience and observation of practice (Danko *et al.*, 1989). Although she had worked for 20 years as a nurse, the development of this theory took place while she was working in the field of maternity care.

In the preface to the second edition of *Family-Centred Maternity Nursing*, Wiedenbach (1967) summarizes her theory of nursing (midwifery):

> The theory of accountability which underlies the concept of nursing presented in this book, envisions the nurse as accountable not only for what she does, but also in large measure for the results she obtains from what she does. Her responses, other than reflex, according to this theory, stem from her perception of the realities which make up the situation in which she finds herself at any given point in time. Assumptions resulting from her perception and the degree of validity she attaches to them, colour the character of her responses and determine not only her immediate action but also, to a large degree, the kind of response she obtains from the recipient of her act. (Wiedenbach, 1967: v)

Wiedenbach's central concern is with the influence of the knowledge, attitudes and theories held by midwives on practice. Her own philosophy of midwifery care and action is demonstrated in her description of the 'ultimate goal of maternity nursing' (Wiedenbach, 1967: 22), which: 'extends beyond the immediate needs of the mother and baby, to the broader needs of the mother and father to develop inner strengths – Power in Reserve – on which to draw with confidence and understanding as they prepare for and assume their roles of parents' (Wiedenbach, 1967: 22).

The goal or purpose of the midwife or nurse, according to Wiedenbach, is to meet a person's need-for-help (Marriner-Tomey, 2006). Danko *et al.* (1989) cite Wiedenbach's (1964) definition of a need-for-help: 'A need-for-help is "any measure or action required and desired by the individual and which has potential for restoring or extending his ability to cope with the demands implicit in his situation"' (Danko *et al.*, 1989: 241).

Needs have to be recognized by the midwife or nurse and, according to this model, must be acknowledged by the individual. Danko *et al.* (1989) comment that this restricts the use of the model as, for example, an infant or a comatose person cannot recognize or express a need-for-help. Wiedenbach (1967) illustrates the utility of this idea in midwifery practice in a description of the identification of postnatal needs:

> Whenever a need-for-help exists, its presence may usually be suspected by behaviour – physical, emotional or physiological – which is different from the normal or usual pattern. The nurse [midwife] who is perceptive will be aware of it. Perceptiveness thus is an important attribute of postpartum nursing. The fact that a need is perceived, however, does not mean that it is met. First it must be identified. To do this requires skilled use of eyes, ears, hands and mind – eyes through which to observe or look intently; ears with which to listen expectantly; hands with which to feel, touch or palpate sensitively; and a mind with which to understand and interpret the observation. Once the need is recognised and has been validated by the one whose need it is, appropriate action may be taken to meet it. (Wiedenbach, 1967: 353–4)

Figure 3.1 illustrates Wiedenbach's model of Need-for-Help.

Wiedenbach's model of the need-for-help focuses on practice, on the process of care, rather than on the outcomes of care and, in terms of this focus, it can be likened to the model developed later by Ela-Joy Lehrman (1981), although both models have potential in terms of the development of outcome measures.

Lehrman (1981) studied the work of certified nurse-midwives. Interestingly, her data is of antenatal visits of women to nurse-midwives who were all providing what would be termed, in the United Kingdom, midwife-led clinics. The underlying question of her study was: 'what are the components of prenatal care provided by certified nurse-midwives?' (Lehrman, 1981: 27). What Lehrman has done is take a step backwards to identify the concepts underlying antenatal care. In Chapter 2, Hayward's (1975) model of preparation for surgery – which brings together the concepts of information, anxiety and pain – was considered. To study these concepts, Hayward had to identify measurable indicators – such as use of analgesia, or the degree of pain shown on a scale – that would provide information about the amount of anxiety or pain being experienced by the individual. Lehrman (1981) is asking the questions: What is it that makes midwifery care important?, what are the components/concepts that make midwifery care important?, and How do these concepts relate to practice? Once these components have been identified, models of the inter-relationship between the components or concepts can be proposed (theorized), and measurable indicators and tools to measure these indicators developed.

Lehrman developed her concepts through a combination of inductive and deductive theorizing. Antenatal visits were audio-taped and, from these, she

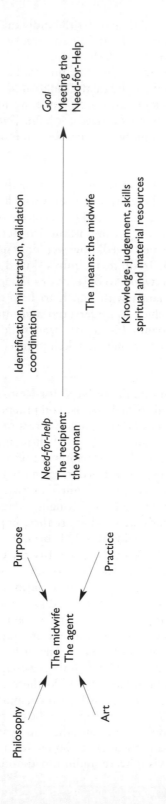

Figure 3.1 Ernestine Wiedenbach's model of nursing (midwifery) practice: need-for-help

Source: Bryar (1995).

developed initial categories or concepts of practice. In addition, Lehrman examined literature covering the preceding 25 years that had been written by nurse-midwives: 'These articles contained a consistent reoccurrence of concepts considered to be aspects of nurse-midwifery practice. These were extracted from the literature and grouped, resulting in eight aspects of 'nurse-midwifery practice' (Lehrman, 1981: 29). The eight concepts describe the underlying philosophy that appeared (from the literature and the grounded theory work undertaken by Lehrman) to underpin nurse-midwifery practice in antenatal care in the USA:

- continuity of care
- family-centred care
- education and counselling as part of care
- non-interventionist care
- flexibility in care
- participative care
- consumer advocacy
- time.

To assess whether these concepts could be demonstrated in practice, Lehrman defined and described the concepts in measurable terms (operationalized the concepts). Her subsequent research confirmed the presence of these concepts in practice. As a result of describing these concepts in measurable terms, relationships between the concepts and outcomes of antenatal care can be examined. Putting these concepts into more familiar language, questions can be asked about the choice (flexibility), control (participative care) and continuity (continuity of care) experienced by a woman, and the social, psychological and physical outcomes of this care. What consequences do the eight concepts individually and collectively have for the actions of midwives and the outcomes of care experienced by a woman, her baby and her family?

This outline of the work of Wiedenbach and Lehrman is foundational and illustrates a number of the elements that combine in the development of theory. In Part II, research from a number of people active in midwifery theory development provides additional information on the processes used to develop and test theory for midwifery practice.

Reva Rubin: attainment of the maternal role

Rubin was a nurse-midwife whose research and theory development influenced the care of childbearing women, and research and theorizing about that care, particularly in the USA. Her research questions were stimulated by role theory and explored the development of the maternal role. This, then, is an example of deductive research: questions were raised in the investigator's mind by role theory, and research was then undertaken to collect data to provide information about the stages and activities involved in the attainment of the maternal role. Inductive reasoning (from the data) was combined with deductive reasoning (from established theory) to develop a theory of maternal role attainment (see Chapter 2).

Rubin (1967a; 1967b) describes the theoretical issues on which her research was based, distinguishing between the concept of position, described as the social status assigned to someone (for example, teacher or mother), and the concept of role, described as the activities and actions carried out by the individual demonstrating occupancy of a certain position. Individuals hold different positions at different stages of their lives and may hold a number of positions at one time – for example, daughter, mother or friend. 'Actions, organised around positions, comprise roles' (Rubin, 1967a: 237). Roles are acquired through a process of learning, achieved through a series of activities. Rubin's work is aimed at identifying how women take on (learn) the role of mother (maternal role) and thus, by implication, what interventions or actions might assist or have a negative effect on this learning process.

The theoretical basis for her work is given in much greater depth in *Maternal Identity and the Maternal Experience* (Rubin, 1984), but the essential questions addressed by her research over a considerable number of years are: 'The problem studied and reported here was how a particular adult role is acquired, specifically the maternal role. What are the processes involved in the acquisition of the maternal role? Who are the models or referrants for maternal role expectations?' (Rubin, 1967a: 237–8).

In the initial study, data were collected by a number of graduate students, as they undertook care of women in antenatal clinics and postnatal settings, through interviews and telephone conversations. The data from these interactions were recorded by the students, following the interaction, which lasted between one and four hours. (Clearly, there are methodological questions that might be asked about such a method of data collection, and it would be neither possible nor desirable to replicate this approach, but the original work is seminal and of historical value). The data relating to the problems of becoming a mother were then coded and analyzed. From this analysis, Rubin identified four tasks that a woman has to complete to achieve the maternal role identity. This analysis was supplemented and modified over the next 20 years with observations of over 6000 women.

Rubin's research and writing covers a period of more than a quarter of century, during which her terminology changed. The following description of the four tasks of pregnancy is taken from Rubin (1984):

> The objectives of the woman's efforts during pregnancy are: a) to ensure safe passage of herself and the baby during pregnancy and childbirth, b) to ensure social acceptance for herself and her child, c) to increase the affinial ties in the construction of the image and identity of the 'I' and 'you', and d) to explore in depth the meaning of the transitive act of giving/receiving. (Rubin, 1984: 10)

These tasks or goals of activity during pregnancy and the puerperium are described more succinctly by Josten (1981) as:

- ensuring the physical wellbeing of herself and the baby
- social acceptance of herself and her child by people who are significant to them both
- attachment to the baby
- understanding of the complexities of mothering.

From earlier data, Rubin (1967a: 240) identified three aspects of the maternal role identity: 'the ideal image, the self image and the body image'. The ideal image comprises all the ideas that the woman had about the positive attributes and activities of women who are mothers. The self image comprises the attributes that the woman saw herself as possessing from her experience: 'Self image was used as the representation of the consistent "myself"' (Rubin, 1967a: 240). The body image is related to changes in the body during pregnancy and the significance of those changes in terms of the progress of the pregnancy.

The maternal identity is achieved by a process of taking-in activities, taking-on activities and letting-go activities. In 1967, Rubin described five operations or means by which the maternal identity is incorporated into the woman's image of herself:

- Taking-on activities: mimicry and role play
- Taking-in activities: fantasy and introjection–projection–rejection
- Letting-go activities: grief-work.

By 1984, mimicry and role play are defined together as replication; fantasy remains as a separate operation, but incorporates grief-work; and introjection–projection–rejection becomes dedifferentiation (Rubin, 1984).

Mimicry involves the replication of actions and behaviours carried out by role-models (for example, other women who are or have been pregnant) and learning from a variety of sources about events in the future: what the delivery will be like, how the baby will be in the first few days. In role play, women act out roles that they will be undertaking in the future; for example, they baby-sit for friends' children, undertake feeding or child care activities. This role-play may be something that actually takes place or something that takes place in the imagination. Replication (taking-on activities) assists the woman in understanding how someone who is pregnant, or a new mother, behaves. Fantasy and the other operations of the taking-in phase enable the woman to develop an understanding of how she will behave. In fantasy, the woman imagines the future for herself: for example, what the birth will be like, what the baby will wear, and the future relationships with other members of the family. In grief-work, the woman reviews her past roles and relinquishes those roles that are no longer appropriate or possible; letting-go takes place:

> Grief-work is a review, in memory, of the attachments and associated events of a former self (role). The experiences, interpersonal and situational, associated with the former self include the actual and the hoped for, the pleasant and unpleasant. The review in the memory of the details of the former-self serve to loosen the ties with the former-self. (Rubin, 1967a: 243–4)

Introjection–projection–rejection is an active process in which the woman compares the available models with her view of herself, and makes active decisions about adopting or rejecting particular models. This activity is differentiated from mimicry, in which an activity, such as wearing maternity clothes, is copied. For example, mimicry may occur postnatally when a woman copies (or is made to follow, in some instances) the bathing 'procedure' with her baby, but introjection–projection–rejection has occurred when, at home, she develops her own approach to bathing based on what she has learnt in hospital and elsewhere.

The maternal role identity described in this model comprises the achievement of the four tasks of pregnancy, which are accomplished by undertaking the operations or activities of mimicry, role play and so on. Rubin (1967a; 1967b) suggests that this model can be imagined as a sphere, with the maternal role identity at the centre, surrounded by the operations. The operations of taking-on (mimicry and role play) precede the operations of taking-in and letting-go, and are thus depicted as the outer rings of the model, as shown in Figure 3.2. The model may also be presented in a linear fashion, as shown in Figure 3.3.

Rubin's model will now be considered in relation to the key concepts of person, health, environment and midwifery, which were discussed in Chapter 2 as four of the central concepts underpinning midwifery care. Other models discussed in this and subsequent chapters can also be analyzed in this way. This model puts greater emphasis on the person and environment than on health and midwifery.

Person: The model developed by Rubin from integration of theory with vast quantities of empirical data has as its focus the person: the woman and the development of the woman and her identity as a woman, mother and member

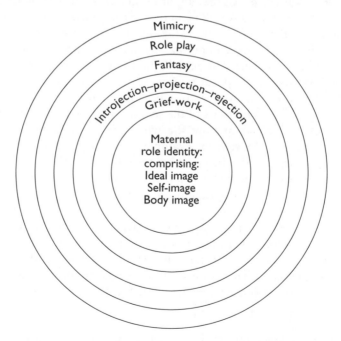

Figure 3.2   Rubin's model of attainment of the maternal role

Source: Bryar (1995).

of society who is a mother – the central concern of the model is with the achievement by the woman of a positive identity as a mother. The achievement of this role can be assessed in terms of attainment of the four tasks of pregnancy. For example, whether the woman has been able to ensure safety for herself and her baby can be assessed in terms of physical outcomes, the health of the baby and the woman. Whether the woman has managed to integrate the baby into her social situation may be assessed in terms of their support systems, financial situation or accommodation.

Health: One of the tasks of pregnancy identified is the maintenance of safety of the woman and baby, including maintenance of health. The maternal identity is described as comprising ideal, self and body images. Throughout pregnancy, the body is seen as being of central concern, so that health and perceptions of health are particularly important during a time when body changes may be alarming or may not have been experienced before.

Environment: The environment, or social system, is the second major focus of this model. Rubin essentially views maternal behaviour as a social activity that is demonstrated in interactions and relationships with others in the woman's social system. Again, the extent to which the woman has achieved the tasks of pregnancy can be assessed in terms of her relationship with the baby, family, friends, colleagues and health professionals.

Midwifery: This model describes the woman as being involved in an active process of growth and development during pregnancy. During this time, she is actively seeking out role-models and integrating these role-models into her picture, or image, of herself. The woman is the central actor in this process. The aim of the midwife, within this model, is to provide interventions that support the operations and achievement of the maternal tasks. For example, by providing information about food and exercise early in pregnancy, the midwife provides a model for the woman to mimic. By providing information about different options for delivery, she provides information that the woman can use in introjection–projection–rejection, and, in undertaking observations in labour, the midwife helps the woman achieve a safe outcome.

This model places the focus clearly on achievement by the woman of a new role and can be classified with other development-focused models, although the basis of Rubin's model is in symbolic interactionism. (Symbolic interactionism is based on the work of G.H. Mead and proposes that: 'people's selves are social products'; '(1) People act towards things based on the meaning those things have for them; and (2) these meanings are derived from social interaction and modified through interpretation' (Blumer, no date)). Rubin thus demonstrates that models may draw on a range of different traditions, or paradigms, rather than being based on only one (see Chapter 2). The model helps to identify factors that indicate the health of the woman (in the terms of the model) in its widest sense. Those indicators may be measured during pregnancy to demonstrate the extent to which the tasks have been achieved (Josten, 1981) or, at the end of the midwife's care, to provide a summative evaluation of care and achievement of maternal role identity. The model can be operationalized to provide a basis for practice, a basis on which to audit practice and a means of generating research questions.

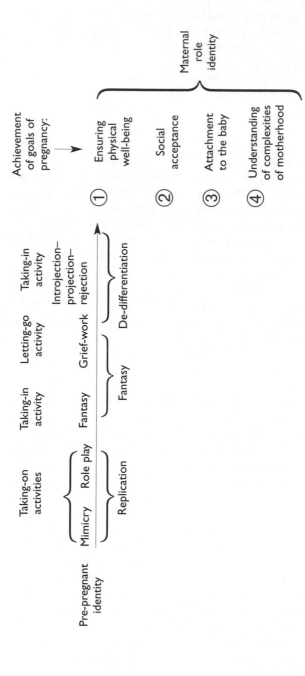

Figure 3.3 Linear representation of Rubin's model of attainment of the maternal role

Source: Bryar (1995).

Cranley (1981), in a study of maternal–foetal attachment during pregnancy, provides an illustration of the need to test the relationships between concepts in all parts of a model. In this study, the concept of maternal–foetal attachment during pregnancy is tested. A measurement tool was developed that women completed during pregnancy and in the early postnatal period. The items in this tool measure six aspects of attachment, including interaction measured by items on the scale such as: 'I poke the baby to get him/her to poke back' (Cranley, 1981: 282), giving of self, and nesting. The results provided support for the activity of maternal–foetal attachment during pregnancy.

Parts of the model have also been used postnatally; indeed, Martell and Mitchell (1984) cite nine maternity textbooks that base postnatal care on the taking-in and taking-hold phases. In her later work, Rubin (1984) describes these processes as taking place throughout pregnancy (see Figure 3.3) but, in 1961, Rubin described, again from observation, taking-in and taking-hold occurring in the immediate postnatal period. Taking-in, where the woman was focused on herself and the immediate past of the labour, dominated in days 1–2, and taking-hold, where the woman was more orientated to others and to becoming more independent, dominated in days 3–10.

Martell and Mitchell (1984) and Ament (1989) describe studies in which they collected data to assess the extent to which taking-in and taking-hold activities occurred. Ament (1989) found that women did display taking-in and taking-hold behaviours, but that taking-in only predominated on day 1, with taking-hold activities predominating from day 2. Martell and Mitchell (1984), on the other hand, found no support for a taking-in phase, but did find support for a taking-hold phase that peaked on day 2.

These studies demonstrate the need to test the findings of observational studies in other settings, as well as the need to test theoretical propositions. The authors of these studies undertaken in the 1980s discuss the cultural and organizational changes that had taken place in labour and postnatal care since the 1960s that could also have had a significant effect on the demonstration of these phases – as, for example, postnatal hospital stay has been reduced. Subsequent changes in maternity care provision indicate the need to further test the propositions of this model in current practice.

Ramona T. Mercer: theories of antepartum stress and maternal role attainment – becoming a mother

Mercer is the only theorist whose work has been exclusively concerned with understanding the process of childbearing that is included in a collection considering the work of the major theorists in nursing (Marriner-Tomey and Alligood, 2006). Bee and Oetting (1989) provide a description of Mercer's distinguished academic career, which has focused on theory building, research and practice applications of research findings in the field of maternity care. Her work was greatly influenced by Rubin, who was the professor in maternity nursing at the university where Mercer obtained her doctoral degree (Mercer, 1995). By 1988, Mercer had published four books, over 55 articles, book chapters and reports: a body of work that, in itself, shows that there has been considerable theory development by nurse-midwives in the care of the childbearing family.

Mercer has been responsible for the development of a number of research measurement tools that have been widely used by other researchers (see, for example, Fawcett *et al.*, 1993; Marut and Mercer, 1979). Mercer has also been concerned to apply the findings of her research and theory building to practice: 'The concepts theorized by Mercer have been used by nursing in multiple obstetric textbooks. She is often cited as taking the work by Rubin and expanding its utilization. Her theory is extremely practice orientated' (Bee and Oetting, 1989: 299). This concern with the utilization of theory is shown in the discussion of implications for nursing intervention in *First-Time Motherhood* (Mercer, 1986) and in articles such as 'The Nurse and Maternal Tasks of the Early Postpartum' (Mercer, 1981a). For example, in this article Mercer comments on the tasks that the woman has to undertake in the early postnatal days, and indicates that these tasks 'encompass far more than "bonding" to her infant' (Mercer, 1981a: 344). One of the tasks that has been identified theoretically and confirmed through research observation is the task of integrating the labour and birth experiences:

> When the nurse asks, 'What was your labor and delivery like?' this requires creative listening to hear what the woman is really saying when she answers. One way to facilitate the work of fitting in the 'missing pieces' and integrating the birth is through a review of the labor and delivery with the nurse who was with her. (Mercer, 1981a: 344)

Another interesting feature of Mercer's work that also applies to many other theorists in the USA is that it has been utilized and built upon by a large number of graduate students who were supervised by Mercer (Bee and Oetting, 1989). Such a programme of ongoing research provides further evidence of the utility of the theory, or provides information that can lead to modification of a theory. The final section of this chapter describes the work of Soo Downe and colleagues, and chapters later in this book demonstrate the value of such programmes of research activity (see, for example, Chapters 4, 5, 11 and 13).

Mercer has undertaken theory building and research in two main areas: the effects of antepartum stress, and attainment of the maternal role.

The effect of antepartum stress on the family

Mercer's research is concerned with a number of measures of the effects of antenatal stress relating to the functioning of the family unit. Mercer and her colleagues have been seeking to understand the effects of antenatal stress on family functioning, as a whole; on functioning of pairs of individuals in a family; and on health status. Mercer *et al.* (1986) identify six variables from research and other literature that are related to the outcome variables of health status, dyadic relationships and family functioning:

- antepartum stress
- social support
- self-esteem

- sense of mastery
- anxiety
- depression.

The outcome variables (dependent variables) were defined; for example, 'health status' was defined as follows: 'the mother's and father's perception of their prior health, current health, health outlook, resistance-susceptibility to illness, health worry concerns, sickness orientation, and rejection of the sick role' (Mercer *et al.*, 1986: 342).

Each of the independent variables – for example, social support and self-esteem – is defined, and the theoretical basis for each variable discussed. Three models are then presented that suggest the relationships between the independent variables and the dependent variables of health status (of the individual), dyadic relationships and family functioning. These models consider antenatal stress in relation to: the individual; the dyads; and family functioning.

In a later article, Mercer *et al.* (1988) present the results of a study that was undertaken to test one of the three models of antepartum stress. This study considered the effects of antepartum stress on family functioning. Within the model, it is suggested that variables have either negative or positive effects on family functioning, as indicated in this description of the model:

Stress from negative life-events and pregnancy risk were predicted to have direct negative effects on self-esteem and health status; self-esteem, health status, and social support were predicted to have direct positive effects on sense of mastery; sense of mastery was predicted to have direct negative effects on anxiety and depression which in turn have direct negative effects on family functioning. (Mercer *et al.*, 1988: 269)

The relationships in the model were tested in a study of women who had been admitted to hospital with high-risk pregnancies. These women were compared with a group of women who had low-risk pregnancies. In addition, the partners of half the women in both groups were also interviewed. Mercer *et al.* (1988) make the point that much research on pregnancy has been from the woman's viewpoint, and that there is a need to consider family functioning from the viewpoint of the male partner as well. Data was collected in relation to each of the six independent variables using a variety of data-collection tools, including an index of general health and measures of social support. The dependent variable, family functioning, was measured using a family-functioning measurement instrument. The data were collected when the women were between 24 and 34 weeks pregnant.

The data were then analyzed using a range of statistical tests to test the study hypotheses:

Hypothesis 1:
High-risk women experiencing antenatal hospitalization and their partners will report less optimal family functioning than low-risk women and their partners.

Hypothesis 2:
Expectant partners will report similar levels of family functioning (Mercer *et al.*, 1988: 269).

The study findings supported the first hypothesis but did not support the second hypothesis in relation to the partners of the low-risk women. The researchers are able to show the impact of each of the variables on family functioning, and to show the different predictive values of the different variables for women in both the low-risk group and the high risk-group. This enabled the researchers to redraw their model of the effect of antepartum stress on family functioning. Two different models emerge from the data, one that demonstrates the relationship of the variables in the case of the low-risk women and one for the case of high-risk women. These models may now be further tested and modified. These findings, derived from testing a model combining the variables of particular importance in predicting antenatal stress and the effects of that stress on family functioning, may also help midwives decide on priority areas for antenatal care.

Maternal role attainment

The underlying concern in Mercer's work is with attainment of the maternal role: 'Becoming a mother means taking on a new identity. Taking on a new identity involves a complete rethinking and redefining of self' (Mercer, 1986: 3). The reason for the interest of American nurse-midwives in attainment of the maternal role may appear to be self-evident, but Mercer indicates that interest in the role is important because some women have difficulty taking on the maternal role which, Mercer suggests, has consequences for their children: 'While most women achieve the role successfully, approximately one to two million mothers [in the USA] experience difficulty with the role, as evidenced by the number of abused or neglected children' (Mercer, 1981b: 73).

Mercer (as does Rubin), takes an interactionist approach to understanding the process by which people take on new roles. The interactionist view is that the way an individual takes on and acts out a particular role is dependent on the reactions and interactions that they have with people in their environment; for example, their partner, the infant, their family and other people.

The expression of a role by an individual will also be affected by their past experiences and view of themselves (Mercer, 1981b; 1986; Dunnington and Glazer, 1991). Mercer (1981b) describes the theoretical base of her research in role acquisition theory, which identifies four stages to role acquisition: anticipatory, formal, informal and personal stages:

> The anticipatory stage is the period prior to incumbency when an individual begins social and psychological adjustment to the role by learning the expectations of the role. The formal stage begins with actual incumbency during which role behaviours are largely guided by formal, consensual expectations of others in the individual's social system. The informal stage begins as the individual develops unique ways of dealing with the role that are not

conveyed by the social system. During the final, or personal, stage of role acquisition, an individual imposes an individual style on the role performance, and others largely accept the enactment. Social adjustment has occurred through role modification, and psychological adjustment has resulted in the individual's feeling a congruence of self and role. (Mercer, 1981b: 74)

While Rubin describes many of the activities associated with taking on the maternal role as occurring in pregnancy and up to six months after the birth of the child (Mercer, 1981b), Mercer's theoretical model indicates that the majority of the role-taking activities occur after the birth of the child, and that attainment of the maternal role may occur between three and 10 months after the birth. Mercer has identified 11 independent variables that influence the attainment of the maternal role (the dependent variable) and a number of confounding variables. Confounding variables include the woman's cultural background, which will have an effect on the way she perceives the maternal role and the way that she adopts the role. Confounding variables affect both the independent and dependent variables (see Box 3.1).

Mercer has undertaken extensive research describing the relationship between the maternal, infant and other/confounding variables and the attainment of the maternal role.

The influence of these variables was investigated by Mercer in a longitudinal study of 242 women aged between 15 and 42 years (Mercer, 1986). The main aim of this research was to identify whether age had any effect on attainment of the maternal role. Secondary aims were to identify the effect of the other variables, either individually or in combination, on the maternal role, and to identify from the data collected whether there were any other factors that appeared to affect the maternal role (Mercer, 1981b; 1986). The study involved the collection of data using a battery of measurement tools from the sample on five different occasions, from the early postnatal period through to the end of the first year.

Mercer (1986) uses the data to present a model of adaptation to the maternal role in the first year that combines four phases of adaptation at three

---

Box 3.1   Variables identified by Mercer related to attainment of the maternal role

Maternal variables
1 Maternal age at first birth
2 Perceptions of the birth experience
3 Early maternal-infant separation
4 Social stress
5 Social support
6 Self-concept
7 Personality traits
8 Child-rearing attitudes
9 Maternal health status

Infant variables
1 Temperament
2 Infant health

Other/confounding variables
1 Ethnic background
2 Marital status
3 Socioeconomic status

levels. The four phases described are: 'physical recovery phase, from birth to 1 month; an achievement phase, from 2 to 4 or 5 months; a disruption phase, from 6 to 8 months; and a reorganization phase that begins after the eighth month and is in process at 12 months' (Mercer, 1986: 300).

The three levels at which adaptation occurs are the biological, the psychological and the social. The biological level includes the woman's physical recovery and her adaptation to the growth and development of the infant. The psychological is concerned with the woman's reactions to and perceptions of being a mother, and the social is concerned with changes in her life and social relationships over the first year. During the course of the year, the achievement of adaptation at the different levels varies, as shown in Figure 3.4. In the physical recovery phase, the biological level predominates, while at later phases the social or psychological levels predominate. Adaptation at later phases may be inhibited if there are unresolved problems from earlier phases; for example, poor physical health in the achievement phase will inhibit the psychological and social achievements that should be occurring then.

These findings have implications for practice. In the achievement phase, for example, Mercer (1986) notes that women need to be advised to have an examination if they have any physical or psychological problems. She found that, at four months, more women reported health problems than at one month postpartum: 66 per cent of the women reported health problems, 44 per cent had one problem and 22 per cent had two problems. While 25 per cent had colds, other problems reported included genital tract infections, chronic illnesses, gastro-intestinal problems, breast problems, joint or muscle problems, emotional tension or headaches, loss of hair, anaemia, injuries and accidents (Mercer, 1986: 164–5). These findings are congruent

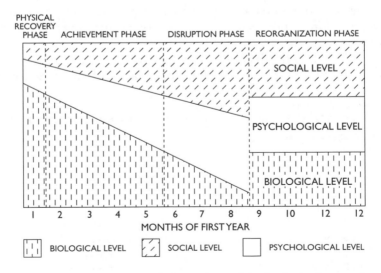

Figure 3.4   A representation of Mercer's model of adaptation to the maternal role in the first year of motherhood

Source: Bryar (1995).

with the findings reported in the United Kingdom by MacArthur *et al.* (1991) and from Jordan by Hatamleh *et al.* (2007) of the high level of postnatal morbidity women experience after the six-week check. MacArthur *et al.* (1991) suggest, as does Mercer (1986), that antenatal prevention of some of these problems may be achieved, and the need to follow up women, possibly at six months, post-delivery.

The role of the midwife that emerges from Mercer's writings is to assist the woman with the work needed to adjust to the maternal role, and to identify and intervene where there are factors that are affecting maternal role attainment or contributing to antenatal stress. This discussion of the work of Ramona T. Mercer has shown the process of theory development, testing and application of the theory and research results in practice.

Rosamund Bryar: the action approach to organizations and midwifery practice

In the late 1970s and early 1980s, Rosamund Bryar was involved in an action research project that aimed to develop individualized care in midwifery in a hospital and community midwifery service. The aim of the project was, therefore, to bring about organizational change. Actions in the study were concentrated on increasing midwives' knowledge of individual care and in changing some of their working practices through the allocation of women to each midwife (Adams *et al.*, 1981; Bryar, 1985; 1991). The evaluation of this study showed that most of the midwives held models of childbearing (their theories-in-action – Agyris and Schön, 1974) that supported the idea of individualized care but, in practice, the type of care that was given was focused on physical needs and on routine needs rather than the individual needs of women (their theories-in-use – Agyris and Schön, 1974). In Chapter 7 in Part II of this book, Hunter provides further evidence in support of these findings, as does the work of Crozier *et al.* in Chapter 11. The organization, the system within which these midwives worked, limited the extent to which they could provide individualized care and actually discouraged individualized care, through the operation of policies and routines that were supported by the structures of the organization, the professional power relationships and management hierarchies. In the study, change was not attempted in other parts of the organization, which limited the care that the midwives could provide. It was concluded that change in care could not be produced simply through a change in the knowledge of the midwives within an organization.

Descriptions of organizations frequently focus on the internal relationships within organizations but, as Handy (1976) acknowledges in relation to the role culture organization, organizations do not exist in isolation but, rather, are part of society and are affected by society. Davies and Francis (1976) argue that the professional organization and bureaucracy models are inadequate to describe the hospital as an organization, and Davies (1979) suggests that organizational theory should consider the inter-relationship of health care with other organizations and aspects of society. Silverman (1970) is similarly critical of organization theory, which separates the organization as a unit from the wider society, and considers that a better understanding of organizations may be achieved if the relationships between the organization and the wider society are specified. Silverman's (1970) action approach to organizations rests on the view that society – and, thus, organizations – are socially constructed and dependent on the meanings attached to them by members of the society or the organization. Berger and Luckmann (1976) describe this as the social construction of reality, a model that describes the theory developed by symbolic interactionists. Each individual experiences reality differently, and constructs their own understanding of their reality, or their environment, differently.

Silverman (1970) contrasts the action approach to organizations, which places the organization within its social context, with the approach of the bureaucratic and systems models, which reify organizations and separate them from the social context. Systems theories describe organizations as biological systems with certain needs and goals that are achieved by taking in inputs and producing end-products. All parts of the system are seen as being interdependent and little attention is given, within these models, to the purposes of individuals within organizations. The professional organization model, in contrast, concentrates on the relationship between individuals and the power held by different professions. Silverman (1970) argues that neither of these approaches is satisfactory, as one emphasizes the formal role structure and role position of members of an organization and ignores their individual values, and the other exaggerates the extent to which individuals seek to achieve their own ends and extend their own power while ignoring the existence of shared values and interdependence (Silverman, 1970).

The model that Silverman (1970) describes as a framework to assist in the analysis and understanding of organizations, such as that of a maternity service, has four elements: the changing stock of knowledge outside the organization, in the wider society; the internal organizational role system; the individual's definition of the situation: values, attitudes, attachments, meanings and the way that the individual understands (constructs) reality, which will be a consequence of their wider experiences and experiences in the organization; and the actions of individuals that result from the interaction of the other elements, as shown in Figure 3.5.

Applying this approach to midwifery care demonstrates that the action – midwifery care – results from the interaction of a number of factors. Some of the factors that are relevant to the care of the childbearing woman are illustrated in Figure 3.6. The values and attitudes in the wider society towards birth, motherhood, women, families, midwives, the medical profession and other factors will have an influence on the organization of maternity services. The structures within the organization will also affect the activities of midwives and the care of women; for example, the relationships between the different professional groups involved in the care of the childbearing woman: midwives, obstetricians, physiotherapists and others, and the management systems, whether these are hierarchical or collegial.

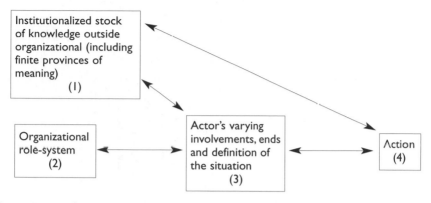

Figure 3.5   The action approach to organizations

Source: Silverman (1970). Reproduced with kind permission of D. Silverman.

The knowledge, skills and models of midwifery care held by the midwives and the women for whom they are caring will also have a significant influence on the type of care that midwives are able to provide. For example, if a midwife lacks communication skills, it may be more difficult for a woman to become an active participant in her care. If a woman expects health care professionals to take responsibility for her care, she may react with hostility when asked to assume this responsibility herself.

This conceptual model brings together the different models held by the different parties involved in the provision of midwifery care: the wider society, the hospital/community unit, the individual practitioners, women and their families. It also suggests ways in which these models may inter-relate to produce the action – the care of the childbearing woman.

In relation to the models held by individuals, Odent (1984) provides an illustration of one model that may be held by some midwives and, as he suggests, has a significant impact on the type of care they give: 'Then there are the others, possibly more of them, who unconsciously protect themselves from over-involvement and will offer more impersonal, technical, brisk, mechanical and ultimately "inhuman" care. They are a bad model for the mother to emulate' (Odent, 1984: 90).

Arms (1981) illustrates the effect that the organizational structures may have on care, even when the nurse-midwives and other health practitioners hold woman-centred models of care:

Despite the personal beliefs and intentions of the residents and midwives alike, both are caught in a system that moves women through birth too quickly to permit closeness with any patient.

If nurse-midwives are ever to function as true midwives, they must be free from the pressure to rush and alter the natural process. The average hospital is not conducive to normal birth experiences, even with the finest nurse-midwives and the finest intentions. (Arms, 1981: 323)

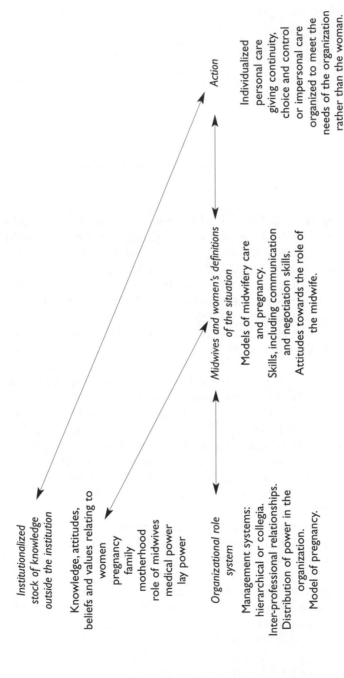

Institutionalized stock of knowledge outside the institution

Knowledge, attitudes, beliefs and values relating to women
pregnancy
family
motherhood
role of midwives
medical power
lay power

Organizational role system

Management systems: hierarchical or collegia.
Inter-professional relationships.
Distribution of power in the organization.
Model of pregnancy.

Midwives and women's definitions of the situation

Models of midwifery care and pregnancy.
Skills, including communication and negotiation skills.
Attitudes towards the role of the midwife.

Action

Individualized personal care giving continuity, choice and control or impersonal care organized to meet the needs of the organization rather than the woman.

Figure 3.6   The action framework and care of the childbearing woman

Source: Bryar (1991).

In Chapter 8, Walsh demonstrates the impact on care when midwives and maternity care assistants are able to express a women-centred model of care in a birth centre.

At the societal level, the World Health Organization model of Health for All (WHO, 1988) illustrates the potential impact that attitudes at this level might have on the care of childbearing women. Figure 3.7 identifies the concepts in this model and the impacts on the action (care) of the model. These underlying concepts have been restated in the World Health Organization Report in 2008 (WHO, 2008), which calls for reform in four areas:

- universal coverage reforms to improve health equity
- leadership reforms to make health authorities more reliable (effective services)
- public policy reforms to promote and protect the health of communities (inter-sectoral collaboration)
- service delivery reforms to make health systems more people-centred (community participation). (WHO, 2008: xvi)

These illustrations show the effects that the models held by midwives, the model structuring the organization, or the model informing health policy, may have on the type of care provided to childbearing women. These illustrations

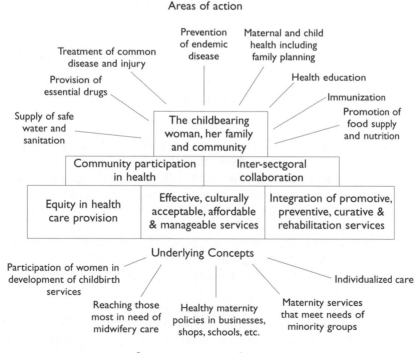

Figure 3.7   The Health for All model: consequences for practice

Source: Bryar (1995).

also indicate that changes in models are required at different levels, if the care women experience is to change. Change at one point, in one part of the organizational system illustrated by the framework, cannot be relied on to produce change in care.

The action approach to organizations demonstrates the need to attend to the constraints on change at the level of society, the organization (and all the groups within the organization) and the individual. Depending on the models held by the policy-makers, midwives, obstetricians, health service managers, women and their families, changes in care will be more or less difficult to attain in different places. The model helps to clarify why it is important that midwives are able to articulate their models of practice. If these models can be articulated, they can then be examined in relation to the prevailing models in society and the models held by other occupational groups, the women and their families. Difficulties in achieving the aims of midwifery care may then be more easily identified, together with ways of seeking to achieve change.

Jean Ball: the deckchair theory of maternal emotional wellbeing

Jean Ball, a British midwife, undertook extensive research into the postnatal needs of women, and the consequences for women of different forms of organization of maternity services (Ball, 1981; 1987; 1989). In *Reactions to Motherhood* (1987), she describes the following aim of postnatal care:

> The purpose of all maternity care is to enable a woman to be successful in becoming a mother, and this success applies not only to the physiological processes involved but also to the psychological and emotional processes which motivate the desire for parenthood and its fulfilment. (Ball, 1987: 127)

This aim can be seen as Ball's personal aim or philosophy of postnatal care, which identifies pregnancy and the postnatal period as a time of adoption of a new role. The literature review for Ball's (1987) study of postnatal care identifies role theory, change theory, theories of stress, coping and support as the theoretical basis for the study. The concepts investigated are drawn from theories of coping and support systems. The variables investigated relate to the woman's personality; life-events, and personal and family circumstances; factors relating to the birth and progress following the birth; and the woman's views of care, support and emotional wellbeing. The hypotheses for the study were that:

> The emotional response of women to the changes which follow the birth of a child will be affected by their personality and by the quality of support they receive from family and social support systems. The way in which care is provided by midwives during the postnatal period will influence the emotional response of women to the changes which follow the birth of a child. (Ball, 1987: 37)

The variables were investigated through collection of information from 279 women. Data were collected using structured interviews administered antenatally, in the early postnatal period and by a postal questionnaire at six weeks. Interviews were held with midwives who were responsible for transferring the women home, and postal questionnaire data were obtained from the community midwives involved with the women. The data were analyzed quantitatively to identify those factors that affected the women's emotional wellbeing and their satisfaction with motherhood. The factors found to contribute to emotional wellbeing are shown in Figure 3.8. Ball (1987) comments:

> Good scores on all these factors would result in a high degree of emotional wellbeing, while poor scores on all of them would result in considerable distress. But as these factors also interact with each other, if poor scores on certain factors are counterbalanced by good scores on others, it might be possible for the potential emotional outcome to be improved. (Ball, 1987: 118)

The analysis supported both hypotheses of the study, which indicated that a woman's wellbeing following delivery is dependent on her own personality,

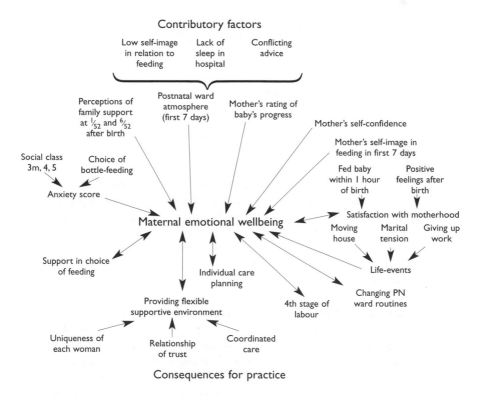

Figure 3.8   Factors identified by Jean Ball as affecting maternal emotional well-being

Source: Ball (1987). Reproduced with permission of J. Ball.

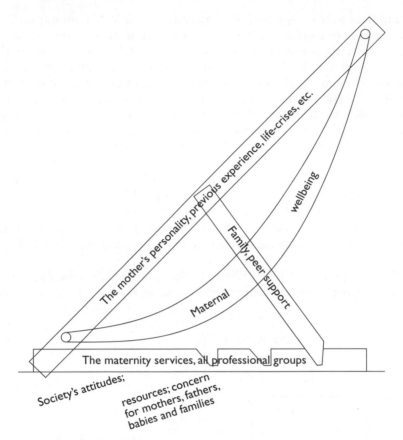

Figure 3.9   Support systems for maternal wellbeing

Source: Ball (1987). Reproduced with kind permission of J. Ball.

her personal support system and the support provided by the maternity services. Ball (1987) illustrates the inter-relationship of these three elements as a deckchair, as shown in Figure 3.9. The base of the chair is formed by the maternity services resting on the views of society regarding families; the side-strut by the woman's personality, life experiences, and so on; and the central strut by her family and support system. The woman's maternal wellbeing (the seat of the chair) is dependent on the effective coming together of all these elements:

> If a deckchair is not erected properly, it will collapse under the weight of its occupant; if it does not stand on a firm base it will fall over with similar results; and if the parts do not fit together well the occupant may be held up, but will become uncomfortable and strained. (Ball, 1987: 120)

The deckchair can be seen to have similarities to the action framework, where the views of society, the individual's definition of the situation and the organization of services all contribute to the action – the woman's maternal wellbeing. Interesting parallels can also be drawn between Ball's work and that of Mercer (1986). Another illustration of the importance of chairs to women and their newborn infants is provided later in this book by Jones and Kendall, in Chapter 6. If the picture or theory of maternal wellbeing that Ball has identified, from empirical data in combination with a theoretical framework, is compared with the key concepts of midwifery described in Chapter 2, it can be seen that this theory addresses each of these of concepts.

- **Women:** The focus of Ball's work is concern for individual women and for their successful emotional, social and psychological development during the childbirth process.
- **Health:** Health is central to this model, being seen in the definition of the aim of postnatal care: 'to enable a woman to be successful in becoming a mother' (Ball, 1987: 127).
- **Environment:** The social and organizational environments, in the form of support systems and postnatal care services (as well as the wider society), are important elements of this model, support having been shown to be crucial for the wellbeing of the woman.
- **Midwifery:** In part, the research on postnatal care was motivated by a concern relating to the lack of information about the effects of midwifery care on emotional wellbeing. The model provides guidance on many areas of intervention by midwives that are discussed by Ball, including patterns of care, support in decisions on feeding methods, help with feeding and individual care planning (see Figure 3.8).
- **Self:** The theory clearly starts from the standpoint that the role of the midwife is to support and assist the woman to become confident in the role of mother. Ball (1987) contends that services and patterns of care must change in response to the needs of women, however painful that may be for the health professionals concerned. The stance underpinning this approach to care is, thus, one of listening, learning and changing.

This theory relates concepts of, for example, anxiety, life-events and emotional well-being, and can be described as a factor-relating theory (Dickoff and James 1992; see Chapter 2) and the relationships between the factors, or concepts, now need to be tested further by research. In addition, there is now a need for midwives to undertake further research to determine what aspects of midwifery practice may modify, for example, women's perceptions of the postnatal ward atmosphere, or the woman's self-image of feeding in the first seven days. It is time to test the deckchair and Ball's DeckChair Theory of Maternal Emotional Wellbeing.

Soo Downe: salutogenesis, complexity theory and authoritative knowledge

Soo Downe may be described as a new midwifery theory activist. Studies undertaken by Downe and colleagues chart a movement towards a new perception of the nature and consequences of maternity care based on salutogenesis and complexity theory (Downe and McCourt, 2008). Their publications have covered expertise (Downe *et al.*, 2007), traumatic and positive birth (Thomson and Downe, 2008; Thomson and Downe, 2010), leadership and the good midwife (Byrom and Downe, 2010), skilled help from the heart (El-Nemer *et al.*, 2006), authentic midwifery (O'Connell and Downe, 2009), and the design and poetics of metasynthesis as a basis for capturing the essence of prior qualitative work (Walsh and Downe, 2005; Walsh and Downe, 2006; Downe, 2008).

The approach that underpins these studies has emerged as a result of encounters with a number of relevant theories. This section describes these theories, and explains how the interconnectivity between them (in complexity theory terms) has enabled the new theoretical turn described in Downe and McCourt (2008) and Downe (2010a).

Authoritative science thinking in medicine and health care has, until very recently, been strongly rooted in positivism. This approach has been very successful in identifying improved treatments for many areas of health care. In maternity care, for example, the use of magnesium sulphate for pre-eclampsia has made a dramatic contribution to improving the outcomes of pregnant women with pre-eclampsia and eclampsia (Altman *et al.*, 2002). However, there is an increasing recognition that this approach to knowledge, based on simple linear thinking at a population level (what is best for the majority) may not provide the solutions for a range of more complex issues at the level of the individual, where most service users interact with most health care staff. In a paper published in 1997, David Sackett and colleagues make it quite clear that evidence-based medicine (EBM), then in its infancy, was: 'the conscientious, explicit and judicious use of current best evidence in making decisions about the care of individual patients ... integrating individual clinical expertise with the best available external clinical evidence from systematic research' (Sackett *et al.*, 1997: 3).

As Jordon (1993) has noted, there is never one culture at work in society. At the same time as normal science EBM has flourished, new movements have been emerging as pretenders to the throne. Baysien theory, for example, has been fighting a rearguard action against frequentist science for at least four decades. Put simply, Bayesian theory proposes that, in cases where the evidence for an intervention is unclear, prior probabilities for the range of effects can be set, based on such evidence as does exist and expert opinion, beliefs, and experience. These so-called 'priors' can then be moderated by data arising from formal investigation, whether the data are generated from a strictly controlled randomized trial of sufficient size or not (Cornfield, 1969; Lilford and Braunholtz, 1996). This approach depends on *post hoc* re-calculations of relative risk and sensitivity analyses. Its value lies in the fact that it does not depend on black and white acceptance or rejection of a null hypothesis, in such a way that other relevant data (such as biological plausibility or implausibility) is not assessed. It also explicitly accepts the fact that most researchers, and most users of research, have strong views about an intervention, and they bring this to their interpretation of new data (that is, they are not in equipoise). It can, therefore, be applied to relatively small trials, or to large trials assessing rare outcomes (Thornton and Lilford, 1996). This approach begins to acknowledge that contextual features of culture and organization can be at least as important as pure trials evidence in determining what works.

Complexity theory offers another interpretation of this phenomenon (Downe and McCourt, 2008; Downe, 2010a; 2010b). One of the features of systems that are complex (and not merely complicated or chaotic) is that they are dynamic, self-organizing and adaptive. They are, therefore, constantly in a state of flux and change, and they are not very amenable to being measured by fixed-state tools or rules. Complexity theorists note the power of interconnectivity within and between systems. Systems (organizations, organisms) that are highly-connected can magnify small stimuli that take place in one part of the system, leading to sudden changes, called 'tipping points'. The rapid change from post-nursing midwifery education to direct entry training in England is an example of this kind of change. Paradoxically, extensive attempts at change might have no effect at all, if the system is not change ready. For example, the multitude of trials and practice development schemes designed to change practice in routine foetal monitoring for low-risk women have had very little effect in many settings.

At the level of the organism, the pregnant and labouring body adapts dynamically to a wide range of hormonal and physiological inputs, with interconnected feedback loops between biochemical, cellular, and (as in labour) muscular signals and responses. It is also a neurologically complex state, as recent evidence on the impact of pathological emotional stress in pregnancy on maternal and neonatal outcomes indicates. Even more intriguingly, it appears to be socio-psycho-neuro-hormonally dynamic (Schmid and Downe, 2010). Recently, it has been suggested that caesarean section might be linked with auto-immune diseases in the infant, such as Type 1 diabetes or asthma (Cardwell et al., 2008; Roduit et al., 2008). This may seem to be a far-fetched claim. However, there have been a number of studies that indicate that a range of variables related to labour and birth might impact on asthma and eczema, and there is an increasing interest in the link between emotional and psychosocial states and the immune response (Solomon, 1987).

This also indicates that an insistence on seeing labour and birth as linear phenomena may lead to erroneous decision-making on the part of care givers. There is anecdotal evidence that some women exhibit patterns of pregnancy (such as very long gestational periods) and of labour (such as slow first phases and rapid second phases) that are like their mother and/or sisters. This may suggest that there are genetic 'initial conditions' (epi-genetics) that might predispose some pregnancy and labour patterns to look unusual to those using an average-woman based linear model, but that are physiological to certain women and/or infants. Again, attention to a complexity model of pregnancy and childbirth might limit unnecessary intervention in these groups, and provide an early warning system for women who have pregnancy and labour patterns that are unusual, with no evidence of prior family physiology that would suggest this is normal for them.

Complexity theory claims that complex systems tend to be fractal, or 'self-similar': that is, that similar phenomena can be observed at all levels of the system. This suggests that optimum environments for birth might be founded, fractally, on calmness, confidence, trust and expertise, and an authentic concern for the health and well-being of women, babies, partners, staff and managers (Downe, 2010a; 2010b). Conversely, toxic environments are likely to be epitomized by fear, and distrust of and distance from colleagues, managers and childbearing women. Moving from the latter state to the former requires an approach that values what is good and positive in the individual and their environment. We have used the theory of salutogenesis to frame work that is designed to do this.

Salutogenesis is a theory that was first proposed by Aaron Antonovsky (1987). Antonovsky began to develop his central ideas while he was undertaking research on the psychological impacts of being a concentration camp survivor. Most individuals in the studies he undertook experienced the expected high levels of psychological pathology. However, some were remarkably positive about their lives, and about the world. Rather than seeing these individuals as inconvenient exceptions to the rule, Antonovsky began to explore how they could be so resilient and so positive when they had been through so much. This question developed into an exploration of what Antonovsky termed the 'Sense of Coherence' concept. This postulated that an individual who can see the world as manageable, comprehensible and meaningful was more likely to see their life as coherent, and to be able to cope with adverse events positively, no matter how extreme their experiences might be. Apart from this specific psychological theory, Antonovsky began to think about what would happen if we saw life generally in terms of how it goes right, rather than what makes it goes wrong: 'A salutogenic orientation facilitates seeing things that experts in a given pathology might well fail to see … it … pressures one to think in systems terms … it leads one to deal with (both) entropic (disorder-promoting) forces and … negentropic (order-promoting) forces' (Antonovsky, 1993: 115; 1996).

This statement has a strong resonance for health care in general, and for maternity care in particular. It has implications for how we understand particular events that might be seen as pathological (such as pain in labour, a long gestation, a slow labour, or the early pushing urge). It also has implications for systems of maternity care. Given that there is disquiet nationally and internationally about high levels of intervention, and about women's views and staff morale, a salutogenic approach might create the energy to make the changes that appear to be elusive at the moment. This would ask: How do some services and systems get it so right, and how can we learn from them? The power of the concepts of salutogenesis and complexity in the context of maternity care was first fully described in Downe and McCourt (2008 [2004]), and has subsequently been extended (Downe 2010a; 2010b)

Recent moves towards realist research (what works, for who, in what context – Pawson *et al.*, 2005), and narrative-based medicine mark a turn towards a more nuanced way of understanding health care issues and solutions. In maternity care, the problems of pathology-based thinking have been increasingly identified, and critiqued (Downe, 1991; Machin and Scamell, 1997; Johanson *et al.*, 2002; Downe, 2007). From about 1994, Downe and colleagues have written about normal birth, building on the theoretical insights described. This has led to an increasing awareness of the need to move away from super-valuation of risk, and from tick box audit in the name of safety, towards concepts of transformation, joy, elation, becoming mother, and well-being as a state of super-health. It has become clear that, in complexity terms, safety in maternity care (clinical, psychological and emotional) is not a state to be imposed but, rather, is an emergent phenomenon, if human systems are seen/treated/coaxed into being fundamentally salutogenic, based on authentically positive relationships. This has been termed 'skilled help from the heart' (El-nemer *et al.*, 2006: 81). This approach has an ethical dimension, with a specific emphasis on Aristotelian virtue ethics, or the value of becoming 'the good (wo)man'.

The current theoretical position adopted by the team builds on archaic constructs of wisdom and vocation (Downe *et al.*, 2007), while integrating modernist concepts of evidence and best possible knowledge with post-modern relativist concepts of realist research and policy. In a challenge to existing meta-discourses of risk in health care, the team proposes that it is as ethically unacceptable to pursue risk-aversion blindly in the design and delivery of health care systems as it is to ignore risk wantonly. This is about (in Aristotelian terms) courage, but not recklessness. These are the poetics of a knowledge–love approach to maternity care, in opposition to a knowledge–power approach. There is emerging (currently anecdotal) evidence that these kinds of approaches have the power both to reduce infant and maternal mortality, and to reduce iatrogenic damage through unnecessary intervention. This, of course, also has a health economic dimension.

All of these theories remain to be tested empirically, but the evidence so far suggests that there is interconnectivity between maternal and foetal physical and psycho-social initial conditions, the 'strange attractors' of the birth environment and care givers' attitudes, behaviours, skills and knowledge, and the values and beliefs of the woman and her family. Shifting the professional gaze so that pregnancy and labour are seen as complex, dynamic, self-organizing systems that are unique to each individual (rather than simple, predictable linear processes) brings this possibility into focus.

Conclusion

This chapter has traced the development of theory for midwifery practice from the late 1940s to the present day. A constant theme throughout has been the efforts made by these theorists to develop theories to best describe and support the most effective midwifery care. Appreciation of the needs of the childbearing woman has resulted in a number of theories that focus on the perception by the individual of their new role. A more recent focus has been on the context of care and the influence of the social, political and policy context on care. Soo Downe and colleagues demonstrate the importance of bringing these two themes together in their current explorations of a strengths-based approach to care.

ACTIVITIES

Undergraduate

From the data, Rubin (1967a) identified three aspects of the maternal role identity: 'the ideal image, the self image and the body image' (p. 240).

Reflect on your current practice and consider ways in which you would explore how Rubin's theory about the maternal role 'fits' or 'reflects' the characteristics of modern women. Select a case study and write it up using a model of reflection.

Postgraduate

Using available literature, personal contacts and historical archives, select one of the major theorists identified within this chapter and map their journey from theory to practice and beyond. Produce a table that shows the timeline, influencing factors, publications and current status.

References

Adams, M., Armstrong-Esther, C., Bryar, R., Duberley, J., Strong, G. and Ward, E. (1981) 'The Nursing Process in Midwifery: Trial Run'. *Nursing Mirror*, 151(9): 26–7.

Agyris, C. and Schön, D.A. (1974) *Theory in Practice. Increasing Professional Effectiveness*. San Francisco, CA: Jossey-Bass.

Altman, D., Carroli, G., Duley, L., Farrell, B., Moodley, J., Neilson, J., Smith, D. Magpie Trial Collaboration Group (2002) 'Do Women with Pre-Eclampsia, and their Babies, Benefit from Magnesium Sulphate? The Magpie Trial: A Randomised Placebo-controlled Trial', *Lancet*. 359(9321): 1877–90.

Ament, L.A. (1989) 'Maternal Tasks of the Puerperium Re-identified', *Journal of Obstetric, Gynecologic & Neonatal Nursing*, 19(4): 330–5.

Antonovsky, A. (1987) *Unravelling the Mystery of Health: How People Manage Stress and Stay Well*. San Francisco, CA: Jossey-Bass.

Antonovsky, A. (1993) 'The Implications of Salutogenesis: An Outsider View', in A.P. Turnbull, J.M. Patterson, S.K. Behr, D.L. Murphy, J.G. Marquis and M.J. Blue-Banning (eds), *Cognitive Coping, Families and Disability*. Baltimore, MD: Paul H. Brookes, pp. 111–22.

Antonovsky, A. (1996) 'The Salutogenic Model as a Theory to Guide Health Promotion', *Health Promotion International*, 11(1): 11–18.

Arms, S. (1981) *Immaculate Deception*. New York, NY: Bantam Books.

Ball, J.A. (1981) 'The Effects of the Present Patterns of Maternity Care upon the Emotional Needs of Mothers: I, II and III', *Midwives Chronicle*, 95(1120): 150–4; (1121): 198–202; (1122): 231–3.

Ball, J.A. (1987) *Reactions to Motherhood. The Role of Postnatal Care*. Cambridge: Cambridge University Press.

Ball, J.A. (1989) 'Postnatal Care and Adjustment to Motherhood', in S. Robinson and A. Thomson (eds), *Midwives, Research and Childbirth, Volume I*. London: Chapman & Hall, ch. 8: 154–75.

Bee, A.M. and Oetting, S. (1989) 'Ramona T. Mercer: Maternal role attainment', in A. Marriner-Tomey (ed.), *Nursing Theorists and Their Work*. 2nd edn. St Louis, MO: C.V. Mosby.

Berger, P. and Luckmann, T. (1967) *The Social Construction of Reality*. Harmondsworth: Penguin Books.

Blumer, H. (no date) Society for the Study of Social Interaction (www.espach. salford.ac.uk/sssi/).

Bryar, R. (1985) 'A Study of the Introduction of the Nursing Process in a Maternity Unit', Unpublished MPhil thesis. London: Southbank Polytechnic.

Bryar, R. (1991) 'Research and Individualised Care in Midwifery', in S. Robinson and A.M. Thomson (eds), Midwives, Research and Childbirth. Volume 2. London: Chapman & Hall, ch. 3: 48–71.

Bryar, R. (1995) Theory for Midwifery Practice, 1st edn. London: Macmillan.

Bryar, R. and Strong, G. (1983) 'Trial Run – Continued', Nursing Mirror, 157(15): 45–8.

Byrom, S. and Downe, S. (2010) ' "She Sort of Shines": Midwives' Accounts of "Good" Midwifery and "Good" Leadership', Midwifery, 26(1): 126–37.

Cardwell, C.R., Stene, L.C., Joner, G., Cinek, O., Svensson, J., Goldacre, M.J., Parslow, R.C., Pozzilli, P., Brigis, G., Stoyanov, D., Urbonaite, B., Sipetić, S., Schober, E., Ionescu-Tirgoviste, C., Devoti, G., de Beaufort, C.E., Buschard, K. and Patterson, C.C. (2008) 'Caesarean Section is Associated with an Increased Risk of Childhood-Onset Type 1 Diabetes Mellitus: A Meta-analysis of Observational Studies', Diabetologia, 51(5): 726–35.

Cornfield, J. (1969) 'The Bayesian Outlook and its Application', Biometrics, 25(4): 617–57

Cranley, M.S. (1981) 'Development of a Tool for the Measurement of Maternal Attachment during Pregnancy', Nursing Research, 30(5): 281–4.

Danko, M., Hunt, N.F., Marich, J.E., Marriner-Tomey, A., McCreary, C.A. and Stuart, M. (1989) 'Ernestine Wiedenbach: The Helping Art of Clinical Nursing', in A. Marriner-Tomey (ed.), Nursing Theorists and their Work, 2nd edn. St Louis, MO: C.V. Mosby, ch. 20: 240–52.

Davies, C. (1979) 'Organization Theory and the Organization of Health Care: A Comment on the Literature', Social Science and Medicine, 13A(4): 413–22.

Davies, C. and Francis, A. (1976) 'Perceptions of Structure in National Health Service Hospitals', in M. Stacy (ed.), 'The Sociology of the NHS', Sociological Review Monograph 22: 120–39. Keele: University of Keele.

Dickoff, J. and James, P. (1992) 'A Theory of Theories: A Position Paper', in, L.H. Nicholl (ed.), Perspectives on Nursing Theory, 2nd edn. Philadelphia, PA: J.B. Lippincott Co, ch. 8 pp. 99–111.

Downe, S. (1991) 'Who Defines Abnormality?', Nursing Times, 87(18): 22.

Downe, S. (2007) 'The Uniqueness of Normality', Midwives, 10(3): 132–3.

Downe, S. (2008) 'Metasynthesis: A Guide to Knitting Smoke', Evidence Based Midwifery, 6(1): 4–8.

Downe, S. (2010a) 'Beyond Evidence-Based Medicine: Complexity, and Stories of Maternity Care', Journal of Evaluation in Clinical Practice, 16(1): 232–7.

Downe, S. (2010b) 'Toward Salutogenic Birth in the 21st Century', in D. Walsh and S. Downe (eds), Essential Midwifery Practice: Intrapartum Care. Chichester: Wiley-Blackwell, ch. 16: 289–96.

Downe, S. and McCourt, C. (2008) 'From Being to Becoming: Reconstructing Childbirth Knowledges', in S. Downe (ed.), Normal Birth, Evidence and Debate, 2nd edn. Oxford: Elsevier, ch. 1: 3–28.

Downe, S., Renfrew, M. and Gerrett, D. (2004) 'The Effect of Position in The Passive Second Stage on Birth Outcome in Nulliparous Women using Epidural Analgesia: A Prospective Randomised Trial', Midwifery, 20(2): 157–68.

Downe, S., Simpson, L. and Trafford, K. (2007) 'Expert Intrapartum Maternity Care: A Meta-synthesis', Journal of Advanced Nursing, 57(2): 127–40.

Dunnington, R.M. and Glazer, G. (1991) 'Maternal Identity and Early Mothering Behaviour in Previously Infertile and Never Infertile Women', Journal of Obstetric, Gynecologic & Neonatal Nursing, 20(4): 309–18.

El-Nemer, A., Downe, S. and Small, N. (2006) ' "She Would Help Me From The Heart": An Ethnography of Egyptian Women in Labour', *Social Science and Medicine*, 62(1): 81–92.

Handy, C.B. (1976) *Understanding Organisations*. Harmondsworth: Penguin Books.

Hatamleh, R., Sinclair, M., Kernohan, W.G. and Bunting, B. (2008) 'Technological Childbirth in Northern Jordan: Descriptive Findings from a Prospective Cohort Study', *Evidence Based Midwifery*, 6(4): 130–5.

Hayward, J. (1986) 'Report of the Nursing Process Evaluation Working Group', NERU Report No 5, Nursing Education Research Unit, Department of Nursing Studies. London: King's College.

Johanson, R., Newburn, M. and Macfarlane, A. (2002) 'Has the Medicalisation of Childbirth Gone Too Far?', *British Medical Journal*, 13 April, 324(7342): 892–5.

Jordon, B. (1996) *Birth in Four Cultures*, 4th edn, revised by Robbie Davis-Floyd. Prospect Heights, IL: Waveland.

Josten, L. (1981) 'Prenatal Assessment Guide for Illuminating Possible Problems with Parenting', *American Journal of Maternal Child Nursing*, 6(2): 113–17.

Kuhn, T.S. (1962) *The Structure of Scientific Revolutions*. Chicago, IL: University of Chicago Press.

Lilford, R.J. and Braunholz, D. (1996) 'The Statistical Basis of Public Policy: A paradigm shift is overdue', *British Medical Journal*, 313(7057): 603–7.

Lehrman, E.-J. (1981) 'Nurse-Midwifery Practice: A Descriptive Study of Prenatal Care', *Journal of Nurse-Midwifery*, 26(3): 27–41.

MacArthur, C., Lewis, M. and Knox, E.G. (1991) *Health after Childbirth*. London: HMSO.

Machin, D. and Scamell, M. (1997) 'The Experience of Labour: Using Ethnography to Explore the Irresistible Nature of the Bio-medical Metaphor During Labour', *Midwifery*, 13(2):78–84.

Marriner-Tomey, A. (2006) 'Nursing Theorists of Historical Significance', in A. Marriner-Tomey and M.R. Alligood (eds), *Nursing Theorists and Their Work*. St Louis, MO: Mosby Elsevier, ch. 5: 50–67.

Marriner-Tomey, A. and Alligood, M.R. (eds) (2006) *Nursing Theorists and Their Work*. St Louis, MO: Mosby Elsevier.

Martell, L.K. and Mitchell, S.K. (1984) 'Rubin's "Puerperal Change" Reconsidered', *Journal of Obstetric, Gynecologic & Neonatal Nursing*, 13(3): 145–9.

Marut, J.S. and Mercer, R.T. (1979) 'Comparison of Primiparas' Perceptions of Vaginal and Caesarean Births', *Nursing Research*, 28(5): 260–6.

Meleis, A.I. (2007) *Theoretical Nursing. Development & Progress*. Philadelphia, PA: Lippincott Williams & Wilkins.

Mercer, R.T. (1981a) 'The Nurse and Maternal Tasks of the Early Postpartum', *American Journal of Maternal Child Nursing*, 6(5): 341–5.

Mercer, R.T. (1981b) 'A Theoretical Framework for Studying the Factors that Impact on the Maternal Role', *Nursing Research*, 30(2): 73–7.

Mercer, R.T. (1986) *First-Time Motherhood: Experiences from Teens to Forties*. New York, NY: Springer.

Mercer, R.T. (1995) *Becoming a Mother: Research from Rubin to the Present*. New York, NY: Springer.

Mercer, R.T., Ferketich, S.L., DeJoseph, J., May, K.A. and Sollid, D. (1988) 'Effect of Stress on Family Functioning During Pregnancy', *Nursing Research*, 37(5): 268–75.

Mercer, R.T., May, K.A., Ferketich, S. and DeJoseph, J. (1986) 'Theoretical Models for Studying the Effect of Antepartum Stress on the Family', *Nursing Research*, 35(6): 339–46.

Nickel, S., Gesse, T. and MacLaren, A. (1992) 'Ernestine Wiedenbach: Her Professional Legacy', *Journal of Nurse-Midwifery*, 37(3): 161–7.

O'Connell, R. and Downe, S. (2009) 'A Metasynthesis of Midwives' Experience of Hospital Practice in Publicly Funded Settings: Compliance, Resistance and Authenticity', *Health: An Interdisciplinary Journal for the Social Study of Health, Illness and Medicine*, 13(6): 589–609.

Odent, M. (1984) *Entering the World. The De-medicalisation of Childbirth*. London: Marion Boyars.

Pawson, R., Greenhalgh, T., Harvey, G. and Walshe, K. (2005) 'Realist Review – A New Method of Systematic Review Designed for Complex Policy Interventions', *Journal of Health Service Research & Policy*, 10 Suppl., 1: 21–34.

Roduit, C., Scholtens, S., de Jongste, J.C., Wijga, A.H., Gerritsen, J., Postma, D.S., Brunekreef, B., Hoekstra, M.O., Aalberse, R. and Smit, H.A. (2008) 'Asthma at 8 Years of Age in Children Born By Caesarean Section', *Thorax*, 64(2): 107–13.

Rose, H. (1994) *Love Power and Knowledge towards a Feminist Transformation of the Sciences*. London: Polity Press.

Rubin, R. (1961) 'Puerperal Change', *Nursing Outlook*, 9(12): 743–55.

Rubin, R. (1967a) 'Attainment of the Maternal Role. Part I. Processes', *Nursing Research*, 16(3): 237–45.

Rubin, R. (1967b) 'Attainment of the Maternal Role. Part II. Models and Referrants', *Nursing Research*, 16(4): 342–6.

Rubin, R. (1984) *Maternal Identity and the Maternal Experience*. New York, NY: Springer.

Sackett, D.L. (1997) 'Evidence-Based Medicine', *Seminars in Perinatology*, 21(1): 3–5.

Sackett, D.L., Straus, S.E., Richardson, W.S., Rosenberg, W. and Haynes, R.B. (2002) *Evidence Based Medicine: How to Practice and Teach EBM*. Edinburgh: Churchill Livingstone.

Schmid, V. and Downe, S. (2010) 'Midwifery Skills for Normalising Unusual Labours', in D. Walsh and S. Downe (eds), *Essential Midwifery Practice: Intrapartum Care*, Chichester: Wiley-Blackwell, ch. 10: 159–90.

Silverman, D. (1970) *The Theory of Organisations. A Sociological Framework*. London: Heinemann.

Solomon, G.F. (1987) 'Psychoneuroimmunology: Interactions between the Central Nervous System and the Immune System', *Journal of Neuroscience Research*, 18(1): 1–9.

Thomson, G. and Downe, S. (2008) 'Widening the Trauma Discourse: The Link Between Childbirth and Experiences of Abuse', *Journal of Psychosomatic Obstetrics and Gynecology*, 29(4): 268–73.

Thomson, G. and Downe, S. (2010) 'Changing the Future to Change the Past: Women's Experiences of a Positive Birth Following a Traumatic Birth Experience', *Journal of Reproductive and Infant Psychology*, February, 28(1): 102–12.

Thornton, J.G. and Lilford, R.J. (1996) 'Preterm Breech Babies and Randomised Trials of Rare Conditions', *British Journal of Obstetrics and Gynaecology*, 103(7): 611–3.

Walsh, D. and Downe, S. (2005) 'Meta-Synthesis Method for Qualitative Research: A Literature Review', *Journal of Advanced Nursing*, 50(2): 204–11.

Walsh, D. and Downe, S. (2006) 'Appraising the Quality of Qualitative Research', *Midwifery*, 22, (2): 108–19.

Wiedenbach, E. (1964) *Clinical Nursing: A Helping Art*. New York, NY: Springer.

Wiedenbach, E. (1967) *Family-Centered Maternity Nursing*. 2nd edn. New York, NY: G.P. Putnam & Sons.

WHO (1988) *From Alma-Ata to the Year 2000. Reflections at the Midpoint*. Geneva: WHO.

WHO (2008) *Primary Health Care: Now More Than Ever*. Geneva: WHO.

Understanding Motivational Theory and the Psychology of Breastfeeding

4

Janine Stockdale, Marlene Sinclair, George Kernohan and John Keller

---

Key points

- Psychological theories can help explain why some women are more likely to start and continue breastfeeding than others
- Motivational theory applied to breastfeeding offers new knowledge about the motivational role of value and expectancy for success
- Understanding breastfeeding persistence from the perspective of personal attributions adds meaning to the socio-demographic and behavioural trends that are commonly associated with breastfeeding cessation
- When providing women-centred care, it is important for breastfeeding practitioners and educators to understand fully what goals women are aiming to fulfil when they commence breastfeeding.

Introduction

Most breastfeeding literature has an accepted and almost expected introduction, such as: 'while the initiation rate of breastfeeding is increasing, national and international data demonstrate that few women are breastfeeding for the recommended duration'. Even though the familiarity of this type of introduction has the potential to limit its effect, writers seem compelled to set the contextual scene: that is, women who choose to start breastfeeding do not always maintain their motivation to sustain this behaviour. Although breastfeeding initiation rates are reportedly rising (Bolling *et al.*, 2005), understanding why maternal motivation commences has been at the fore of breastfeeding research for over two decades. Perspectives on the phenomenon have been both psychological and socio-demographical. Psychologically the behaviour has been explained in terms of constructs such as maternal self-efficacy (Dennis, 2003), intrinsic and extrinsic motivation (Wells *et al.*, 2002), attitudes, social norms and perceived control (Dick *et al.*, 2002), self-identity (McMillan *et al.*, 2008), and pain and depression (Hatton *et al.*, 2005). Socio-demographically, women who are younger, less educated and possibly single with lower incomes are also associated with failing to breastfeed (Dennis, 2002). While practitioners are aware of these different factors, few find the time or the impetus to explore how these factors might converge to explain breastfeeding cessation; yet, recent recommendations suggest that health professionals should be motivationally screening women before offering breastfeeding advice and support (Racine *et al.*, 2009). Before doing this, it seems imperative that practitioners first begin to understand the role of human motivation and the psychological theories that can help explain why some women are more likely to start and continue breastfeeding than others.

This chapter and Chapter 5 are designed to introduce midwives to the role of motivation in relation to breastfeeding.

In this chapter, we introduce the key aspects of motivation associated with breastfeeding behaviour. Motivational theories will be used as a framework for enabling practitioners and breastfeeding educators to contextualize what is now a rapidly growing 'psychology-orientated' evidence base for breastfeeding behaviour. While the focus of this chapter is on breastfeeding behaviour, the principles of motivation are representative of the general field of achievement (learning) psychology and have application to many aspects of health and midwifery practice, including health promotion, health education and person-centred care.

Defining motivation

Many of us would find it difficult to define 'motivation' without relying on some familiar image such as 'the carrot before the donkey's nose'. While this image represents one aspect of motivation, often referred to as 'approach'-orientated motivation, it fails to capture times when our motivation is 'avoidance' in nature; for example, when we find ourselves motivated to flee from a crowded place. The debate as to how health professionals should influence women's motivation to breastfeed could easily rest on this level of understanding: we explain the benefits of breastfeeding as something that should be approached and the disadvantages of bottle feeding as something that should be avoided. While discussion as to whether practitioners should depend upon approach-orientated messages or include 'risk-based' avoidance messages continues (Heinig, 2009), these conceptualizations alone cannot sufficiently define motivation to breastfeed.

In 2000, psychologists Sansone and Harackiewicz (p. 1) defined motivation as that which: 'energises and guides behaviour towards reaching a particular goal', Unlike other definitions of motivation, this conceptualization suggests that, when a person is motivated, they experience an energy or force that has the ability to guide them in the pursuit of their goal(s). The relationship between the energy experienced and the goal pursued implies that motivation involves knowing exactly what it is you want to achieve (a personal goal or goals) and how you plan to achieve it (plan of action). Of course, the 'how' part of motivation involves regulation of your thoughts, behaviours and resources towards the successful attainment of your goal (often referred to as self-regulation). The goal itself also has motivational properties. Theorists Deci and Ryan (2000) comment that, when a behaviour satisfies a person's sense of competency and self-determination (sometimes referred to as higher-order goals), that person is more likely to experience 'intrinsic' motivation and well-being.

Intrinsic motivation has most often been described in breastfeeding research as a sense of enjoyment or satisfaction (Wells *et al.*, 2002; Racine *et al.*, 2009). At a personal level, this aspect of motivation is easily recognized. When we feel competent in our ability to do something, we are more likely to feel a sense of enjoyment/satisfaction and our commitment for future engagement in the behaviour is energized. Likewise, when we believe ourselves to be incompetent or failing, negative feelings are experienced that can deplete the energizing effect of intrinsic motivation. Although intrinsic motivation is often considered paramount, our motivation to achieve a goal can also be extrinsic in nature. Extrinsic motivation introduces the idea of motivation that is energized by some type of reward external to the behaviour or to the person (back to the carrot in front of the poor donkey!). For example, if the only motive a woman had for breastfeeding was because she was being paid to do so, we could consider her to be extrinsically motivated.

However, there are problems with extrinsic motivation. For example, when the reward is removed, there is a strong possibility that the behaviour will stop or that focusing on the reward will interfere with the creativity the person invests in the experience (Amabile *et al.*, 1986). Rarely is a person only intrinsically or extrinsically motivated; in fact, an intricate relationship exists between these two constructs. (See Stockdale *et al.* (2010) for a more detailed explanation of intrinsic and extrinsic motivation related to breastfeeding behaviour.) By adopting the definition of motivation provided by Sansone and Harackiewicz (2000), our thinking is opened up to consider many different aspects of human motivation, including those of goals, satisfaction, enjoyment, perceived competency and self-regulation.

As each theorist has added to our understanding of 'motivation', it becomes apparent that no one magical key exists that can unlock women's motivation to sustain breastfeeding. In fact, motivation is a multi-factorial phenomenon that requires a multi-factorial approach. Therefore, rather than thinking of 'motivation' as a single construct, motivation is best thought of as a diamond, which can only be fully appreciated when viewed from many different perspectives. Although many motivational theories and models could be explored, key theories are purposely introduced as a theoretical starting point for the understanding and contextualization of sustained breastfeeding behaviour.

Motivation, meaning and breastfeeding

Within current practice, breastfeeding is most often introduced to women as an instinctive, natural behaviour that does require a degree of 'learning'. Even though success requires that both mother and baby are involved in the learning process, the motivational energy required is exclusively maternal. Of course, the behaviour of the baby can influence the energy experienced within the complexity of the mother/baby dyad. Nevertheless, it is still the woman who interprets her baby's behaviour, adds meaning to her breastfeeding experience and self-regulates her behaviour accordingly. To appreciate how the motivational process associated with breastfeeding might unfold in relation to perceived breastfeeding success and failure, three theoretical dynamics of motivation must be considered:

- motivational balance between value for the behaviour and expecting that you can succeed
- motivational impact of experience and goals
- motivational impact of personal persistence.

It is only when these three foundational dynamics of motivation to breastfeed are understood, that health professionals can begin to manage the individual uniqueness surrounding women's breastfeeding behaviour.

Motivational balance between value for the behaviour and expecting that you can succeed

According to many theorists, the two significant determinants of motivated behaviour are the subjective value that the person places on the behaviour, and their perception concerning the probability they will succeed – referred to as 'expectancy for success'. Fishbein (1967) has elaborated the concept of expectancy value (E-V) and used it to describe the nature of different theories. For example, the Theory of Reasoned Action (Fishbein and Azjen, 1975) and its later version the Theory of Planned Behaviour (Ajzen and Madden, 1986) are referred to as E-V theories, as is Rotter's (1945) Social Learning Theory. Building on social learning, other familiar theories such as the Theory of Self-Efficacy (Bandura, 1994) has, at its heart, the idea of expectancy coupled with value: for example, the stronger a person's perception of self-efficacy (expectancies), the more challenging their adopted goals and their commitment to achieve their goals (value). While different theories can be classified as E-V theories, Feather (1982), in his book *Expectations and Actions: Expectancy-Value Models in Psychology*, explains that central to all E-V theories and models is the idea that our actions are embedded in a complex means-to-an-end goal structure; that is, a goal structure that includes our perception not only of what the behaviour will be like, but also what the person believes to be the potential short- and long-term consequences.

In other words, before adopting or re-adopting any behaviour such as breastfeeding, women will consider how valuable they believe breastfeeding to

---

Box 4.1   Value as defined and classified by Jacobs and Eccles (2000)

Value can be conceptualized as 'a set of stable, general beliefs about what is desirable … a class of motives that affect behaviour by influencing the attractiveness of different goals and consequently, motivation to attain these goals' (Jacobs and Eccles (2000) citing Feather (1988)). The four motivational components of value include:

- attainment value – personal importance of doing well on the task (linked to aspects of one's self-identity)
- intrinsic value – enjoyment the person gets from achieving the desired outcome (linked to the concepts of intrinsic motivation and interest)
- utility value – determined by the degree to which the behaviour is linked to the person's current and future goals
- cost value – the negative aspects of the behaviour, which can include fear of success or failure.

Source: Jacobs and Eccles (2000: 408).

---

be for them and their baby, not just in a general sense, but what value it holds for them personally (see Box 4.1).

Placing value on a behaviour does not, in itself, generate the motivational energy required to make it happen. For example, I might place different aspects of value on cycling to work every day; however, when I consider the distance involved, my current level of fitness and time available to me, I might quickly conclude that I have little chance of being successful! To find the motivational energy I need to perform the behaviour therefore requires me to have some sense of competency, control or expectancy that I can achieve what I believe to be valuable (see Box 4.2).

Of course, while it is easier to consider value and expectancy for success as separate components of motivated behaviour, theorists recognize that the type

---

Box 4.2   Expectancy for success as defined by Maddux (1995)

Expectancy for success – There are many theorists who explain the role of competency, control and expectancy related to task motivation; for example, *The Theory of Self-Efficacy* by Bandura (1977). Self-efficacy theory operates on the premise that *initiation* of behaviour and *persistence* to sustain it are determined primarily by 'people's beliefs about their capabilities to exercise control over events that affect their lives and their beliefs in their capabilities to mobilize the motivation, cognitive resources and courses of action needed to exercise the control over task demands' (Maddux, 1995: 7). Self-efficacy beliefs are therefore judgements that people make about themselves that answer the questions:

- I know I have the knowledge, but can I transfer that knowledge into action?
- Do I have the thinking, the resources and the persistence to really do this?

Source: Maddux (1995: 7).

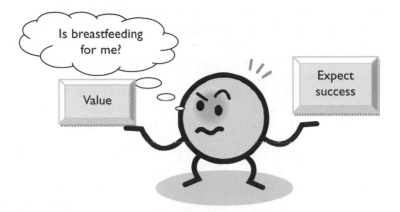

Figure 4.1   An interactive balancing between a sufficient amount of value and expectancy for breastfeeding

and amount of value placed on a behaviour interacts with how much the person believes they can succeed. For example, cost value – such as fear of failure – will affect the degree of self-efficacy the person is likely to experience. In other words, when women consider commencing or continuing a behaviour such as breastfeeding, they will add to one side of their motivational scales what they consider to be valuable about it and, to the other, their assessment of whether or not they are likely to be successful. If a sufficient amount of value and expectancy for success exists for the behaviour, then the behaviour is likely to occur (see Figure 4.1).

Using the analogy of a set of motivational scales is very helpful in visualising the motivational processes associated with breastfeeding behaviour. When a woman places sufficient value on breastfeeding and the belief that she can succeed, she experiences a motivational balance that creates the energizing force described by Sansone and Harackiewicz (2000). The motivational energy is directed or channelled towards achievement of her personal goal(s). Conversely, when a woman places little personal value on breastfeeding or lacks belief in her ability to be successful, her motivational balance is compromised and the degree of motivational energy experienced is limited. Seldom have breastfeeding researchers or educators considered motivation to breastfeed as a motivational balancing between value and expectancy for success. Nonetheless, when evidence to date on breastfeeding is considered from this perspective, a clearer picture of motivation to sustain breastfeeding begins to emerge.

Low expectancy for success: Researchers and practitioners have known for some time that women who stop breastfeeding tend to be those who lack expectancy for success (low maternal confidence). The most compelling evidence has been provided by application of the Breastfeeding Self-Efficacy Scale (Dennis and Faux, 1999; Dennis, 2003). The same phenomenon can also be easily detected throughout qualitative research such as that reported by Mozingo *et al.* (2000) and Schmied *et al.* (2001). The measure of self-efficacy clearly demonstrates that women who stop breastfeeding are those whose motivational scale is tipped in the direction of a low expectancy for success. However, this is only one side of the motivational balance. To understand women's motivation to breastfeed, we must take into consideration the influence of the 'value' component.

Low value coupled with low expectancy for success: Due to the interactive nature of these two motivational components, most researchers, when investigating women's motivational persistence towards breastfeeding, measure the value component in conjunction with their expectancy for success. One E-V theory, the Theory of Planned Behaviour (TPB) by Azjen and Madden (1986) has provided considerable evidence concerning motivation to breastfeed (Wambach, 1997; Duckett *et al.*, 1998; Dick *et al.*, 2002; Dodgson *et al.*, 2003; McMillan *et al.*, 2008). Measuring the key variables of the theory, (perceived control, influence of significant others, attitudes towards breastfeeding) in relation to attrition, women who stop breastfeeding have been found to lack confidence in their ability to breastfeed and hold less positive attitudes (low value) towards breastfeeding (Avery *et al.*, 1998) – findings that are reminiscent of those reported by Janke (1994).

Understanding the significance of low value on a woman's motivation towards breastfeeding can be challenging for practitioners and educators. The most tempting assumption to make is that these women have always lacked utility value towards breastfeeding, and so the negative attitudes they reported on breastfeeding cessation are a direct reflection of the amount of value they first placed on the behaviour. Yet, when the evidence is considered more closely, two important indicators of their motivational state emerge:

- Women who lack value at the point of cessation are often those who previously valued breastfeeding and so had adopted a personal goal to sustain breastfeeding for much longer (Avery *et al.*, 1998); that is, a future goal had been created that was indicative of a degree of utility value
- Low value may be preceded by a low expectancy for success. (Duckett *et al.*, 1998)

Piecing together the evidence from an E-V perspective suggests the probability that a distinct and directional motivational shift seems to be occurring between the time women commence breastfeeding and the point of early cessation. As outlined in Figure 4.2, women may start breastfeeding with a high sense of value and expectancy for success; however, if breastfeeding problems are perceived and experienced, there is a possibility that, as their expectancy for success begins to deplete, value for the behaviour will also be lost.

Researchers have been able to detect the key points in this process; for example, high value and low expectancy for success was found in first-time mothers who were in the process of learning to breastfeed (Stockdale *et al.*, 2008). However, pinpointing exactly where an individual woman might be on this continuum is difficult. This is not surprising because motivation, as previously stated, is multi-factorial. However, one indication of a woman's motivational state is the different emotional responses to the challenge of breastfeeding; that

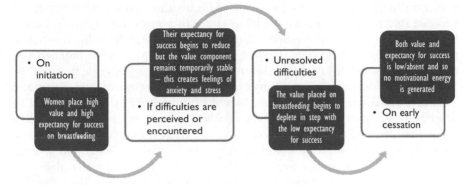

Figure 4.2   Diagrammatic representation of the proposed motivational shift associated with early breastfeeding cessation

is, different emotional outcomes often accompany the different stages of the de-motivational process. Authors such as Hegney *et al.* (2008) suggest that screening the level of women's psychological distress is an indicator of their breastfeeding experience, but caution is needed here as motivation is highly individualized and complex. Describing this complexity, psychologists Linnenbrink and Pintrich (2000: 209) state: 'the literature on affect and emotions is exceedingly complex and there is not even complete agreement on a basic taxonomy of emotions or the underlying theoretical models'. However, it is nonetheless worthwhile considering the following emotional outcomes as potential indicators of the overall process of de-motivation to breastfeed.

Emotions of high value and high expectancy for success: When women value breastfeeding highly and believe they can succeed, they are more likely to experience feelings of satisfaction and/or enjoyment when breastfeeding successfully (intrinsic motivation): this, in turn, energizes their future commitment and persistence to breastfeed.

Emotions of high value and low expectancy for success: When women value 'breast as best' but do not believe they 'have-what-it-takes' to be successful, their satisfaction is negatively affected, and feelings of anxiety and stress are likely. Shakespeare *et al.* (2004) describe the emotional complexity that occurs when women's expectations for breastfeeding are not matched by their experience. The source of anxiety, according to Martin and Tesser (1996: 45), is related to the unexpected aspects of an experience: 'self-discrepancy theory holds that the discrepancy between the actual and the ought is what determines anxiety'. Imagine how you might feel if you really thought you 'ought' to be able to secure that ideal job but, secretly, you felt that you could not succeed at interview. It is this discrepancy between the 'ought' and the 'actual' of women's breastfeeding experience that leads to the associated stress and anxiety so often reported by researchers – not just directly in relation to women (Clifford *et al.*, 2006), but also indirectly in relation to the response of health care professionals whose role it is to support and instruct women at these difficult times (Cloherty *et al.*, 2003).

Motivationally, women must find a way of resolving the anxiety or distress associated with a motivational position of high value and low expectancy for success. Two basic options are available: either they must manage their distress by finding a new level of confidence, or they must lower the value they originally placed on breastfeeding. Finding the confidence to proceed requires that they effectively self-regulate their behaviour: they must assess exactly what the situation will demand in congruence with their self-resources. As Ryan and Deci (2000: 47, citing Sheldon and Elliot, 1999) point out, people can only be described as: 'truly regulating when they are able to freely process current needs and demands and spontaneously generate actions based on the match between available behaviours and current needs'. If no obvious and spontaneous behavioural match is available, lowering the value originally placed on breastfeeding may, for some individuals, be the better option. Breastfeeding literature indicates that many women will experience a period when they attempt to self-regulate their behaviour towards sustained breastfeeding. For example, women will often introduce soothers or supplementation as strategies for managing a difficult breastfeeding experience. Health professionals may differ in their belief as to whether these strategies are appropriate or not (Victora *et al.*, 1997; Righard, 1998). Nevertheless, it should not be presumed that a simple cause-and-effect relationship operates where early cessation is motivationally thought to be dependent on inappropriate strategies. As breastfeeding is still highly valued, the strategies women adopt are a window into their self-regulatory processing and their attempts to self-resolve the perceived problems, such as their inability to produce sufficient milk.

Emotions of low value and low expectancy for success: As increasing self-confidence is not altogether straightforward or automatic, many women will eventually opt for a lowering of the value component and the behaviour will be abandoned. The emotions associated with the point of attrition can vary from guilt to relief. To understand the source of these emotions, we need to consider the nature of personal persistence in greater depth: this will be addressed in the section on the motivational impact of personal persistence.

Even though the emotions that women exhibit may indicate something of their motivational state when learning to breastfeed, there is a need to consider what it is that women are motivated towards, so as to increase our understanding of personal persistence. We must consider the impact of the goal towards which women's motivational energy is directed before we can be sure that the success they hope to achieve is what we, as practitioners, presume it to be.

The motivational impact of experience and goals

Albert Einstein is credited with having said: 'The only source of knowledge is experience.' However, the idea that people learn by doing is an ancient one. Over two millennia earlier, Sophocles (495–406 BC) stated: 'One must learn by doing the thing. For though you think you know it you have no certainty until you try'. Evidence that women's motivation to persist with breastfeeding is directly related to the feelings of expectancy generated by their learned experience of breastfeeding appears throughout the literature.

The most insightful account that links a lack of motivational energy with women's breastfeeding experience, rather than their breastfeeding knowledge *per se*, is found in the paper by Fowler and Lee (2007). These authors report a case of a midwife/lactation consultant whose intention to breastfeed, although not described in motivational terms, was supported antenatally by a strong sense of value and personal expectancy for success. As her personal experience of breastfeeding progressed, she began to sense that breastfeeding was not as she had expected, and so she found herself motivationally compromised to the point of considering stopping. While previous researchers had provided evidence that experience of breastfeeding problems and a lack of motivation to persist were inextricably linked (Coombe *et al.*, 1998), this paper was unique in questioning two assumptions often made by practitioners and educationalists: that is, if women had the correct breastfeeding knowledge they would not experience breastfeeding difficulties and so would continue confidently.

Few researchers or educators would disagree that breastfeeding knowledge is an important element in goal attainment; nevertheless, as already pointed out, having knowledge does not necessarily transfer into confidence (self-efficacy). The case reported by Fowler and Lee (2007) demonstrates that motivational persistence has more to do with a woman's self-assessment of her ability to fulfil her own personal goal/s than possession of the correct knowledge. In other words, the degree of motivational energy generated by value and expectancy for success for breastfeeding does not operate within a vacuum; it is influenced by a woman's personal goal(s), her experience and personality. As women practise breastfeeding, they make self-evaluations of their competency, based on their interpretation of their experience. This information tells them how close to they are to achieving their goal, or how likely they are to succeed.

There are various definitions and conceptualizations of 'goals'. Molden and Dweck (2000: 133) define goals simply as: 'the specific purposes toward which a person's efforts are directed'. This positive and directed relationship between the goal set and the effort employed to achieve the goal has been well-established (Locke and Latham, 1990); yet, for many as health educators, our understanding of 'goals' is to some degree incomplete. Within the hierarchy of goals, the means by which a goal is obtained has historically been considered less motivationally significant than the goal itself. Take, for example, when a person sets a goal to become physically fit. Different means of attaining this goal are available and, although the person might choose to swim or run, their motivational energy is normally thought to be related to their overall goal to get fit, and not necessarily the mean or means they have adopted. As theorists expanded the conceptualization of goals, it became apparent that the mean or means of attaining a goal could also have motivating properties, in that the means selected could increase the likelihood of goal success and so generate further commitment to the goal and the mean(s). In fact, psychologists Shah and Kruglanski (2003) suggest that a person's experience of the mean(s) can be powerful enough to create what they call a 'bottom-up' effect on the person's primary goal structure. They conclude that persistence to perform any behaviour can be dependent upon perceiving that the particular goal is accessible through a given mean(s).

When providing women-centred care, it is important for breastfeeding practitioners and educators to understand fully what goals women are aiming to fulfil when they commence breastfeeding. Interestingly, little is known about the actual goal structuring that underpins breastfeeding behaviour; however, current literature does suggest that the goal is not as simple as wanting to attain the associated health benefits (Racine *et al.*, 2009). Evidence demonstrates that women's breastfeeding behaviour is likely to be part of a more complex goal structure that can be as multifarious as having a desire for self-control (Wells *et al.*, 2002), wanting to feel important (Kong and Lee, 2004), needing some independence and/or a sense of freedom (Stewart-Knox *et al.*, 2003). Rarely have health educators thought of breastfeeding separate from the simple goal structure: 'my goal is to breastfeed so I will breastfeed'. Yet, to understand the impact of women's experience and subsequent commitment to breastfeeding, it is important to consider that breastfeeding may not necessarily be a woman's overall goal but, rather, may be the means by which she is aiming to attain some other overarching goal. (The term 'means' from this point forward will be understood within the context of goal structuring where breastfeeding as a behaviour is the 'means' by which a person attains some related goal. The word 'means' will therefore be used interchangeably with the term 'experience'.) Even though the established evidence as to the exact nature of the goal structure that surrounds breastfeeding is largely unknown, it remains that, if women create higher-order goals (such as the need to attain maternal competency or self-determination), the potential that breastfeeding remains the 'means' by which they fulfil their goal increases.

Selection of the type of 'means' adopted is most often on the basis of what might be called a 'best fit' principle. Women will consider the different means available to them and, if breastfeeding is still considered the 'best' option, they will continue to commit to it as the most likely way of securing their overall goal success. Although, initially, there may be what Shah and Kruglanski (2003) refer to as a strong 'associative link' between the goal and the means selected, a negative experience can challenge that association, and the person may find themselves reconsidering the role of the means in relation to successfully attaining their overall goal. Take, for example, a woman whose primary goal is to be independent. She believes that the best way of achieving that goal is to secure her own career while ensuring that her baby remains as healthy as possible. To achieve these goals, she assumes that breastfeeding is the most effective means and commences the behaviour. As she experiences unexpected breastfeeding difficulties, her overall goal attainment begins to feel threatened, and she starts to contemplate other potential means that could secure her independence. Figure 4.3 illustrates how the commitment to breastfeeding, as a means by which to obtain her primary goal, shifts towards the option of 'breast and bottle' feeding as a more effective means.

Based on their high value and expectancy for success, women at first create a strong associative link between their goal and breastfeeding as a means of

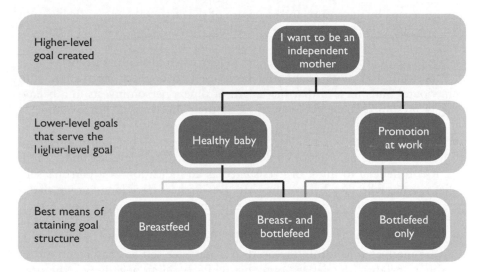

Figure 4.3   One example of potential goal structures where breastfeeding competes with alternative means of goal attainment

attaining their goal. Unfortunately, a negative personal experience of breast-feeding can threaten their goal accessibility and lowers their self-efficacy – and, subsequently, the type of value they had placed on breastfeeding. Ultimately, the link or association between the goal (in this example, to be independent) and the original means (to breastfeed) begins to weaken and, eventually, an alternative means will come to the fore. The nature and the velocity of this process are complex and individual. Until researched, it can only be surmised that, if a more complex goal–means structure exists, the potential for competing means and goals can interfere with women's commitment to sustain the behaviour.

Not all women who experience breastfeeding difficulties will abandon the behaviour. Similarly, not all women who experience low expectancy for success will lose the value they once placed on breastfeeding. Viewing motivation from the perspective of value, expectancy for success and goals has, no doubt, increased our understanding of motivational persistence and breastfeeding. However, the question must be asked: Why are some women more likely to persist and adapt to the challenge of breastfeeding, while others do not? To understand why individual responses to breastfeeding difficulties may occur, we need to consider a third motivational dynamic: the motivational impact of persistence related to the person's perception of 'self'.

The motivational impact of personal persistence

The idea of persistence is almost always viewed as a strong and commendable trait that can be summed up in 'if at first you don't succeed try, try again'. Nevertheless, not all people do try and try again, so it is important to consider what factors might combine to influence the amount of persistence an individual is willing to exercise. As discussed, motivation and persistence are influenced by the nature and structure of the goals women set, the amount and type of value placed on breastfeeding (low valence results in reduced persistence) and the expectations women have for success (a person with a strong sense of self-efficacy will persist longer when difficulties occur).

Persistence has most commonly been used to connect motivation with behavioural outcomes, in that the length of time a person invests in a behaviour is presumed to be an indication of their motivation. For example, a woman who is still breastfeeding at six months is presumed to be motivated, and her persistence is considered a demonstration of her continuing goal attainment. While persistence could be restricted to this level of understanding, it is beneficial to think of persistence as an indication of a person's self-belief system: who they believe they are. Researchers have long known that a person's feelings of self-worth and self-esteem significantly impact upon their willingness to persist. Citing the work of Connell and Wellborn (1991), Jacobs and Eccles (2000: 413) assert that all individuals have three fundamental needs they are motivated to fulfil; 'the need to experience self as competent and so be able to produce the desired outcome while avoiding negativity', 'the need to be autonomous and so able to make meaningful choices', and 'the need for relatedness and to feel socially connected, self-worthy and respected'.

As already discussed in relation to the higher-order goals women set, it is consistent with the nature of human motivation that researchers who continue to investigate motivation to breastfeed find that maternal issues of low self-esteem and self-identity are associated with early breastfeeding cessation (McMillan *et al.*, 2008; O'Brien *et al.*, 2009). In 2001, Schmied *et al.* reported that breastfeeding was so intricately interwoven into womanhood itself, that women equated breastfeeding with an overall sense of 'good mothering'. Recognizing that women's 'self' cannot, in a sense, be separated from the goals they have set, it then follows that we must ask: What does it mean to a woman when she perceives herself to be succeeding or failing to achieve her personal goal and what difference will the conclusion she draws make to her future engagement in the behaviour?

To begin answering these questions, we turn to the work of attribution theorists Weiner (1986) and Feather (1982). These theorists contended that, as individuals, we find it necessary to add 'meaning' to our successes and failures throughout life; that is, people will always ask themselves Why am I succeeding or why am I failing? How we answer this question dictates how willing we are to persist, not just in relation to our current goals, but also in relation to future goals. That is, people use particular 'meaning sets' to conclude why they are succeeding or failing. If the answer suggests that success is still possible, persistence is more likely. In fact, the conclusion reached subsequently impacts upon their emotions and self-regulation process (including coping strategies adopted and subsequent behaviour). To understand the role of attributions in relation to persistence, three dimensions come into play as a person attempts to make sense of their experience:

- whether or not the locus is internal or external to them
- the degree of stability/instability involved

- whether or not they believe that the reason for their perceived success/failure is within or outside their control.

Through application of attributions, it then follows that two women could set the same goal for breastfeeding, experience the same difficulties and yet demonstrate very different responses to their experience. Of course, it is the potential diversity of the individual response that makes experiences and responses to those experiences in life 'individual'. Consider the following examples of how attributions of 'meaning' attached to the experience of breastfeeding can influence breastfeeding persistence.

Perceived ability within this context is thought to be an internal, stable, uncontrollable attribution, in that ability is something that one thinks they either have or do not have. If a woman perceives that her breastfeeding difficulties are due to a lack of her own ability, then her persistence is likely to be negatively affected. She does not have control over the amount of ability that she owns and so it is outside her control; she cannot magically increase her ability. Interestingly, not only will this internal stable attribution have a negative effect on her persistence, it will also influence the motivational impact of the support provided. Consider the scenario in Figure 4.4.

The woman experiences breastfeeding difficulties and perceives these to be attributed to her own fixed inability to breastfeed successfully. Even though support may resolve the physical difficulties experienced, psychologically she remains lacking in self-confidence because the solution has come from outside of herself, from the midwife. On the other hand, when effort is considered the main attribution for failure, a very different response is likely to occur. As an internal attribution, effort differs from ability in that it is an unstable attribution; a person can decide to increase the amount of effort they apply to a task. As a result, women who conclude that their breastfeeding failure is the result of their lack of invested effort are more likely to experience feelings of guilt and regret at having abandoned the behaviour too soon (Hegney et al., 2008). Interestingly, research demonstrates this regret phenomenon also in relation to adolescent mothers' experience of breastfeeding (Wambach and Cohen, 2009). However, researchers investigating breastfeeding failure from a phenomenological perspective (although not in motivational terms) often report a range

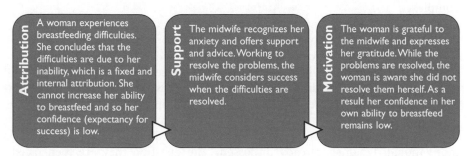

Figure 4.4   An example of how a fixed attribution of personal ability can negatively affect perception of breastfeeding support and success

of expressions that indicate different attributions, for example: ' "I just felt like I couldn't do it … it just wasn't working" is indicative of a fixed ability attribution while: "I think maybe I could have tried a little harder" reflects an attribution suggestive of failed "effort" (Mozingo *et al.*, 2000: 123, 125). The attributions people assign to their perceived success or failure demonstrate their motivational persistence and something of their motivational personality. When a person tends to perceive failure to be due to a lack of their ability (a stable factor), then their expectations for further successes, when in a learning situation, are likely to be negatively affected. Understanding breastfeeding persistence from the perspective of personal attributions adds meaning to the socio-demographic and behavioural trends that are commonly associated with breastfeeding cessation: for example, why women's past experiences when learning to breastfeed affect future behavioural engagement (Da Vanzo *et al.*, 1990; Nagy *et al.*, 2001), and why women who are young, socially deprived and have not achieved academically are least likely to persist with breastfeeding (Avery *et al.*, 1998).

Conclusion

Ryan and Deci (2000: 69) state: 'in the real world, motivation is highly valued because of its consequences; motivation produces' and when it comes to breastfeeding, motivation still 'produces', in that:

- Women who perceive themselves to be breastfeeding competently are more motivationally secure because their experience positively energizes their goal commitment and increases their persistence
- Women who perceive themselves to be incompetently breastfeeding are motivationally compromised, in that their experience of breastfeeding negatively influences their goal commitment and willingness to persist.

While it is true that motivation produces, it is equally true that motivation is both complex and personal. Even with the necessarily limited view of motivation as is described in this chapter, it becomes apparent that women's experience of breastfeeding, and how they process that experience, is extremely complex.

To understand the complexity of motivation, we could view this process as cyclical (Figure 4.5). Prior to commencement of breastfeeding, women may foresee value in the behaviour and expect to succeed; so they commence with the anticipation that it will be a fulfilling and successful experience. As they encounter breastfeeding difficulties, their personal experience of breastfeeding provides informational feedback that it is not going well and a degree of perceived incompetency results. Women then filter this information back through their original goal structure and breastfeeding is assessed using the motivational dynamics already discussed. The question they are then faced with is: If I persist with breastfeeding will I attain my personal goals? Of course, to answer this question, they must consider why they have experienced

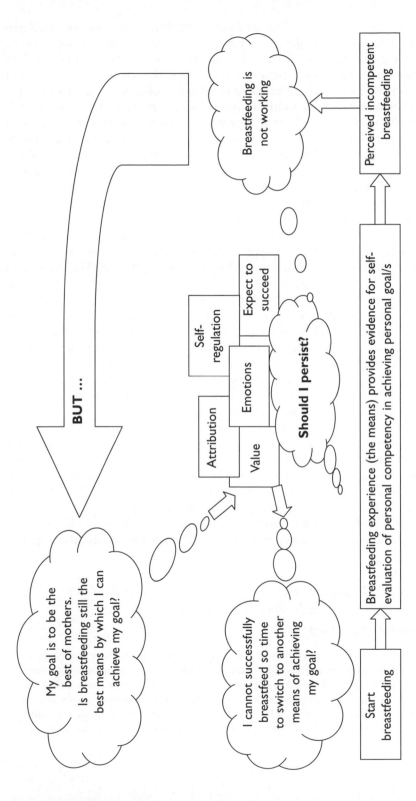

Figure 4.5 Motivational framework for understanding the aetiology of failure to breastfeed when women perceive themselves incapable of resolving perceived difficulties

difficulties in the first place. The attributions adopted, the emotions generated and the resources they believe they have, directly affect the balance between their value and expectancy for success, and they move closer to making their conclusive decision about breastfeeding. In other words, as value and expectancy for success are re-adjusted to account for a person's current experience of breastfeeding, the motivational energy generated dictates the person's willingness to persist. If sufficient value and expectancy for success remains on breastfeeding as a 'mean' to their personal goal attainment, then the individual is likely to commit and persist with breastfeeding (and so the cycle continues). However, if expectancy for success remains low and value begins to deplete then there is a greater likelihood that the behaviour will be abandoned for a more desirable mean.

While it is helpful to think of this process as cyclical, the interaction that occurs between the different motivational dynamics already discussed cannot be completely explained in this way. To the contrary, all the key psychological factors introduced can and do interact to influence each other. For example, a reciprocal effect can occur, in that low expectancy for success can affect our mood and emotions, which, in turn, has an unfortunate effect on the self-regulatory strategies adopted and our belief that we can succeed. This then affects the value placed on the behaviour and our willingness to persist. Although not described using motivational theories, researchers Nelson and Sethi (2005) begin to capture the motivational processing of sustained breastfeeding. Using a grounded theory approach, they described the core variable related to adolescent mother's experiences of breastfeeding as 'continuously committing to breastfeeding' (Nelson and Sethi, 2005: 618).

As this motivational processing is contemplated, it can be concluded that not only is motivation to sustain a behaviour like breastfeeding complex, it is also highly individual and personal (see Box 4.3).

While increasing our theoretical understanding of motivation in relation to breastfeeding is an important starting point, it is only a starting point. To empower women to sustain breastfeeding successfully requires that health professionals, (including midwives) not only consider the motivational power attached to women's perceived experience of the behaviour, but also begin to

---

Box 4.3   **Importance of developing an understanding of the nature of human motivation in relation to persistent breastfeeding behaviour**

Developing a basic understanding of the nature of human motivation in relation to persistent breastfeeding behaviour is an important starting point for educators, researchers and practitioners. Keeping the complexity of motivation at the fore of our thinking has two major advantages; first, it prevents health professionals from prematurely profiling or categorizing women and their behaviour; and, secondly, it compels health professionals to consider the *personal* nature of women's motivation to breastfeed

consider their role in contextualizing women's experience. Breastfeeding experience does not happen within an experiential vacuum: to the contrary, the instruction provided by health professionals and the way in which that instruction is communicated has a critical role to play in how women will motivationally view their experience. Historically, the shift from theory to practice has not always been straightforward or automatic, yet, the need to create routine instruction that is theoretically designed and motivationally sensitive is paramount. Therefore, Chapter 6 describes how routine breastfeeding instruction may be redesigned using motivational strategies and, in doing so, move one step closer to increasing women's overall motivation to sustain the behaviour.

ACTIVITIES

Undergraduate

It has been stated (p. 100): 'women will often introduce soothers or supplementation as strategies for managing a difficult breastfeeding experience. Health professionals may differ in their belief as to whether these strategies are appropriate or not (Victora et al., 1997; Righard, 1998)'.

Search the literature to answer the following questions:

1   What strategies do breastfeeding women use in order to self-regulate their behaviour in order to sustain breastfeeding?
2   How do midwives interpret women's self-regulatory behaviours?

Postgraduate

Connell and Wellborn (1991) and Jacobs and Eccles (2000) identify three fundamental needs underpinning motivation:

* the need to experience self as competent and so be able to produce the desired outcome while avoiding negativity
* the need to be autonomous and so able to make meaningful choices
* the need for relatedness and to feel socially connected, self-worthy and respected.

Design a research study to explore whether or not these assertions are true.

References

Ajzen, I. and Madden, T.J. (1986) 'Prediction of Goal Directed Behavior: Attitudes, Intentions and Perceived Behavioral Control', *Journal of Experimental Social Psychology*, 22: 453–74.

Amabile, T.M., Hennessey, B.A. and Grossman, B. (1986) 'Social Influences on Creativity: The Effects of Contracted-for Reward', *Journal of Personality and Social Psychology*, 50: 14–23.

Avery, M., Duckett, L., Dodgson, J., Savik, K. and Henly, S.J. (1998) 'Factors Associated with Very Early Weaning among Primparas Intending to Breastfeed', *Maternal and Child Health Journal*, 2(3): 167–79.

Bandura, A. (1977) *Social Learning Theory*. Englewood Cliffs, NJ; London: Prentice-Hall.

Bandura, A. (1994) 'Self-Efficacy', in V.S. Ramachaudran (ed.), *Encyclopedia of Human Behavior Volume 4*. New York, NY: Academic Press: 71–81. (Reprinted in H. Friedman (ed.), *Encyclopedia of Mental Health*. San Diego, CA: Academic Press, 1998).

Bolling, K., Grant, C., Hamlyn, B. and Thorton, A. (2007) *Infant Feeding Survey 2005*. United Kingdom: NHS, The Information Centre (www.ic.nhs.uk – accessed 1 August 2010).

Clifford, T.J., Campbell, M.K., Speechley, K.N. and Gorodzinsky, F. (2006) 'Factors Influencing Full Breastfeeding in a South Western Ontario Community: Assessments at 1 Week and at 6 Months Postpartum', *Journal of Human Lactation*, 22(3): 292–304.

Cloherty, M., Alexander, J.and Holloway, I. (2003) 'Supplementing Breastfed Babies in the UK to Protect their Mothers from Tiredness or Distress', *Midwifery*, 20(2): 194–204.

Connell, J.P. and Wellborn, J.G. (1991) 'Competence, Autonomy and Relatedness. A Motivational Analysis of Self-system Processes', in M.R. Gunnar and L.A. Sroufe, *Minnesota Symposia on Child Psychology. Systems and Development*, 23: 43–77. Hillsdale, NJ: Erlbaum. Cited in J.E. Jacobs and J.S. Eccles (2000) 'Parents, Task Values, and Real-Life Achievement-Related Choices', in C. Sansone and J.M. Harackiewicz (eds), *Intrinsic and Extrinsic Motivation. The Search for Optimal Motivation and Performance*. San Diego, CA: Academic Press, ch. 14: 408–33.

Coombs, D.W., Reynolds, K., Joyner, G. and Blankson, M. (1998) 'A Self-help Program to Increase Breastfeeding among Low-income Women', *Journal of Nutrition Education*, 30(4): 203–9.

Da Vanzo, J., Starbird, E. and Leibowitz, A. (1990) 'Do Women's Breastfeeding Experiences with their First-borns Affect Whether they Breastfeed their Subsequent Children?', *Social Biology*, 37: 223–32.

Deci, E.L. and Ryan, R.M. (2000) 'Self-Determination Theory and the Facilitation of Intrinsic Motivation, Social Development and Well-being', *American Psychologist*, 55(1): 68–78.

Dennis, C.L. (2002) 'Breastfeeding Initiation and Duration: 1990–2000 Literature Review', *Journal of Obstetric, Gynecologic, and Neonatal Nursing*, 31(1): 12–32.

Dennis, C.L. (2003) 'Breastfeeding Self-efficacy Scale – Psychometric Assessment', *Journal of Obstetric, Gynecologic, and Neonatal Nursing*, 32(6): 734–44.

Dennis, C.L. and Faux, S. (1999) 'Development and Psychometric Testing of the Breastfeeding Self-efficacy Scale', *Research in Nursing and Health*, 22(5): 399–409.

Dick, M.J., Evans, M.L., Arthurs, J.B., Barnes, J.K., Caldwell, R.S., Hutchins, S.S. and Johnson, L.K. (2002) 'Predicting Early Breastfeeding Attrition', *Journal of Human Lactation*, 18(1): 21–8.

Dodgson, J.E., Henly, S.J., Duckett, L. and Tarrant, M. (2003) 'Theory of Planned Behavior-based Models for Breastfeeding Duration Among Hong Kong Mothers', *Nursing Research*, 52(3): 148–58.

Duckett, L., Henly, S., *et al.* (1998) 'A Theory of Planned Behavior-based Structural Model for Breast-Feeding', *Nursing Research*, 47(6): 325–36.

Einstein, A. 'Albert Einstein Quotes' (www.brainyquote.com accessed 1 August 2010).

Feather, N. (1982) *Expectations and Actions: Expectancy-Value Models in Psychology*. Hillsdale, NJ: Lawrence Erlbaum.

Fishbein, M (1967) 'Attitude and the Prediction of Behaviour', in M. Fishbein (ed.), *Readings in Attitude Theory and Measurement*. New York, NY: Wiley: 477–92.

Fishbein, M. and Ajzen, I. (1975) *Belief, Attitude, Intention and Behavior: An Introduction to Theory and Research*. Reading, MA: Addison-Wesley.

Fowler, C. and Lee, A. (2007) 'Knowing How to Know: Questioning "Knowledge Transfer" as a Model for Knowing and Learning in Health', *Studies in Continuing Education*, 29(2): 181–93.

Hatton, D.C., Harrison-Hohner, J., Coste, S., Dorato, V., Curet, L.B. and McCarron, D.A. (2005) 'Symptoms of Postpartum Depression and Breastfeeding', *Journal of Human Lactation*, 21(4): 444–9.

Hegney, D., Fallon, T. and O'Brien, M.L. (2008) 'Against All Odds: A Retrospective Case-controlled Study of Women who Experienced Extraordinary Breastfeeding Problems', *Journal of Clinical Nursing*, 17(9): 1182–92.

Heinig, M.J. (2009) 'Are There Risks to Using Risk-based Messages to Promote Breastfeeding?', *Journal of Human Lactation*, 25(1): 7–8.

Jacobs, J.E. and Eccles, J.S. (2000) 'Parents, Task Values, and Real-life Achievement-Related Choices', in C. Sansone and J.M. Harackiewicz (eds), *Intrinsic and Extrinsic Motivation: The Search for Optimal Motivation and Performance*. San Diego, CA: Academic Press, ch. 14: 408–33.

Janke, J.R. (1994) 'Development of the Breastfeeding Attrition Prediction Tool', *Nursing Research*, 43(2): 100–4.

Kong, S.K.F. and Lee, D.T.F. (2004) 'Factors Influencing Decision to Breastfeed', *Journal of Advanced Nursing*, 46(4): 369–79.

Linnenbrink, E.A. and Pintrich, P.R. (2000) 'Multiple Pathways to Learning and Achievement', in C. Sansone and J.M. Harackiewicz (eds), *Intrinsic and Extrinsic Motivation: The Search for Optimal Motivation and Performance*. San Diego, CA: Academic Press, ch. 8: 196–222

Locke, E.A. and Latham, G.P. (1990) *A Theory of Goal Setting and Task Performance*. Englewood Cliffs, NJ: Prentice-Hall.

Maddux, J.E. (1995) *Self-efficacy, Adaptation and Adjustment: Theory, Research and Application. Springer Series in Social/Clinical Psychology*. New York, NY: Plenum Press.

Martin, L.L. and Tesser, M. (1996) *Striving and Feeling: Interactions Among Goals, Affect and Self-Regulation*. Hillsdale, NJ: Lawrence Erlbaum.

McMillan, B., Conner, M., Woolridge, M., Dyson, L., Green, J., Renfrew, M., Bharj, K. and Clarke, G. (2008) 'Predicting Breastfeeding in Women Living in Areas of Economic Hardship: Explanatory Role of The Theory of Planned Behaviour', *Psychology and Health*, 23(7): 767–88.

Molden, D.C. and Dweck, C.S. (2000) 'Meaning and Motivation', in C. Sansone and J.M. Harackiewicz (eds), *Intrinsic and Extrinsic Motivation: The Search for Optimal Motivation and Performance*. San Diego, CA: Academic Press, ch. 6: 131–53.

Mozingo, J., Davis, M.W., Droppleman, P.G. and Merideth, A. (2000) 'It Wasn't Working – Women's Experiences with Short-term Breastfeeding', *American Journal of Maternal and Child Nursing* (MCN), 25(3): 120–6.

Nagy, E., Orvos, H.A., Pa, I., Kova, C.S. and Loveland, K. (2001) 'Breastfeeding Duration and Previous Breastfeeding Experience', *Acta Paediatric*, 90(1): 51–6.

Nelson, A. and Sethi, S. (2005) 'The Breastfeeding Experiences of Canadian Teenage Mothers', *Journal of Obstetrics Gynecologic Neonatal Nursing*, 34(5): 615–24.

O'Brien, M., Buikstra, E., Fallon, T. and Hegney, D. (2009) 'Exploring the Influence of Psychological Factors on Breastfeeding Duration, Phase 1: Perceptions of Mothers and Clinicians', *Journal of Human Lactation*, 25(1): 55–63.

Racine, E.F., Frick, K.D., Strobino, D., Carpenter, L.M., Milligan, R. and Pugh. L. (2009) 'How Motivation Influences Breastfeeding Duration Among Low-income Women', *Journal of Human Lactation*, 25(2): 173–81.

Righard, L. (1998) 'Are Breastfeeding Problems Related to Incorrect Breastfeeding Technique and the Use of Pacifiers and Bottles?', *Birth*, 25(1): 40–4.

Rotter, J.B. (1945) Social Learning and Clinical Psychology. Englewood Cliffs, NJ: Prentice-Hall.

Ryan, R.M. and Deci, E.L. (2000) 'When Rewards Compete with Nature', in C. Sansone and J.M. Harackiewicz (eds), *Intrinsic and Extrinsic Motivation: The Search for Optimal Motivation and Performance*. San Diego, CA: Academic Press, ch. 2: 13–54.

Sansone, C. and Harackiewicz, J.M. (eds) (2000) *Intrinsic and Extrinsic Motivation: The Search for Optimal Motivation and Performance*. San Diego, CA: Academic Press.

Schmied, V., Sheenan, A. and Barclay, L. (2001) 'Contemporary Breastfeeding Policy and Practice: Implications for Midwives', *Midwifery*, 17(1): 44–54.

Shah, J.Y. and Kruglanski, A.W. (2003) 'When Opportunity Knocks: Bottom-up Priming of Goals by Means and its Effects on Self-regulation', *Journal of Personality and Social Psychology*, 84(6): 1109–22.

Shakespeare, J., Blake, F. and Garcia, J. (2004) 'Breastfeeding Difficulties Experienced by Women Taking Part in a Qualitative Interview Study of Postnatal Depression', *Midwifery*, 20(3): 251–60.

Sheldon, K.M. and Elliot, A.J. (1999) 'Goal Striving, Need-satisfaction, and Longitudinal Wellbeing: The Self-concordance Model', *Journal of Personality and Social Psychology*, 76 (3) 482–97. Cited in R.M. Ryan and E.L. Deci (2000) *When Rewards Compete with Nature*, in C. Sansone and J.M. Harackiewicz (eds), *Intrinsic and Extrinsic Motivation: The Search for Optimal Motivation and Performance*. San Diego, CA: Academic Press, ch. 2: 13–54.

Sophocles 'Quotes on Learning' (http://quotations.about.com – accessed 1 August 2010).

Stewart-Knox, B., Gardiner, K. and Wright, M. (2003) 'What is the Problem with Breastfeeding? A Qualitative Analysis of Infant Feeding Perceptions', *Journal of Human Nutrition and Diet*, 16(4): 265–73.

Stockdale, J., Sinclair, M., Kernohan, W.G., Dunwoody, L., Cunningham, J.B., Lawther, L. and Weir, P. (2008) 'Assessing the Impact of Midwives' Instruction: The Breastfeeding Motivational Instructional Measurement Scale', *Evidence Based Midwifery*, 6(1): 27–34.

Stockdale, J., Sinclair, M., Kernohan, W.G. and Lavender, T. (2010) 'What Do We Mean When We Talk about Intrinsic and Extrinsic Motivation to Breastfeed: A Short Commentary', *Journal of Human Lactation*, 26(1): 15–17.

Victora, C.G., Behague, D.P., Barros, F.C., Olinto, M.T. and Weiderpass, E. (1997) 'Pacifier Use and Short Breastfeeding Duration: Cause, Consequence or Coincidence?', *Pediatrics*, 99(3): 445–53.

Wambach, K.A. (1997) 'Breastfeeding Intention and Outcome: A Test of the Theory of Planned Behaviour', *Research in Nursing & Health*, 20: 51–9.

Wambach, K.A. and Cohen, S.M. (2009) 'Breastfeeding Experiences of Urban Adolescent Mothers', *Journal of Paediatric Nursing*, 24(4): 244–54.

Wells, K.J., Thompson, N.J. and Kloeblen-Tarver, A.S. (2002) 'Intrinsic and Extrinsic Motivation and Intention to Breastfeed', *American Journal of Health Behaviour*, 26(2): 111–20.

Weiner, B. (1986) *An Attributional Theory of Motivation and Emotion*. New York, NY: Springer-Verlag.

PART II

Theoretical Application in Practice

Motivation, Breastfeeding and Midwives: Theory in Action

5

Janine Stockdale, Marlene Sinclair, George Kernohan and John Keller

---

Key points

- Motivational theory applied to breastfeeding promotion
- Demonstration of the utility of the ARCS Model of Motivational Instructional Design (Keller, 1983)
- Process of motivational diagnosis and design of optimally motivating breast feeding instruction
- Testing the motivationally-designed intervention.

Introduction

As far back as 1974, Jacox proposed that theory in action is when: 'given this nursing goal (producing some desired change or effect in the patient's condition), these are the actions the nurse must take to meet the goal (produce the change)' (cited by Walker and Avant, 2005: 14). When it comes to motivation to breastfeed, the principle of theory-in-action remains the same; the motivational action taken by health professionals has an important contextual role to play in the amount of motivational energy women experience when breast-feeding. Even though many health professionals agree with this call for action, to create a culture of sustained breastfeeding behaviour, the 'know-how' of facilitating this cultural shift from breastfeeding cessation to one of sustained breastfeeding behaviour is anything but straightforward. United Kingdom national data reveal that, while the prevalence of breastfeeding may have increased since 2000, the proportion of women sustaining breastfeeding at key points such as six weeks, has at best remained static (Bolling *et al.*, 2007).

Building on the theoretical foundation of Chapter 4, Chapter 5 describes a five-year research project that aimed to put motivational theory into action (Stockdale, 2007; Stockdale *et al.*, 2007; 2008a; 2008b; 2008c). A motivational instructional design model was applied to all routine antenatal, intranatal and postnatal breastfeeding instruction provided by midwives in a Baby Friendly Initiative (BFI) accredited hospital and community facility (Baby Friendly Initiative, 1998). Following a brief introduction to motivational instructional design, this chapter explains the process of how routine breastfeeding instruction was motivationally enhanced. The main three phases of the research study are described in relation to:

- motivational diagnosis of current instruction
- motivational design of current instruction
- testing of the motivationally enhanced version of instruction.

The purpose of this chapter is to provide readers with a general overview of the process involved in introducing motivational strategies into routine breastfeeding instruction.

What is motivational instructional design?

Although the motivation theory described in Chapter 4 explains personal motivation to achieve, educationalists have long recognized that an individual's motivational state can be positively or negatively influenced by the nature of the instructional environment to which they are exposed. When reflecting on our personal learning experiences throughout life, few of us would disagree that our motivation to learn is influenced by the way in which the instructor communicates the information. In other words, motivational instructional design is not concerned so much with the content of an instructional programme but, rather, asks: How can the same content be presented so that learners are more likely to experience optimal, personal motivation to learn?

Originating in educational theory, motivational instructional design models are 'theory-based, practically-orientated' models that have been specifically designed to guide educators in their attempt to create the optimal motivational learning environment. As pointed out by Ertmer *et al.* (2009), expertise in instructional design requires a deep and connected domain knowledge that is guided by the theories of learning and motivation (see Chapter 4). Through the application of motivational instructional design, educators can begin to close the gap between the theories of motivation and the process of learning. Recognizing that breastfeeding is a learned behaviour and that midwives are often the main educators (Bolling *et al.*, 2007), one such model, the ARCS Model of Motivational Instructional Design by Keller (1987a), was applied to the routine breastfeeding instruction provided by midwives. The aim was to create the optimal learning environment so that women's motivation to sustain breastfeeding was more likely to increase.

The ARCS Model of Motivational Instructional Design

The ARCS Model of Motivational Instructional Design (Keller, 1987a; 1987b) is a widely applied model that is both simple and powerful in its approach. The conceptual foundation for the model (Keller, 1979, 1983) is based primarily on an expectancy-value (E-V) approach to motivation (see Chapter 4). As an E-V model, it presumes that: 'people are motivated to engage in an activity if it is perceived to be linked to the satisfaction of personal needs (the value aspect) and if there is a positive expectancy for success (the expectancy aspect)' (Keller, 1987c: 3). Recognizing that educators may not be fully aware of the theoretical underpinnings of the motivation to learn, the author of the ARCS model synthesized the main theories of motivation into four concise components. It is these four components that guide the instructor in the process of creating an optimally-motivating instructional environment. Based on the acronym 'ARCS', the four motivational components developed are Attention, Relevance, Confidence and Satisfaction. When educators are designing instruction/learning materials, these four components must be addressed. For example, if women are going to be motivated to sustain breastfeeding the instruction provided must be relevant to them. Underpinning each of these components are the important motivational theories associated with successful attainment and a set of practical strategies that guide the educator in the overall design process (Figure 5.1).

In other words, the ARCS model operates as a bridge between the theoretical and practical (action). Even though women differ in their motivational profile, when the ARCS Model is applied the: 'assumption is that the group as a whole will be responsive if an effective set of motivational strategies is applied' (Keller, 1987c: 6). Motivational effectiveness does not always require each of the ARCS strategies. However, it is necessary to undertake a motivational diagnosis of the learning environment, to determine the inherent motivational strengths and weaknesses.

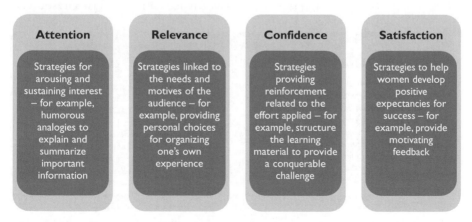

Figure 5.1   Illustration of the four components of the ARCS Model by Keller (1987a), and the focus of the associated motivational strategies built into the design and delivery of learning approaches

A motivational diagnosis of routine breastfeeding instruction

In this research, the purpose of the diagnostic phase of the ARCS model was to establish the motivational strengths, weaknesses and deficits of current breastfeeding instruction routinely provided by midwives. As breastfeeding is a complex behaviour that can be influenced by antenatal, intranatal and post-natal instruction, it was necessary to examine all environments where women were likely to receive breastfeeding instruction/advice. A series of structured observations was undertaken to identify the motivational content of current instruction in relation to any suggested purpose and target goals, as defined by Harackiewicz and Sansone (2000). Suggestions offered to women as to why they should value breastfeeding were recorded as purpose goals, while instruc-tion related to 'how to breastfeed' was recorded as target goals. As a result, all breastfeeding instruction was mapped from the time that women first attended the antenatal clinic until three weeks postnatal using the ARCS model (infor-mational analysis) across nine settings:

- The antenatal booking visit to the hospital
- 20-week parentcraft talk
- 34-week antenatal visit
- 34–40 weeks antenatal parentcraft class
- Delivery suite
- Postnatal ward (day)
- Postnatal ward (night)
- Postnatal community midwife support
- Postnatal support groups.

Subsequently, all verbal and written instruction was analyzed to determine the transfer of a breastfeeding goal structure to women as they progressed through the different instructional environments. Recognizing that women often rely on the Internet for confirming professional instruction (Dickerson, 2006), an additional diagnostic study was carried out of Internet resources.

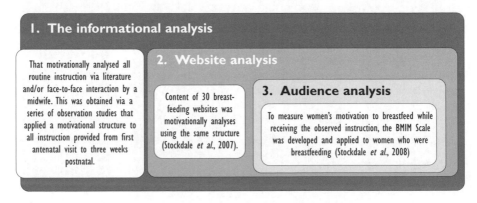

Figure 5.2   Three phases of the diagnostic analysis of current best breastfeeding practice that explores motivation in relation to information provided and its effects

This resulted in a three-level approach to understanding women's motivation to breastfeed (see Figure 5.2).

As each stage of the diagnostic phase was completed, the findings began to reveal a clear picture as to why women who, although motivated to start breastfeeding, often lost their motivation and gave up on breastfeeding. A short summary of the main findings associated with the different levels of the diagnostic phase follows.

Informational analysis

Application of a simplified version of Harackiewicz and Sansone's (2000) goal structure revealed that midwives routinely and consistently worked to motivate women to breastfeed. 'Purpose goals' were defined as the reasons given to women as to why they might want to breastfeed and 'target goals' as the things they must do or learn to be successful. A series of structured observations were carried out that explored routine breastfeeding instruction.

Antenatal observation: During the antenatal phase women were routinely offered many reasons why they might want to breastfeed (purpose goals). The main purpose goals offered to women clearly communicated the health and bonding benefits of breastfeeding. For example, a midwife explained at an antenatal session:

'Breastfeeding is the best start and helps you lose weight' (AN session 3).

Midwives' enthusiasm to encourage women to create value for breastfeeding was not limited to a simple factual transfer of the benefits of breastfeeding. The following examples demonstrate how (although unaware of the theoretical underpinnings) midwives passionately attended to the value component of motivation to breastfeed:

'If your baby could choose it's likely he or she would choose to be breast-fed' (AN session 3)

'Less constipation and smelly nappies' (AN session 4)

'Did you know that bottle milk is made up of fish oil mixed with cow's milk?' (AN session 4)

'Quality of breast milk remains high even if you are ill or smoke' (AN literature)

From time to time, the effort applied by the midwives to encourage women to adopt purpose goals for breastfeeding appeared to move towards that of a 'hard sell':

'You could get breast cancer – is that not a good reason?' (AN session 3)

'Ear aches can get so bad your baby could end up needing vents or something' (AN session 2 ['vents' also known as 'grommets'])

'Breastfed babies get lots of chain fatty acids, so your baby's intelligence will be above his potential' (AN session 1)

Literature distributed during AN classes also added to the suggested reasons why women might consider breastfeeding. One image of a mother and baby carried the caption: 'I am so glad I did it. It is a great bond' (Health Promotion Agency for Northern Ireland, 2004).

The frequency of the purpose goals during pregnancy appeared to be directed more towards first-time mothers (15 episodes) than experienced mothers (9 episodes). It was therefore not surprising that, when measured (audience analysis), first-time mothers placed greater value on breastfeeding than women who were already mothers. Nevertheless, as pointed out in Chapter 4, value alone cannot motivate a person to sustain a behaviour such as breastfeeding; a sense of expectancy for success (maternal confidence) must also be experienced.

Knowing how to breastfeed successfully is, in itself, confidence building and so the observation of antenatal purpose goals coincided with the observation of 'target goals'. The term 'target goal' refers directly to the instructions that women were given in relation to what they had to do to breastfeed successfully. When target goals accompany purpose goals, women can develop a long-term goal for breastfeeding, feel confident they have the necessary knowledge to succeed, and be able to use this information to measure their own success. Target goals therefore not only provide the 'know-how' of successful breastfeeding, but also provide learners with some form of performance indicator that signals to them whether or not they are being successful. Although less frequent than purpose goals, midwives routinely communicated target goals during the antenatal phase. Table 5.1 provides examples of the main target goals communicated by midwives during the antenatal phase.

By the end of the antenatal phase, midwives were observed providing women with many purpose goals (positively influencing their value for breastfeeding) and fewer, but important, target goals (positively influencing their expectancy for success). Perhaps unknowingly, at least from a theoretical perspective, by the transfer of these two types of goals midwives were routinely providing what seemed like motivating instruction that would have a consequential effect on women's (especially first-time mothers') intention to initiate and sustain breastfeeding.

A distinct instructional shift appeared to occur in the postnatal phase. Purpose goals for breastfeeding were no longer the dominant goals; target goals came much more to the fore as midwives tried to troubleshoot women's breastfeeding experience. Not only did target goals make up the majority of midwife instruction in the postnatal phase, observations revealed that the postnatal target goals were not necessarily those observed in the antenatal phase. Instead, the postnatal target goals could be categorized according to 'When to, when not to breastfeed' and what might be called 'Midwife-led breastfeeding' (see Table 5.2).

Few purpose goals were observed in the postnatal phase, in that their use

Table 5.1   Examples of categorisation and frequency counts related to target goals observed in the antenatal period

Target goal suggested	Count of 'how' aspect of target goal	Count of 'performance feedback' aspect of target goal
Breastfeed in first half-hour	13	
Demand feed your baby	33	
Learn to attach your baby properly	24	
Breastfeed exclusively – no teats, dummies or formula	19	
Baby will be content if breastfed properly		12
It shouldn't hurt if your baby is latched properly		28
It will be easy and straightforward		7
You will feel confident (before you leave hospital)		3
You will see a satisfactory nappy output (wet and dirty nappies)		8
Your baby will gain weight and grow		11
Ask your midwife to resolve your problem	27	

Table 5.2   Examples of target goals emerging from observation of postnatal instruction

When to feed, when not to	Midwife-led breastfeeding
'You need to lift her and feed her' (PN session 1)	'You have a graze, she must have slipped, don't feed till I check you are doing it right' (PN session 2)
'Okay we need to get this baby fed' (PN session 1)	'Do it like this, okay?' (PN session 2)
'No let sleeping babies lie' (PN session 3)	'I'll put him on for you' (PN session 3)
'If he hasn't fed, you need to lift him' (PN session1)	'that one (meaning the woman's breast) is easier for me (the midwife)' (PN session 1)

was mainly restricted to the messages communicated by wall posters; for example, the World Health Organization poster depicting the benefits of breastfeeding was displayed in the postnatal corridor. It was only when a woman reported a desire to stop breastfeeding that purpose goals were introduced by the midwife by conversation offering women reasons for sustaining breastfeeding.

Internet analysis
Although the observation studies disclosed distinct patterns of purpose and target goals as part of health care service provision, it was considered possible that women would source breastfeeding advice on the Internet. Using the same structure of purpose and target goals, 30 commonly accessed breastfeeding websites were analyzed for motivation (Stockdale *et al.*, 2007). Although developed by health professionals, health care associations and other parents, the emphasis on breastfeeding was similar, in that the sites gave many reasons for breastfeeding and instructions as to how women might be successful (including troubleshooting instruction). Little difference existed in the overall motivational structure between breastfeeding instruction accessed on the internet and that provided routinely by midwives.

By the end of the informational and Internet analyses, it seemed that routine instruction aimed mainly to motivate women by encouraging them to value breastfeeding (through purpose goals) and by providing them with instruction that would build their confidence in their ability to breastfeed (expectancy for success). In relation to postnatal instruction, target goals became more person-centred as midwives attempted to solve each woman's breastfeeding difficulties.

Audience analysis
While the observation studies provided evidence concerning the motivational content of current instruction, it was important to determine whether the observed instruction positively influenced women's value and expectancy for success in relation to breastfeeding. To analyze the impact of best practice breastfeeding instruction on women's value and expectancy for success (confidence), the Breastfeeding Motivational Instructional Measurement Scale (BMIMS) was developed and tested. Informed by the motivational theories introduced in Chapter 4 and the informational analysis, four motivational theories were incorporated into the BMIMS (Stockdale *et al.*, 2008a). Using a structured interview approach, this new 51-item scale was applied to a convenience sample of 202 breastfeeding women. Factor analysis, as a statistical procedure, revealed important motivational information concerning women's motivation to sustain breastfeeding.

Although (from an IT perspective) factor analysis seems complex, conceptually the procedure is straightforward. Using correlation (-1 to $+1$), the computer is asked to determine which variables go together to form a concept or construct (called a factor) related to the subject matter. The correlation coefficients (called 'factor loadings') indicate the direction and strength of the relationship between the item and the factor that it is placed in. For example, a factor loading of .70 indicates a strong positive correlation between the item and factor, while $-.70$ indicates a strong negative correlation. Factor loadings of less than .35 are normally excluded from the results. As illustrated by the example factor loadings in Table 5.3, first-time mothers were found to place a high value on breastfeeding and a low expectancy for success while learning to breastfeed.

As illustrated by the first four factor loadings in Table 5.3, first-time mothers placed a very high value on breastfeeding. This was not surprising as the

Table 5.3   Example of factor loadings related to the application of the Breastfeeding Motivational Instructional Measurement Scale using first-time mother as a selection variable

No.	Survey items	Factor loading
1.	Breastfeeding is important to me	.65
2.	I would be upset if I did not manage to breastfeed	.64
3.	The amount of effort I put into breastfeeding is worthwhile to me	.65
4.	Breastfeeding is very meaningful to me	.80
5.	I frequently think of quitting breastfeeding	.75
6.	Overall I am no good at breastfeeding	.73
7.	I can find out how good breastfeeding is going just by doing it	−.44
8.	As a result of feedback from my midwives I know I am breastfeeding well	−.73
9.	Breastfeeding itself provides little information as to how well it is going	.42
10.	The feedback I get from my midwives is not very useful	.72
11.	Breastfeeding is quite simple and repetitive	−.47
12.	I have trouble figuring out whether breastfeeding is going well or not	.69
13.	There are things I would like to know about my breastfeeding experience that I am not being told	.73

antenatal education programme was designed mainly for this specific user group. While the purpose goals introduced in the antenatal phase appeared to impact on the value women place on breastfeeding, the observed target goals did not seem to have the same positive effect in relation to their confidence level. In fact, women reported a low sense of confidence and expectancy for success; for example, describing themselves as being no good at breastfeeding (see factor loading 6). Breastfeeding was also described as neither simple nor straightforward (factor loading 11). Additionally, women admitted that they had trouble working out whether breastfeeding was going well or not (factor loading 12). As indicated in Chapter 4, low expectancy for success can challenge a person's motivation to continue breastfeeding and, as indicated in factor loading 5 (Table 5.3), women were already contemplating cessation.

While it was diagnostically important to describe women's motivational state in relation to value and expectancy for success, the more important question was: Why did the observed target goals fail to increase women's confidence? That is, why did first-time mothers who had been exposed to an immense amount of antenatal and postnatal target goals begin to lose their confidence when the time came to put that instruction into action? On closer examination, it became apparent that, although women were given many target goals (including detailed instructions such as when and when not to breastfeed), these target goals were insufficient in helping women understand and take control of their own breastfeeding experience. Based on their personal experience of breastfeeding, women admitted that they were unsure about how they should interpret their experience, and the information provided by midwives did not answer their questions (see Table 5.3 factor loadings 7, 8, 9, 10, 13).

As the free-text comments volunteered by women at the end of the questionnaire were analyzed, it became progressively more evident that the expectations created by the antenatal goal structure had not, for many women, been realized in the postnatal phase. In fact, when women's postnatal comments were mapped alongside the different antenatal target goals to which they had been exposed, the degree of incongruency between what women were told to expect as successful breastfeeding and what they actually experienced became strikingly obvious, as illustrated in Table 5.4.

It was only when this all-encompassing view of the diagnostic information was taken into consideration that it became apparent that the instruction provided in the antenatal period, by midwives, was an important source of women's lack of confidence in their ability to breastfeed. That is, the definition

Table 5.4   Examples of comments from BMIMS by women currently breastfeeding and those who had recently stopped breastfeeding

Antenatal goal set by midwives	*Postnatal phase women reported that*
'You'll be confident before you leave hospital'	'I am just totally unable to see the day when I would be confident enough to look after the baby by myself' (Q39)
'Learn how to correctly position your baby'	'I feel I always need to be convinced that baby is latched properly – I'm not sure' (Q39)
'Breastfeeding creates a special bond between you and your baby'	'the trauma that my inability to breast feed was causing me and the baby every meal time was just too much to bear' (Q132).
'It shouldn't be painful if your baby is attached properly'	'I was in a lot of pain and it was distressing for everyone so I switched to bottle feeding'(Q36)
'Breastfed babies are content babies'	'My baby is feeding all the time and I feel she is not getting enough' (Q87)
'Let your baby tell you when he/she is hungry and follow their lead'	'At the class I was told to demand feed in hospital but now they're telling me to wake him, I need more information' (Q89)

of 'normal' breastfeeding adopted and communicated routinely by health professionals (Mulder, 2006) was the standard by which women measured their success. If their experience of breastfeeding directly matched this conceptualisation of 'normality', then their confidence would remain intact and they would continue breastfeeding. If, however, their experience deviated from this picture of breastfeeding, then they could only surmise that breastfeeding was 'abnormal' and, subsequently, their confidence in their ability to breastfeed successfully would be compromised. In other words, at the heart of women's breastfeeding cessation was a dilemma that is characterized by high value, low confidence and associated maternal stress, as one woman described clearly:

'the past days of trying to learn and manage breastfeeding have been incredibly difficult – very stressful … . Breastfeeding was (and still is) important to me … but the trauma that my inability to breastfeed was causing me and the baby every meal time was just too much to bear' (Q 132).

With this more complete motivational diagnosis, new light began to shine on the findings of prior studies that were considered key to understanding women's motivation to breastfeed, such as that carried out by Coombs *et al.* (1998). This research team reported the testing of a motivationally-enhanced version of current breastfeeding instruction. The intervention incorporated many of the motivational strategies necessary to move someone towards a successful experience. However, when tested, the results demonstrated that, although the initiation rates of breastfeeding increased (indication of increased value), women continued to lack confidence in their ability to breastfeed (low expectancy for success). Coombs *et al.*, (1998) reported a significant relationship between breastfeeding behaviour and the perception of breastfeeding difficulties; that is, women who experienced difficulties were more likely to report low confidence and stop breastfeeding.

In summary, the diagnostic application of motivational theory through the ARCS model to breastfeeding instruction provided an overall synthesis of the main reasons why women fail to sustain their motivation to breastfeed. Women use the information provided by health professionals in the antenatal phase as a measure of their own success in the postnatal phase. In other words, the routine breastfeeding instruction provided by midwives is the standard by which women assess their competency and embark upon the cyclical process of perceived failure described in Chapter 4. As a midwife summed it up for the women attending an antenatal session:

'a breastfed baby is a content baby … it's important you learn how to correctly position your baby to the breast … if this is not done well, feeding is painful and your baby will not be satisfied' (AN session 3).

While diagnosing the nature of women's lack of motivation is an important step in application of the ARCS model, motivationally managing this phenomenon is equally important.

Designing a motivationally-enhanced version of routine breastfeeding instruction

There has been some debate in the literature as to whether antenatal education should address the realities of breastfeeding or continue to create expectations of breastfeeding as natural, easy and straightforward. Authors such as Schmied *et al.* (2001) and Mozingo *et al.* (2000) proposed more than 10 years ago that, by telling pregnant women the truth about breastfeeding, women would have an opportunity to prepare psychologically for what might lie ahead. Most health professionals, however, continue to opt for a more traditional approach to breastfeeding instruction that depicts 'normal' breastfeeding as a problem-free experience but, at the same time, problem-solving information is made freely available. For example, the NHS Choices (2009) website informs women that they will know breastfeeding is successfully progressing and baby is receiving sufficient nourishment when the performance indicators outlined in Box 5.1 are met.

When it came to the application of the ARCS strategies of motivational instructional design, a decision had to be made as to whether the motivational strategies should be embedded into routine instruction that introduced women to the potential difficulties of breastfeeding (see Figure 5.3).

Different factors influenced the research team's thinking in relation to these similar, but significantly diverse, models of routine breastfeeding instruction. It was concluded that, if women used the normality of breastfeeding as their measure of success, there was no theoretical evidence to suggest that introducing problems into the antenatal phase would be motivationally advantageous. To the contrary, from a theoretical perspective, the potential of introducing women to a measure of 'abnormality' before problems occurred could negatively sensitize women towards an 'avoidance-orientated' type of motivation. In other words, women might set a goal to breastfeed that focused on avoiding the problems of breastfeeding, rather than approaching the behaviour confidently with a sense of success.

As a further determinant as to whether it would be theoretically expedient to introduce women to problems before they actually occurred, information was sought from the corresponding author of the work completed in 1998 (Dr Coombs, Psychologist at the University of Alabama, USA). With permission kindly granted, a motivational appraisal of the intervention materials developed by Coombs *et al.* (1998) confirmed that, even when women had easy

---

Box 5.1   Performance feedback indicators provided by the NHS Choices (2009) website

- 'your baby is healthy and gaining weight'
- 'your breasts and nipples shouldn't be sore'
- 'your baby will appear content and satisfied after most feeds'
- 'your baby will come off the breast on his/her own'

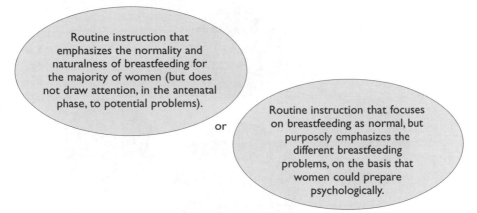

Figure 5.3   Models of breastfeeding antenatal promotion: normal and natural versus normal and sometimes problematic breastfeeding

access to information about potential breastfeeding difficulties, their motivation was not necessarily protected if the problems did subsequently occur. Subsequent trials, such as that by Lavender *et al.* (2005), have continued to suggest that introducing breastfeeding problems as part of routine antenatal instruction does not necessarily increase women's motivation to sustain breastfeeding. In this trial, partnered with a community midwife, women attended a seven-hour BFI workshop which was facilitated by a lactation consultant. At the workshop, women were not only introduced to the nature of breastfeeding, but were also pre-warned of potential breastfeeding problems and how to deal with them. Admittedly, the trial was not designed to test the efficacy of pre-warning pregnant women of breastfeeding problems. Nevertheless, the findings reported by Lavender *et al.* (2005) indicated that, even with additional support, this approach could not be presumed to increase breastfeeding outcomes.

As the theoretical and evidential factors pointed towards the insufficiency of both approaches, it became apparent that an alternative approach had to be designed – an approach that would facilitate women in their need to prepare psychologically for breastfeeding, and yet prevent an unhealthy focus on potential breastfeeding problems. This motivational approach would have to be capable of achieving the objectives of preparing women for different breastfeeding experiences, while protecting their expectancy for success.

Designing motivationally-enhanced breastfeeding instruction
To address what seemed to be two opposing objectives, all breastfeeding instruction introduced to women through suggested purpose and target goals was examined and re-adapted at a macro-level. The five most common breastfeeding problems reported by women that interfered with their motivation to sustain breastfeeding were re-introduced into the antenatal period, not as 'potential problems' but as normal 'challenges' associated with the normal process of learning to breastfeed. In other words, what health professionals often labelled as 'problems' were carefully and motivationally embedded into

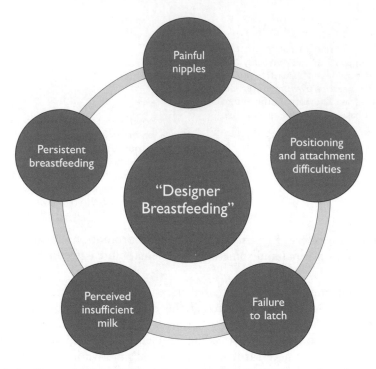

Figure 5.4   Breastfeeding difficulties motivationally-enhanced and introduced to antenatal education as normal breastfeeding challenges

routine instruction, so that they would not be an indicator of perceived failures. The problems that were motivationally re-designed and embedded into routine antenatal instruction as part of an overall instructional design process were as shown in Figure 5.4.

This motivational shift in the overall way in which these challenges were communicated resulted in a new breastfeeding curriculum called 'Designer Breastfeeding'. Theoretically, the programme was designed to facilitate:

- women's psychological preparation and motivation, if challenges were to occur
- the motivation of 'the typical breastfeeding audience' through routine instruction
- the potential diversity of women's breastfeeding experiences.

However, motivational enhancement was not only necessary at a theoretical or macro-level, it was also important that the observed motivational strengths of current instruction were capitalized, weaknesses strengthened, and instructional deficits met at a micro-level. Within the limitations of this chapter, it is not possible to provide readers with a full account of the complete motivational design process at macro- and micro-levels (for further information, see Stockdale, 2007 and Stockdale *et al.*, 2008c). However, the following examples are provided as a means of illustrating how motivational instructional design can occur at a micro-level.

Motivational strengths

Current instruction was noted to be strong in relation to the consistent and enthusiastic transfer of purpose and target goals by the midwives. Women were introduced to reasons for considering breastfeeding early in their pregnancy and, as their pregnancy progressed, target goals were introduced. This already existing motivational structure (observed purpose and target goals) was considered to be a significant motivational strength of current instruction, in that additional motivational strategies could be easily embedded without incurring additional instructional cost. In other words, current instruction could be motivationally enhanced without the introduction of extra instructional workshops and staff. With the pre-existing purpose/target goal framework, the appropriate motivational strategies could be easily embedded as a means of addressing the observed motivational weaknesses and deficits of current instruction.

Motivational weaknesses

While, at a macro-level, it was important that problems such as 'failure to latch' were re-introduced into the antenatal period, how this and other challenges were motivationally designed was critical to the overall success of the motivationally-enhanced version of instruction. Although, this instruction was considered strong in relation to the consistency with which women were introduced to the 'learning to latch target goal', a number of motivational weaknesses were noted as to how this instruction was routinely communicated. The main instructional episode occurred at the antenatal educational class. Facilitated by a midwife, couples were asked to visualize how a breastfed baby should be positioned for optimal attachment to occur. The process was demonstrated by the midwife using a doll and prosthetic breast as teaching aids. The demonstration of the learning content was also supported by the provision of literature that provided women with a written account and pictures of how a baby latches. The excerpt in Box 5.2 is taken from the instructional literature, and the subtitle reads 'Here is what to do'.

As this target goal was motivationally assessed from the perspective of potential learners, it became apparent that:

- the instruction was introduced at approximately eight weeks prior to the opportunity to use the information. This had the potential for a negative effect on women's confidence in their ability to recall the information and subsequently use it.
- performance feedback indicators incorporated into the target goal encouraged a performance-orientated approach to breastfeeding, rather than that of a 'learning' or mastery-orientated approach. For example, the goal warned that if the instructions were not followed: 'he will not get enough breast tissue in his mouth to ensure an effective feed'.
- the language used to describe the process of learning to latch could appear contradictory for women who had never seen a baby latch. For example,

> ### Box 5.2   Excerpt from breastfeeding instructional literature provided to women in relation to positioning and attachment
>
> Here is what to do:
>
> – Hold your baby with his body and head in a straight line. He will be uncomfortable and unable to feed effectively if he is twisted.
> – He needs to be in close. He will reach for the breast with his nose rather than his chin if he is too far away from you. Depending on your breast and nipple shape and size, his body may be turned towards you or tucked slightly under the breast – your midwife or health visitor will help with this.
> – His neck needs to be extended very slightly – not tucked into his chest. Think of the way you tip your own head back a little to drink from a glass.
> – The nipple needs to be pointing to his nose. If you try to put your nipple into his mouth too low down he will not get enough breast tissue in his mouth to ensure an effective feed. If he is ready to feed, his mouth opens. You can encourage this by gently stroking his bottom lip with your nipple or a finger.
> – When his mouth is wide open, and his tongue is down and forward (almost like a yawn), bring him even closer. Do this swiftly but gently, so he can scoop up the nipple with his tongue and get a good mouthful of your breast. His chin will come to the breast first, and his nose will probably remain free.
>
> *Source:* Health Promotion Agency for Northern Ireland (2004).

  the instruction warns: 'He will reach for the breast with his nose rather than his chin if he is too far away from you' but, later in the same set of instructions, it states: 'The nipple needs to be pointing to his nose'.
* to enhance this target goal at a micro-level, a number of motivational strategies were embedded that incorporated the appropriate Attention, Relevance, Confidence and Satisfaction building strategies (for examples, see Box 5.3).

Through embedding each of the motivational strategies to the current target goal, the way in which positioning and attachment were communicated during the antenatal phase was changed by introducing the familiar analogy of biting a swinging apple without using hands. Using humour as one of the many motivational strategies, couples were placed in groups and asked to observe someone trying to take a bite from a swinging apple. Key questions accompanied the observations they made (see Box 5.4).

As each step in the process of learning to position and attach was introduced through the analogy, further instructional information was communicated that would help participants internalize the instruction that they would need to recall months later. For example, a short video that showed the action of a newborn first latching on was shown, and couples were encouraged to recognize the key steps as the baby engaged in the process of latching on. Through embedding the suggested strategies, this target goal was motivationally enhanced so that women's attention would remain on breastfeeding while their baby learned how to master the behaviour.

Box 5.3   Examples of the ARCS motivational instructional strategies applied to positioning and attaching instructional literature

Attention strategies
–   to provide a sense of 'Concreteness', 'Inquiry' and 'Participation':

A2:1   Show visual representations of any important object or set of ideas or relationships
A4:3   Use of humorous analogies to explain and summarise
A5:1   Use creativity techniques to have learners create unusual analogies and associations to the content
A6:1   Use games, role plays or simulations that require learner participation

Relevance strategies
–   to connect with people's past experience:

R1:2   Use analogies familiar to the learner from the past

Confidence-building strategies
–   including the re-adjustment of women's expectations and criteria for success:

C1:3   Explain the criteria for evaluation of performance
C3:1   Include statements about the likelihood of success with given amounts of effort and ability
C4:1   Attribute success to effort rather than luck, ease of task when appropriate (i.e. when true!)

Satisfaction strategies
–   such as:

S4:1   Avoid the use of threats as a means of obtaining task performance

---

Motivational instructional deficits

Women reported problems when their baby simply would not follow the expected feed/sleep pattern that they were told, antenatally, to expect. Although some babies did develop this systematic approach to the feed/sleep cycle, others would persistently breastfeed and refuse to settle, or would refuse to wake up and take the breastfeeding lead. Although midwives were observed providing multiple postnatal target goals for each of these situations, from a performance feedback perspective women's motivation was compromised as their baby's behaviour was interpreted as 'failure to breastfeed'. The introduction of a new target goal, one that empowered women to identify their baby's unique breastfeeding pattern, was deemed necessary to help prevent this negative psychological response: this required the creation of a different set of motivational strategies. Therefore, specific confidence strategies (see Box 5.5) were incorporated into practice.

The new target goals introduced couples to three different, but common, feeding patterns. Couples were empowered to recognize and navigate their way

Box 5.4   Motivational enhancement of instruction concerning positioning and attachment as an example of the role of motivational instructional design applied to breastfeeding

How easy is it for her to bite the apple if it is at a distance?
You can make it easier for your baby to learn by holding him/her close to you

How does twisting around complicate what she has to do to be successful?
By lining your baby up so that he/she doesn't have to twist around to latch on, as twisting makes it more difficult to learn how to latch

What touches the apple first?
Her nose and it's the same for your baby, his/her nose starts off touching your nipple

What happens to her head? – It goes back and her chin comes up from below. Her nose moves away from the apple.

This is exactly the action your baby has to master when learning to breastfeed. It takes time for your baby to learn how to do this just like he/she will take their time when learning to walk.

What do you need a lot of while your baby is learning? – PATIENCE!

Source: Designer Breastfeeding © 2007.

Box 5.5   Confidence building ARCS Strategies selected to correct observed motivational deficits

C1:1   Incorporate clearly stated appealing learning goals into instructional materials
C1:2   Provide self-evaluation tools which are based on clearly stated goals
C1:3   Explain the criteria for evaluation of performance

---

through each of these as 'normal' phases. To reduce the harmful effects of social normalization, the instruction emphasized that each baby is unique in the order and timing of his/her sleeping/feeding patterns. However, to ensure that the different feeding patterns remained within the range of 'normal to challenging', a lactation consultant was involved in the motivational-embedding of safety mechanisms into this particular target goal structure. It was predicted that this

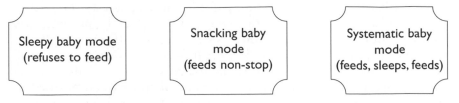

Figure 5.5   Infant breastfeeding patterns/modes of behaviour introduced to women in the antenatal period

target goal would further increase women's confidence in their ability to breast-feed, as they would no longer be reliant on individual midwives in the postnatal phase. Clear guidelines, as to when breastfeeding advice should be sought, were also considered to be confidence building and highly relevant to new parents. The three patterns introduced through this new set of target goals included instruction concerning the three modes shown in Figure 5.5.

Table 5.5   New and enhanced breastfeeding resources

The Designer Breastfeeding Book
This resource book covers all aspects of breastfeeding instruction in a clear and user-friendly way.

The book was designed to help individuals and couples explore breast-feeding, distinguish between essential and non-essential knowledge, and develop personal breastfeeding goals that were congruent with their lifestyle. The book was designed not only as an antenatal educational tool, but also as an important postnatal map and reference source.

The book is motivationally divided into three sections:

- What every woman needs to know about breastfeeding
- What you choose to know about breastfeeding
- Navigating breastfeeding – your breastfeeding map.

Breastfeeding CD-Rom
In addition to the printed book, an electronic version has been developed to enhance visual learning through the use of animation and video.

Breastfeeding antenatal workshop
Couples were invited to a specially designed breastfeeding workshop that lasted for two-and-a-half hours.

As one of a four-part antenatal parenting series, the purpose of this workshop was to introduce women to the essentials of breastfeeding using the motivationally-enhanced learning strategies.

Breastfeeding postnatal support
Midwives supporting the motivationally-enhanced instruction are offered a one-day course on the nature of motivational support.

Summarizing the design phase, breastfeeding instruction was motivationally adapted at a macro-level, in that common breastfeeding problems were introduced into the antenatal period as common breastfeeding challenges. At a micro-level, each part of routine instruction was motivationally enhanced or inserted as directed by the diagnostic phase of the research. The resulting motivationally-enhanced version of current best practice was renamed as 'Designer Breastfeeding'.© The motivational purpose of this name was twofold:

- first, it introduced curiosity as to how breastfeeding could be 'designed'
- second, the name emphasized that breastfeeding behaviour was uniquely experienced by the mother and baby dyad.

In preparation for the testing of the motivationally-enhanced programme, new and enhanced resources were developed (Table 5.5).

Testing the effects of the motivationally-enhanced breastfeeding instruction

At this stage, the key question facing the reader may be: How do we know if this motivational approach will make any difference to women's motivation to sustain breastfeeding? In order to answer this question, Designer Breastfeeding© had to be tested and compared in relation to the non-enhanced version of instruction. The most rigorous approach to such a research question is the randomized controlled clinical trial. Accordingly, recruitment to a randomized control trial was commenced of primigravida women who intended to have their baby within the Trust. Recruitment specifically focused on women who had no personal experience of breastfeeding, as past experience is known to have a motivational impact. A full account of the trial is available (Stockdale *et al.*, 2008a). However this summary highlights the importance of motivational instructional design as a starting point for shifting towards a more sustainable breastfeeding culture.

As a motivationally-enhanced intervention, it was important that the main outcome measure was women's motivation to breastfeed. This was measured using the BMIMS (Stockdale *et al.*, 2008a) that had been developed during the diagnostic phase of the research. The three essential motivational components associated with duration to breastfeed were therefore measured:

- total value placed on breastfeeding ($r = .86$),
- total perceived midwife support ($r = .85$) and
- total expectancy for success ($r = .87$).

In particular, it was predicted that, within the experimental group, there would be a significant increase in participant's total expectancy for success and perception of the relevancy of instruction (referred to as 'midwife support').

Table 5.6   The breastfeeding behaviour within the experimental and control groups: demonstration of a significant increase in the proportion of women breastfeeding at discharge and at three weeks

	Initiated breastfeeding	Breastfeeding 100% on discharge	Breastfeeding 100% at 3 weeks
Control group	53 (n = 75) 70%	33 44%	15 20%
Experimental group	57 (n = 69) 82%	44 64%	37 53%
χ^2	Not significant	p < 0.01	p < 0.001

As the diagnostic phase had revealed that first-time mothers place very high value on breastfeeding, no significant increase was expected in relation to this motivational component. Measuring motivation as a primary outcome is advantageous when testing a motivationally-designed intervention, as it enables ongoing development. Of course, if the motivationally-enhanced instruction has the desired effect, the secondary outcome of sustained breastfeeding would also be evident in the experimental group.

Of the 182 women who consented to participate, 144 completed the research. On an 'intention to treat' basis, breastfeeding behaviour was assessed prior to discharge and at three weeks postnatal by telephone follow-up. If women initiated breastfeeding, their motivation was also measured shortly prior to discharge using the BMIMS: this was the primary outcome measure. A significant increase was noted within the experimental group in relation to women's expectancy for success (p< .001) and in their perception that the instruction received was relevant to their breastfeeding experience (p<.001). Theoretically, when expectancy for success is coupled with value, through perceived relevant instruction, persistence to perform the behaviour should increase. As predicted, proportionate breastfeeding differences were noted between the two groups, both on discharge from hospital (χ^2 test p = .01) and at three weeks postnatal (χ^2 test, p < .001) (see Table 5.6).

Completion of the trial marked the achievement of the first cycle in the action research project that aimed motivationally to enhance routine breastfeeding instruction. Although the findings demonstrated that motivational instructional design had the power to close the gap between theory and action, as with many research projects, the results created as many questions as it did answers. For the effective move closer to the creation of a stable breastfeeding culture, future research and development is required.

Further research and development
Although the predicted findings demonstrated that motivational instructional design was effective at an operational level, unexpected phenomena emerged that suggested that the power of motivational instructional design

goes beyond that which was first conceptualized. Supplementation of breast-fed babies has often been associated with failure to sustain breastfeeding (Bolling *et al.*, 2007); yet, as the behaviour of women whose babies had received supplementation was explored, an interesting phenomenon came to the fore. It was noted that, once formula was introduced (whether warranted or not), women in the control group were more likely to tend towards breastfeeding cessation than women in the experimental group. Women in the experimental group were more likely to persist with breastfeeding, working steadily towards being classified as 'fully breastfeeding'. The small incidence of supplementation within both groups did not make it possible to test the level of significance; however, theoretically, the observed response was in step with the nature of an effective learning environment. In other words, it is likely that as women in the experimental group continued to interpret their breastfeeding experience as part of the 'normal' process of learning to breastfeed, their confidence was protected from the unexpected challenges. It seemed that their expectancy for success continued to grow and their persistence to work towards fulfilment of their purpose goal actually increased. Introduction of formula within the control group, from a theoretical perspective, was likely to have a very different outcome. Women, whose success was measured according to the criteria of 'natural and straightforward' breastfeeding, were more likely to interpret the introduction of formula as a further indicator of their failure, so having a negative effect on their persistence. Until tested formally, this can only be surmised; but the unexpected findings of the feasibility trial were suggestive of the presence of this phenomenon.

It is important to point out that these findings are not advocating that breastfed babies should receive infant formula. To the contrary, these results are proposing that, through the introduction of motivational instructional design, an unexpected opportunity has arisen that has the potential to increase our understanding of the motivation, nature and management of supplementation of the breastfed baby. It is this additional phenomenon, when combined with the initial positive effects of motivational instructional design on women's sustained breastfeeding behaviour, that has warranted the ongoing research and development of motivational theory in action: Designer Breastfeeding©.

Conclusion

Application of the ARCS Model of Motivational Instructional Design resulted in an empirically robust research study and a programme of instruction (Designer Breastfeeding©) that, when tested using a randomized controlled design, provided evidence that motivation to breastfeed can be increased through routine instruction by midwives. Although cost-effectiveness was not measured in this instance, the enhancement of the already existing instruction suggests that the intervention has the potential to be cost-effective within a health service environment. More importantly, however, the findings from this research project demonstrate the value of a theoretically-derived breastfeeding instructional programme: essentially, 'theory in action'.

ACTIVITIES

Undergraduate

Undertake a structured search of the literature and critically appraise the concept 'Designer Breastfeeding'.©

Postgraduate

Design a research study to compare the motivational content of current breastfeeding instruction offered by a range of service providers, using the BMIMS tool.

References

Baby Friendly Initiative (1998) 'Implementing the Ten Steps to Successful Breastfeeding – A Guide for UK Maternity Service Providers Working Towards Baby Friendly Accreditation UK'. London: Committee for UNICEF. (http://www.babyfriendly. org.uk – accessed 1 August 2010).

Bolling, K., Grant, C., Hamlyn, B. and Thorton, A. (2007) *Infant Feeding Survey 2005.* UK: NHS, The Information Centre (www.ic.nhs.uk – accessed 1 August 2010).

Coombs, D.W., Reynolds, K., Joyner, G. and Blankson, M. (1998) 'A Self-Help Program to Increase Breastfeeding among Low-income Women', *Journal of Nutrition Education*, 30(4): 203–9.

Dickerson, S. (2006) 'Women's Use of the Internet: What Nurses Need to Know', *Journal of Obstetrics, Gynaecological & Neonatal Nursing*, 35(1): 151–6.

Ertmer, P.A. and Stepich, D.A., Flanagan, S. and Kocaman-Karoglu, A. (2009) 'Impact of Guidance on the Problem-Solving Efforts of Instructional Design Novice', *Performance Improvement Quarterly*, 21(4): 117.

Harackiewicz, J.M. and Sansone, C. (2000) 'Rewarding Competence: The Importance of Goals in the Study of Intrinsic Motivation', in C. Sansone and J.M. Harackiewicz (eds), *Intrinsic and Extrinsic Motivation: The Search for Optimal Motivation and Performance*. San Diego, CA: Academic Press, ch. 4: 82–96.

Health Promotion Agency for Northern Ireland (2004) 'Off to A Good Start: All You Need to Know about Breastfeeding Your Baby' (www.healthpromotionagency. org.uk – accessed 1 August 2010).

Jacox, A. (1974) 'Theory Construction in Nursing: An Overview', *Nursing Research*, 23(1): 4–13. Cited in L.O. Walker and K.C. Avant (2004) *Strategies for Theory Construction in Nursing*, 4th edn. Englewood Cliffs, NJ: Prentice Hall.

Keller, J.M. (1979) 'Motivation and Instructional Design: A Theoretical Perspective', *Journal of Instructional Development*, 2(4): 26–34.

Keller, J.M. (1983) 'Motivational Design of Instruction', in C.M. Reigeluth (ed), *Instructional-Design Theories and Models. An Overview of their Current Status*. Hillsdale, NJ: Lawrence Erlbaum, ch. 11: 383–434.

Keller, J.M. (1987a) 'Strategies for Stimulating the Motivation to Learn', *Performance & Instruction*, 26(8): 1–7.

Keller, J.M. (1987b) 'The Systematic Process of Motivational Design', *Performance & Instruction*, 26(9): 1–8.

Keller J.M. (1987c) 'Development and Use of the ARCS Model of Instructional Design', *Journal of Instructional Development*, 10(3): 2–10.

Lavender, T., Baker, L., Smyth, R., Collins, S., Spofforth, A. and Dey, P. (2005) 'Breastfeeding Expectations versus Reality: A Cluster Randomized Controlled Trial', *British Journal of Obstetrics and Gynaecology*, 112(8): 1047–53.

Mozingo, J., Davis, M.W., Droppleman, P.G. and Merideth, A. (2000) ' "It Wasn't Working": Women's Experiences with Short-term Breastfeeding', *American Journal of Maternal and Child Nursing (MCN)*, 25(3): 120–6.

Mulder, P.J. (2006) 'A Concept Analysis of Effective Breastfeeding', *Journal of Obstetric Gynecological and Neonatal Nursing*, 35(3): 332–9.

Keller JM (1987c) 'Development and Use of the ARCS Model of Instructional Design', *Journal of Instructional Development*, 10(3): 2–10.

NHS Choices 'Your Health, Your Choices' (www.nhs.uk – accessed 1 August 2010).

Schmied, V., Sheenan, A. and Barclay, L. (2001) 'Contemporary Breast-Feeding Policy and Practice: Implications for Midwives', *Midwifery*, 17(1): 44–54.

Stockdale, J. (2007) 'Successful Breastfeeding Promotion – A Motivational Model of Informational Design Applied and Tested', Unpublished PhD Thesis, University of Ulster, Northern Ireland.

Stockdale, J., Sinclair, M., Kernohan, W.G. and Keller, J.M. (2007) 'Exploring the Potential of the Internet to Motivate Breastfeeding', *Evidence-Based Midwifery*, 5(1): 10–5.

Stockdale, J., Sinclair, M., Kernohan, W.G., Dunwoody, L., Cunningham, J.B., Lawther, L. and Weir, P. (2008a) 'Assessing the Impact of Midwives' Instruction: The Breastfeeding Motivational Instructional Measurement Scale', *Evidence-Based Midwifery*, 6(1): 27–34.

Stockdale, J., Sinclair, M., Kernohan, W.G., Keller, J.M., Dunwoody, L., Cunningham, J.B., Lawther, L. and Weir, P. (2008b) 'Feasibility Study to Test Designer Breastfeeding:™ A Randomised Controlled Trial', *Evidence-Based Midwifery*, 6(3): 76–82.

Stockdale, J., Sinclair, M. and Kernohan, W.G. (2008) 'Designer Breastfeeding: Personal, Powerful and Successful. A Research Summary', Belfast: University of Ulster. ISBN 978-1-85923-227-9, Trial Registration Number: ISRCTN47056748 - http://www.controlled-trials.com/ISRCTN47056748.

Walker, L.O. and Avant, K.C. (2005) *Strategies for Theory Construction in Nursing*. 4th edn. Englewood Cliffs, NJ: Prentice Hall.

The Research, Design and Development of a New Breastfeeding Chair

6

Lynn Susanne Jones and Sally Kendall

Key points

- Theory from other disciplines, such as ergonomics, can inform midwifery practice
- Practical solutions can be offered from breastfeeding mothers and should be considered by midwives
- A well-designed, fit-for-purpose chair is one component of what is required to support successful breastfeeding
- Comfort and feeling 'cared for' by the environment also contribute to successful breastfeeding.

Introduction

This chapter provides unique data on the design of a 'fit-for-purpose' chair for breastfeeding mothers and demonstrates the value of multi-disciplinary team working. In this chapter, the work undertaken by one of the authors (Lynn Jones) for her PhD, supervised by Sally Kendall, is presented. The aim of the research was to develop an understanding of the needs of breastfeeding women in terms of a chair to provide the best support for them when they were breastfeeding. The work brought together theory and knowledge from the discipline of furniture design with theory relating to breastfeeding and case study research, making use of qualitative methods of data collection. The chapter demonstrates the necessity for a holistic and comprehensive assessment of a human problem, and the process of development of solutions for subsequent design and testing of a product that meets the assessed need.

Background

In 1996, it was becoming evident that one of the factors that makes breast-feeding difficult was the way in which domestic and institutional furniture design did not correspond with women's bodies or with the posture they needed to adopt comfortably in order to breastfeed successfully. A working group of the Community Practitioners' and Health Visitors' Association, together with the Royal College of Midwives, had identified this issue while working with one of the authors (SK) on professional training materials aimed at supporting practitioners in breastfeeding practice. It became clear that the design of the furniture and the space within which women breastfeed needed to be considered much more carefully in relation to the promotion of breast-feeding. These events led to the development of a PhD proposal by a professional furniture designer (LJ) and the design of a fit-for-purpose breastfeeding chair built to take account of the anthropometrics and ergonomics in relation to breastfeeding posture.

> There are histories of breastfeeding, wet-nurses, etc. but I can't think of one that discusses the furniture. (Greer, 2000)

Research and design process

The research to develop the design of the chair involved a number of stages:

- examination of literature concerning breastfeeding
- examination of design literature on chair design for various uses
- interviews with experts in the field of breastfeeding
- case study research comprising observations, interviews and measurement of a number of women who were breastfeeding.

One midwife asked, as women in other cultures do not need breastfeeding chairs, why, then, do we? In most Western societies, the position for breast-feeding is sitting upright on a chair. We have evolved with the chair as a fundamental accessory to our daily lives. We are brought up with chairs. We go to school, to work, to the doctor's and to the cinema: it is hard to imagine these places without chairs. It is from this culture that the necessity for a chair in which to breastfeed arises.

The example in Box 6.1 demonstrates the challenge facing the research team: finding ways to make the activity of breastfeeding more comfortable, enjoyable and, ultimately, more successful. The personal motivation must be bracketed so that the story of how the medium of furniture can effect change in the lives of people who breastfeed can be told, acknowledging the fact that the first author (LJ) had her own child during the project and, therefore, her personal 'lived experience' is intricately woven into the very fabric of this text.

The key question for this research was: 'Can we design a practical, creative and pleasurable chair for breastfeeding women?' Answering this question

---

Box 6.1   A new mother's account of breastfeeding problems encountered

Often, sutures (stitches) in the perineum prevent comfortable sitting for the initial weeks after birth.

Feeling uncomfortable is the general picture … My partner that evening rushed out to buy the dreaded formula milk, bottles and sterilizing fluid and I watched, sobbing yet again, as our little daughter appeared to snatch the bottle from his hand and milk it dry. I felt that my breasts, though swollen and very sore, were useless. I was useless.

During this time, other discomforts I had suffered all along came to the fore: backache; headaches, due to general discomfort and lack of fluids; warmth, especially when feeding during the long winter nights; poor posture … I had been advised to get up out of bed to feed and to go downstairs, as my baby on more than one occasion had suffered near suffocation when I awoke hours after sitting up in bed to feed her, to find her seemingly choking on my breast. Sitting downstairs on a very inclined sofa offered other dangers; my baby fell off my knee when I fell asleep again. There seemed a never-ending spiral of problems.

Finding a comfortable posture was the most difficult of these and, perhaps, not getting this right early on, proliferated other problems …

(Mother interviewed by LJ, the Infant Feeding Centre, John Radcliffe Hospital, Oxford, 1998).

---

required the support of a team of experts including furniture designers, fabric designers, midwives, researchers and a range of experts in the field of social anthropology. There is nothing like breastfeeding in comfort. In this chapter I hope you will gain an insight into the world of the breastfeeding mother: it is a place in which we should all feel at home. Furniture must support us, making life more manageable and more pleasurable: pleasure is a function not a bonus and an essential criterion for good design.

Postural considerations and observations

Mothers can feed babies in three different positions: sitting up, lying down, and standing (see Illustration 6.1). Some people believe that incorrect positioning is one of the most serious causes of breastfeeding failure (Inch *et al.*, 2003). Positions that are appropriate for later feeding, when the infant is well-established on the breast, may not be appropriate for initiating breastfeeding or for the early feeds.

Breastfeeding is not an instinct; it has to be learned. Non-human primates, such as chimpanzees, have to learn about both sex and suckling by observation when they are young and, if deprived of this, have problems with both activities when they reach maturity. This is why expecting breastfeeding to happen, by telling women to do it, is such an unrealistic goal. It is rather like expecting good performances from choirboys who have always been forbidden to listen to music (see Chapters 4 and 5 for further discussion of these issues).

Observation of our parents, siblings and friends breastfeeding is obviously likely to be a good way of learning how to do it but, as we no longer see

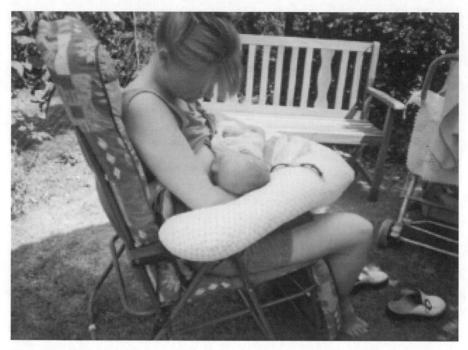

Illustration 6.1   Carly breastfeeding in the garden using a garden chair

breastfeeding as an everyday activity, the role models are increasingly hard to find. Portrayals of breastfeeding women in the media are rare or misleading. Art can, however, provide some startlingly strong positive images of breast-feeding women and clues about posture can be found. For example, Henry Moore's stone *Seated Figure* (1928) depicts the universal theme of mother-hood, with the mother figure seated with her infant on her high lap, as it would be on a low seat, and her back erect at almost 90 degrees from her lap, which depicts the ergonomically correct breastfeeding posture (Henry Moore Foundation, 2010).

As a way of recording posture, paintings and sculpture can illustrate some very useful examples. One of the most informative and moving of these is seen in a painting by Diego Rivera (1916) entitled *Motherhood – Angelina and the Child Diego*, depicting Rivera's partner in Paris with their son Diego (all-art.org). She is seated on a chair on which she leans slightly forward, with her breast falling forward. Her right leg is raised up on her left so raising the height of her lap to support the child. The gaze of the woman forms a trian-gular sequence to the eyes of her baby and over to her left shoulder, a position that promotes mother–child attachment. This painting epitomizes the issue of posture, and indicates the form a breastfeeding chair would need to take in order to function ergonomically. Although the cubist style blurs our perception of the chair, the impression the painting offers is one that meets the key crite-ria of the design brief evolving from this study: it is low-seated, has a high and erect back, and it could have a variety of aesthetic styles and colours.

To achieve correct positioning of the baby at the breast while seated, the mother should be encouraged to lean forward slightly so that the breast falls forward, facilitating attachment. Leaning back flattens the breast making attachment much more difficult. Chloe Fisher, writing in *Successful Breastfeeding*, suggests:

> She may need additional pillows to support her back or arms, or raise the baby to a more comfortable level. Having attached the baby correctly the mother can then be encouraged to relax her back and shoulders against the supporting chair. A footstool may also be a useful aid to relaxation. Modern furniture does not lend itself to good breastfeeding positioning. Often it is too soft, has obstructive armrests and/or sloping backs. Hospital beds and backrests which encourage the mother to lean back are similarly unhelpful. (Fisher, 1991: 5)

Fisher is describing here the scenario of a midwife trying to support initiation of breastfeeding in the very early stages after the birth of a baby. Sometimes, this will happen in the hospital where the baby was born, but often, especially when a mother leaves hospital within a few hours of the birth, the initiation of breastfeeding takes place in the home, sometimes with the help of a midwife, but often not. During these early stages, the requirements of a breastfeeding chair might be different to those of a chair to be used once breastfeeding has been established. For example, mothers learning to breastfeed in special care baby units can be observed sitting on chair seats covered with plastic sheeting, as a mother might be bleeding from her perineum. Getting into a good breast-feeding position quickly is important to instil confidence in the mother.

As the mother's confidence grows, so too does her ability to feed in differ-ent places. Illustrations 6.1 to 6.4 show several examples of breastfeeding in a variety of places: in the garden, on the floor and in the car. The image of the Himba woman (Illustration 6.5) is of particular interest in terms of breastfeed-ing posture: the erect angle of the wall she leans against and the low height of the wall she is sitting on suggest that she has selected this place to sit for its ergonomic appropriateness.

Similarly, if ever you notice a woman breastfeeding in a car or on an aero-plane, she will have adjusted the angle of the seat back into its most upright position (see Illustration 6.4).

The physiological and anatomical aspects of breastfeeding discussed here are of interest to a designer because we can begin to see, anthropometrically, what a woman is doing when she breastfeeds. When her milk is 'let-down' (the initial flow of milk), how does she tend to position herself, where is the gaze of her eyes, and so on? These are the first clues we can use to establish any ergonomic criteria for the chair. Psychologically, similar considerations can be taken into account and can be useful to the process of ergonomic decision-making. For example, how do ambience and spatial factors influence a mother's mental state? How is the psychological pleasure of breastfeeding rele-vant to design? There is plenty of evidence to suggest that chairs can affect us physiologically and psychologically, particularly in the office setting (Berry,

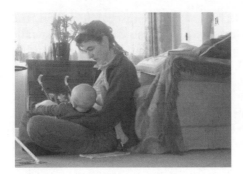

Illustration 6.2   Breastfeeding on the floor with back support

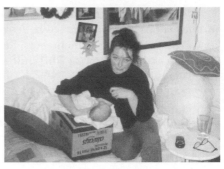

Illustration 6.3   Using a box to raise the baby to help with breastfeeding

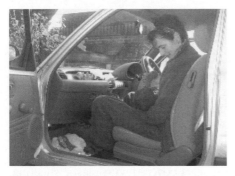

Illustration 6.4   Breastfeeding in the car with back support

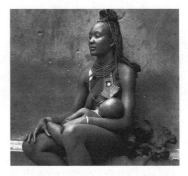

Illustration 6.5   Himba Woman and Child (*Mark Hakansson/Panos Pictures*)

Box 6.2   Design factors from theory and observations

- The psychological preparation of the environment in which a woman intends to feed does evidently affect a woman's ability to produce milk.
- Historical observations offer an understanding of emotional attachment (for example, Bowlby, 1969) that could help mothers and designers to understand the need for skin-to-skin contact and the breastfeeding instinct.
- Breastfeeding for many women is a highly sensual activity. Confidence can be improved by the response of the mother to the objects and the environment around her when she feeds. The feel of a fabric against her skin and the satisfaction of using her chair, for example, will evidently affect her mood and her emotional and physical responses.
- An understanding of physiology, what is happening to her, may help a mother to feel less stressed.
- An understanding of the benefits of breastfeeding will promote a mother's confidence.
- Positive role models, being able to observe more women breastfeeding in everyday life and in art and sculpture, will inspire women to feel less alienated and more confident in their own ability to breastfeed.

2005). However, there is no evidence of what happens in this respect when women breastfeed in chairs. Whether by instinct or by nurture, how do mothers behave? What do they do with their feet and their arms? Do they realize that they are doing it? How do they feel when their milk is released and their infant suckles? How do they re-arrange the objects around them to effect change in their posture or their mental state?

It is evident that an understanding of psychology, anatomy and physiology is more than useful for the designer of a breastfeeding chair. Box 6.2 summarizes the key design conclusions from theory and observations.

These wide-ranging theories and observations were taken into consideration as part of the research process.

A chair for breastfeeding mothers: research and development

In most Western societies, the position for breastfeeding is sitting upright on a chair. We have now evolved with the chair as a fundamental accessory to our daily lives. Correct positioning of the baby at the breast while seated will be the position now investigated and will serve to introduce the design project. 'Modern furniture does not lend itself to good breastfeeding positioning' (Fisher, 2000).

If you were asked to do research about sofas, take some photos of dining chairs, or talk to people about how they feel about their car seat, relatively quickly you could achieve your aim. But, in the United Kingdom, it is almost as difficult to find someone breastfeeding as it is to find a breastfeeding chair. It is possible to find nursing or breastfeeding chairs but, from observation, it would appear that these were not always designed with successful breastfeeding as the goal. Apart from the psychological and physiological factors that a designer needs to take into account, other considerations are also necessary:

- comfort is an ambiguous concept: one woman's comfort is another woman's discomfort
- many chairs are too big for a large number of women, especially for those women needing to breastfeed comfortably in a chair
- not many chairs are offered in more than one height
- many upholstered fireside chairs designed during the 1950s and 1960s were close to being ergonomically correct for breastfeeding, but were not specified for this purpose
- a new breastfeeding chair can only be designed well in the light of the primary research and the secondary research conducted for this study – primary research is imperative to this kind of design project
- industrial collaboration can have a positive effect on the design development process
- industrial collaboration can have a positive effect on the educational process for designers
- designing chairs in isolation of the end-user increases the risk of mistakes and misinterpretations of use.

Research design

The research design was exploratory and descriptive, using data from interviews, original drawings, photographs and video records with consenting breastfeeding women. The main aim of the research was to observe and discuss how people sit when they breastfeed, and how they felt about the sitting positions they adopt. Data were collected while women breastfed, and this was analyzed to determine the ergonomic, aesthetic, social, economic and psychological requirements for a breastfeeding chair. A sample of 16 women took part in the primary research; six of these women were willing to take part in case studies for in-depth observation and interviews that continued for up to 6 months. Women were recruited as volunteers from the community and were informed about the study by maternity specialists or by other women known to the authors. They came from a wide geographical area of England, ranging from Durham to Bristol. Semi-structured interviews lasted up to one hour and, during that time, field notes and sketches of breastfeeding activities and positions were made, as well as eight to ten photographs being taken. The women were all community volunteers and, at the time of data collection, ethics approval was not required for this group. Nevertheless, ethical principles of confidentiality and consent were maintained. Particular care was taken to obtain consent for the use of images. For publication purposes, pseudonyms have been used.

Summary of case study observations

The interviews and observation provided rich data, which are summarized and illustrated here. The photographic evidence showed women using a variety of 'bits and pieces' – from ironing boards to adjustable garden chairs – in an effort to establish a comfortable posture. Observations of what women actually do and the way they move, the way they reach for things and the way they struggle to get comfortable while holding a small infant (often crying for food) demonstrated the actual problems encountered while breastfeeding behaviour was taking place. As Clear comments: 'For breastfeeding to succeed the woman needs to be able to sit down with the baby several times a day, sometimes every hour and sometimes for an hour.' (Clear, 2001: 135).

Each case study was analyzed independently to identify the seating positions of the mothers, and can be summarized as:

- recognition of the need for external support and direction; for example, from midwives, health visitors, breast care nurses and other mothers
- the emotional ownership and psychological security a particular chair evoked gave mothers confidence in their breastfeeding ability
- every mother used more than one pillow or cushion to raise their lap height
- every mother used pillows or cushions to bring the angle of the back forward
- all of the mothers owned and used a 'v' shaped cushion to raise lap height or to breastfeed in bed
- every mother raised her toes on tiptoe to raise the height of her lap
- an optimum, desired seat height of 360 mm was estimated

Box 6.3   Objects mothers had near them when breastfeeding

- Muslin square
- Water to drink
- TV remote control
- Telephone
- Cushions and pillows
- Breast pads
- Breast milk collection cups
- Food, for example, chocolate
- Something to read
- A small lamp
- Nipple cream

- an optimum angle of the mother's back position of 90 degrees to the seat was recorded
- every mother was observed to drink one or more glasses of water or cups of tea whilst breastfeeding
- every mother used a muslin square whilst breastfeeding
- every mother needed some objects next to them
- an arm or side-table attached to the chair obstructs the movements of the mother and baby.

Mothers typically had a number of objects near to them while breastfeeding, as shown in Box 6.3

There is clearly a correlation between the concepts of satisfaction and comfort and duration of feeding period, as the following extracts from the observations show.

Issues of comfort
Interviews with the women demonstrated their physical and psychological needs:

> *Carly*:
> 'You feel raw, cold, uncomfortable, sweaty, sticky, revolting and sore, often all at the same time. The chair should give you that feeling you got from your own mother: lovely and snugly. It should also give you the opportunity for repose.'

Carly had established for herself an ergonomic seated position absolutely in line with that advised by the Infant Feeding Clinic at the John Radcliffe Hospital, Oxford. She sat no higher than 360 mm from the ground, adopting a straight back/flat lap posture in a 1950s fireside chair. Although the seat height was appropriate, the angle or rake of the back of the chair was obtuse, which forced Carly to use cushions and pillows to bring her back into a functional and ergonomically correct position. As cushions and pillows are fluid or dynamic in their form, it is difficult to maintain the correct back angle using cushions in this way, although all the women in the case studies used them:

Carly:
'I think because all my cushions are filled with feathers it's difficult to get them to stay in the right place. You can see they're falling all over! I do have a favourite one but find it's too big and bulky to take anywhere. I do feel happier to have it with me and take it in the car when I remember. It's become a bit like a comfort blanket for me.' (Case study 1, Co. Durham)

The interviews with Carly totalled eight and provided the most comprehensive evidence of the five case studies. She could reflect on the experiences of three different babies and was able to talk of how her ability to relax when feeding improved with each child:

Carly:
'My experiences of breastfeeding the three of them have been different. My confidence definitely improved, probably because experience taught me not to be so anxious and to recognize a bad midwife. ... My chair is great! It has been my best friend, and I keep it just in case we have any more! I used to regret being unable to take it with me shopping or just visiting, which is when I felt people stared at me the most, particularly in the supermarket.' (Case study 1, Co. Durham)

Susan:
'By the time Harriet was two days old, she had fallen out of bed with me on two separate occasions whilst I was trying to get to grips with the feeding, which threw any confidence I had completely out of the window. I had very little help and didn't, on reflection, have a clue what I was doing. I had had an extraordinarily long labour and was very, very tired. When I did have the energy to get out of bed the chair provided, by the bed, was plastic covered, sticky to the touch and too high, so much so that my feet didn't touch the ground. I never felt the feeding would work in there, and decided that it would all come right when I got home. Inevitably, it didn't.' (Case study 2, Aylesbury)

Hattie:
'Feeding in the garden is always better. I am more relaxed and less distracted. It always takes me a while though to get settled. I'll sit down thinking I have everything I need within arms reach and then realize I have forgotten my water, or the phone. Now I try to have everything I need on the pushchair, which is great because then I have everything with me if I need to feed whilst I am out. He is feeding so much at the moment I some-times feel I am having to look for somewhere comfortable to sit every half and hour, which if you're shopping or on a bus can be difficult.' (Case study 3, St Albans)

Julie:
'It took me eight weeks to find a comfortable position to breastfeed in. The best position in the end was sitting up on the floor against the sofa because you need your thighs up don't you?' (Case study 4, Bristol)

Janet:
'I love going out and about ... and sometimes I miss having my cushion with me and find it impossible to get properly comfortable, oh, and the chairs are always too high.' (Case study 5, Thame)

It was evident from the research conducted that, without exception, the issues of lap height, a drink of water, and muslin squares were problematic.

Ergonomics and anthropometrics
An important aspect of the primary research was measuring the women's height when standing and sitting. The anthropometric measurements of their legs when seated – the distance from their buttock to their knee (popliteal length) and the distance from their knee to their ankle bone (popliteal height) – were used to determine the new ergonomic criteria for the breastfeeding chair.

As with most naturally-occurring phenomena, people's sizes follow a normal distribution. That is, when a characteristic such as popliteal height is plotted against its frequency, it forms a bell-shaped curve with the three measurements of the average coinciding (Walker and Almond, 2010). Thus, the median value (the middle value when all are arranged in numerical order) is the same as the modal value (the most frequently occurring value), which is, in turn, the same as the mean value (the sum of all the sizes divided by the number of sizes). Percentile values are a useful way of expressing characteristics of people. They are determined by dividing any number of quantities into 100 equal groups in order of their size, from the least to the greatest, in an orderly sequence. Extreme values of size are therefore represented by small or large percentile figures: the smaller or larger the percentile figure, the more remote is the chance of the occurrence of that value.

According to Pheasant and Haslegrave (2006: 53), the mean average popliteal height of women is 400 mm, with a 5th percentile value of 355 mm and a 95th percentile value of 445 mm, and a standard deviation of 27 mm. The shape of the distribution of the female popliteal height is, thus, a narrow bell-shaped curve with most of the values clustered around the average. It was therefore unsurprising that the statistical analysis undertaken for this research found values very similar to those of Pheasant and Haslegrave, despite the small sample used.

Finding similar values provided confidence in the small sample of women in this study. However, further data were collected at Buckinghamshire New University, where women could volunteer to measure their own popliteal height (Cobb, 2001). A seat designed by the student was provided and, next to it, a measuring tape was glued to a baton fixed onto a wall panel. A box was also fixed to the wall so women could post their results into it. Pencils and paper were provided. A notice on the wall informed participants to remove their shoes and showed an illustration of the part of the leg they were being asked to measure. Seventeen women took part in the exercise. The range of popliteal height in millimetres was between 323 and 480.

Taking into account all of these dimensions, an average seat height for the breastfeeding chair was confirmed, using the test-rig (see Illustration 6.6), to be 360 mm from the floor to the top of the front of the seat. Thus, a chair

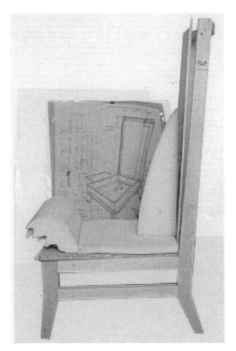

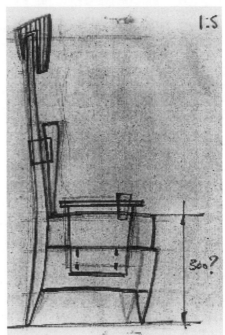

Illustration 6.6   Breastfeeding chair test-rig

Illustration 6.7   Sketch of breastfeeding chair showing optimum seat height

dedicated to breastfeeding women would require a seat the optimum height of which would be considerably lower than most chairs demanding a task or activity (see Illustration 6.7).

This research suggests that the optimum seat height for a breastfeeding chair for a woman of average height is 360 mm. Although research in future testing may dictate otherwise, currently three seat heights are proposed: 340 mm, 360 mm, 380 mm. It is foreseen that women who fall into other percentile groups (that is, those who are unusually tall or unusually short in stature) may require a chair with shorter or longer legs.

Breast size also had some relevance to the relationship of a woman's breasts to the position of her lap, although this was minimal. The primary research concluded that:

- in relation to the backrest, a positive seat angle will help the woman maintain good contact with the backrest and so counteract any tendency to slide forwards out of the seat. The angle of the back in relation to the seat should therefore be 95 degrees.
- too steep an angle of the seat will affect the user's ability to stand up and, because of the vertical nature of the back, discomfort will be immediately apparent.
- if the height of the seat is equal to or higher than the popliteal height of the woman, pressure will be felt on the underside of the thighs and the angle

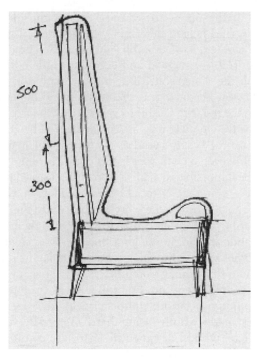

Illustration 6.8   Sketch of breastfeeding chair showing lumbar support

of the 'lap' will not be flat. A flat lap is imperative for the most satisfactory functioning of a breastfeeding chair (Inch, 2000).

- the height of the backrest is not critical and could be anywhere between 1000 mm and 1500 mm from the floor. However, the position of the lumbar support is the more critical dimension and should be placed between 200 mm and 300 mm from the top of the seat (see Illustration 6.8).

The size and weight of the infant also needs to be considered carefully. Carly's 12-month-old son measured 720 mm from head to toe which, relative to the width of the seat of the test-rig, is approximately 300 mm wider. This is an approximate measurement; it cannot be recorded as a static dimension, as the infant moves quite considerably. When considering arms on the chair, this is one of the factors determining the decision to incorporate one or two armrests, if any (or removable armrests). It was the interaction of all dimensions in a dynamic sense when breastfeeding that was the most closely observed dimension. Commonly, body dimensions suggested in ergonomic texts are static. For example, the recommended ergonomic height of an office desk might be 720 mm from the floor, but this assumes a static seat height of, usually, 440 mm from the floor. As breastfeeding is such a dynamic activity, with a baby who moves and a mother who moves in response to her baby moving, it is difficult to determine the most ergonomically suitable position. Therefore, some unusual dimensions were recorded: the space occupied by a constantly moving baby helped determine the need for chair arms, and the changing position of the upper torso and head of the mother immediately following a 'feed' period helped determine the height of the seat back. From studies of these six women, it was established that a 5 degree incline of the seat was the most comfortable, practical and ergonomically 'correct' angle.

In conclusion, all the dimensions of a proposed solution are ergonomically critical, but it is the seat height that is the most critical dimension, as observed during testing using the test–rig. Cushions can remedy incorrect back rake angle. A footstool could be the simplest way of remedying seat height, or a copy of the Yellow Pages (will suffice) – as was used to solve the problem in the Breastfeeding Clinic in Oxford. However, a chair that is too high will simply render that chair useless, and it will be impossible to achieve correct breastfeeding posture. Croney (1980) argues that a seat that is too low will lead to a woman adopting a crouched position, and all postural benefits will be lost. In this sensitive situation, it is not only the seating benefit that can be lost, but also the behaviour of breast-feeding may be abandoned. So, although a breastfeeding chair may be of lower height than many other seats with which we are familiar, its dimensions are that way to be of optimum functioning potential, as is a car seat.

Surface will affect movement too. Friction will either help or hinder the user in achieving the optimum position. Upholstery can give deceptive impressions of comfort. Chairs made wholly using hard materials, such as the Eames L.C.W. (Lounge Chair Wood), designed in 1940, are comfortable because the contours of the seat form provide a useful distribution of pressure beneath the buttocks: softness rarely results in satisfactory support (see Illustration 6.9).

Many chairs such as the L.C.W., or even the traditional Windsor chair, are surprisingly comfortable in the seat despite a lack of upholstery. Therefore, it seemed reasonable to conclude that upholstery should be firm rather than soft. Tests designed to test breastfeeding posture carried out using the test-rig (see

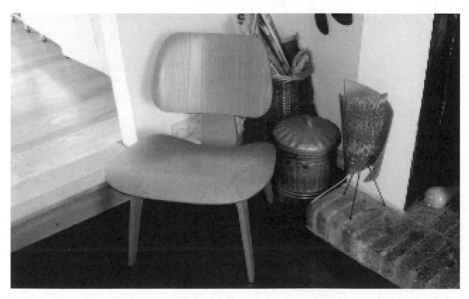

Illustration 6.9   Eames L.C.W.

Illustration 6.6) clearly showed that a user should not be able to deform the upholstered surfaces by more than 20 mm, otherwise the height of the seat effectively will become too low ergonomically. The shape of the backrest of a breastfeeding chair needs to be less contoured than most office chairs or car seats, as the erectness of the angle of the back needs to discourage the sitter from slumping. The angle of the back in relation to the seat should therefore be 95 degrees. The height of the backrest is less critical, but should not exceed 1100 mm from the floor. The position of the lumbar support should be set by the mother or the assisting midwife or health visitor at a supportive height (normally within the range of 200 mm and 300 mm from the top of the seat).

Finally, the placing of accessories will inevitably influence the ergonomics of the chair. As stated earlier, sitting down and breastfeeding is a dynamic activity. Contact with the immediate environment – for example, the surface that holds a glass of water, the surface on which the telephone sits, or the siting of the box storing breast pads – needs to be aligned sensitively in order to optimize the ergonomic performance of the chair.

All over the world people do things with their hands whilst breastfeeding: reading, writing, drinking, watching TV, using the telephone, working in many cases to keep the money coming in. When I wrote my first book 'The Experience of Childbirth' in 1962 I would write in between feeds picking my daughter up to feed her and putting her down to write the book intermittently. Virtually the whole book was written in this way! (Kitzinger, 2000)

By comparing and contrasting already established ergonomics with those that have evolved from this study, it was possible to inform the design of breastfeeding chairs with a set of new ergonomic information that could be employed usefully by designers of such chairs in the future. The application of this newly acquired ergonomic data was applied to the first prototype breastfeeding chair.

In addition to the physical ergonomic data that was collected during the primary research stage, matters of psychological comfort were discussed with each case study woman and with specialists in the field of breastfeeding. 'The chair should be lovely and snugly' and 'it should feel like you felt in your own mother's arms' were two suggestions from breastfeeding women expressing their psychological preferences. Therefore, a woman's first contact with the surface of the chair – the appearance and feel of the upholstery fabric, for example – was to be an important aspect of the design criteria. For many of the women, sheepskin was the favoured comfort material. Its properties are well-known: it holds heat, is warm to the touch, and comforting to feel on the skin. However, it can only be dry-cleaned and therefore it is not practical. Natural and synthetic fleece and wool composite fabrics were consequently investigated.

The prototype fabric proposed is functionally and aesthetically suited for use by clinics and hospitals, and conforms to British Standards for contract furniture in that:

- it is contract quality upholstery fabric that is flame retardant (BS EN 1021, 1&2), cleanable and hardwearing; it is also DS Certified (Danish Systems – environmental management) as environmentally safe fabric

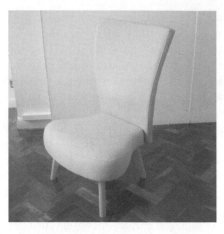

Illustration 6.10   The breastfeeding chair

- the way in which the tubular steel legs support the chair from the floor makes it very easy to clean underneath
- the chrome finish on the metal components (the legs and the hanger on the backrest) is more acceptable from a hygienic point of view
- the chair is extremely stable.

However, there is a critical point that needs emphasizing again: the chair produced as an end product of this research takes a particular form, but it is not the only form that such a chair need take (see Illustration 6.10). The ergonomic data revealed by the research is a critically useful end result, aiding the production of an almost infinite variety of chairs to satisfy the infinite variety of consumer tastes.

Discussion

Without doubt, the most valuable research for this study was that done in collaboration with midwives, health visitors, key figures within the field of breastfeeding, and the women themselves. The decision to conduct case study research proved to be the most useful research approach to provide information to inform the design of the chair. The observation that many women breastfeed with their feet on tiptoes, need a glass of water or wine or a bar of chocolate close at hand, or desire emotional security while breastfeeding might have gone unnoticed had questionnaires been used, rather than observation. Such research also indicated that chairs currently being used in hospitals and baby clinics in the United Kingdom were adapted versions of chairs designed for other uses. These chairs were the starting point for the design: there is clearly a desperate need for a chair that meets breastfeeding needs without needing to be adapted. Mothers were discovered breastfeeding in toilet cubicles because they had nowhere else to go, in their homes balancing their babies on boxes and ironing boards, and feeling humiliated and embarrassed in hospitals.

Midwives adapted their own furniture and spent extraordinary amounts of time highlighting the problems they encounter with furniture every day.

These informal interview techniques proved to be the most suitable for this project. An in-depth insight into the feelings of the women as they breastfed was gained by using conversational techniques. Using design skills such as drawing and model-making skills while employing conversational interview techniques was a useful asset to the research.

Design is always a compromise. Decisions about taste and cost are always difficult to make. Research shows that users of sample breastfeeding chairs in clinics in low income areas would pay between £70 and £80 for such a chair for the home, whereas the midwives and other specialists who work in the field of breastfeeding put a figure of between £200 and £300 for institutional use. Interestingly, women from high-income areas said they would pay between £200 and £300 for the chair for their homes. Taste has also influenced the range of upholstery fabrics and colours offered. It will be interesting to evaluate which are the most popular choices. One baby clinic has asked for fabric upholstery that is easier to wipe on the seat than the back, which is feasible due to the fact that the seat and back are made of two separate components.

It was evident throughout the research that this understanding of psychology, anatomy and physiology is more than useful for the designer of a breastfeeding chair. The psychological preparation of the environment in which a woman prepares to feed does evidently affect a woman's ability to produce milk. The historical observations made by Bowlby (1969), for example, offer an understanding of emotional attachment, which could help mothers and designers to understand the need for skin-to-skin contact and the breastfeeding instinct. More recent research by Strathearn et al. (2009) has clearly shown the relationship between breastfeeding and child neglect, demonstrating the strength of the emotional bond that develops in the first four months of breastfeeding. Breastfeeding is a highly sensual activity. Confidence can be improved by the response of the mother to the objects and the environment around her when she feeds. The feel of a fabric against her skin and the satisfaction of using her chair will affect her mood and her emotional and physical responses.

In its form, the chair is supportive and ergonomically correct for the activity for which it is designed. Moreover, in particular, the form of the seat is shaped to give pleasure: stroking the curves and feeling the warm tactile qualities of the fabric is comforting as well as comfortable. Psychologically, it is important for women to feel confident and attractive while they breastfeed. The sensual, skin-to-skin quality of chairs is rarely addressed by the discourse of design, yet it is often the first and most immediate critical observation to be made. It is an added bonus that you do not need to be breastfeeding to enjoy this chair.

A further consideration is that of role models: positive breastfeeding role models are simply not evident in many western countries. If women, men and children, most importantly, could observe more women breastfeeding in everyday life, on television, in art and in sculpture, they would feel less alienated and more confident in their own ability to breastfeed. The breastfeeding chair acknowledges breastfeeding. It informs the user that it is 'OK' to breastfeed and, moreover, that it is acceptable to those who have put it there, in their clinic, their home, their place of work, beside their hospital bed or in a café. What the chair communicates is a positive message to everyone: not only those who use it, but also those seeing it, manufacturing it, advertising it, and those passing it on to their daughters and sons.

Conclusion

In this study, we have brought together theory from the disciplines of furniture design, psychology, physiology and women's health. As with most research projects, this research raises as many questions as it provides answers. Future research on this chair would need to address the impact of the use of the chair on breastfeeding attitudes, behaviour and promotion. Research questions include therefore:

- What is the effect of using the breastfeeding chair on women's attitudes, behaviour and satisfaction?
- What is the effect of the chair on professionals trying to promote breastfeeding?
- To what extent does the chair change public attitudes towards breastfeeding?
- How does the cost of the chair affect breastfeeding initiation rates?
- Is the chair cost effective in public health terms?

We firmly believe that the chair resulting from this research will be desirable, affordable and practical, and will have a long life in the home of the women who use it.

Acknowledgements

The research enabled contact with such inspirational figures as Sheila Kitzinger, Germaine Greer, Sally Inch and Chloe Fisher, who have committed lifetimes of research to women's issues. Britain's most celebrated living furniture designer, Robin Day, is always delighted to hear about the after-life of his chairs. Now in his nineties, he kindly thanked me for informing him that some of his chairs, designed in the 1960s, were, at the time of the research, being adapted and used on a daily basis by breastfeeding women in the special care baby unit at Gloucestershire Royal Hospital. We would also like to acknowledge the Community Practitioners' and Health Visitors' Association and the Royal College of Midwives for their original support for the research.

Finally, we would like to thank all the women and their babies who volunteered to take part in the study.

Note: Robin Day died on 9 November 2010 during the preparation of this book

ACTIVITIES

Undergraduate

Designing appropriate, functionally relevant and aesthetically pleasing furniture for maternity settings is a real challenge. Based on your understanding of this chapter, select a common item of furniture in the birthing room (bed, beanbag, chair and such like) and analyze its design, functionality and aesthetic value.

Postgraduate

Design a research study to test one of the following features associated with the breastfeeding chair:

- the functionality,
- aesthetic appeal,
- cost effectiveness or
- acceptability of the chair.

References

all-art.org *Diego Rivera*. *www.all-art.org/art_20th_century/rivera2.html* *(Accessed 28th November, 2010)*.

Berry, J.R. (2005) *Herman Miller: Classic Furniture and System Designs for the Working Environment*. London: Thames & Hudson.

Bowlby, J. (1969) *Attachment and Loss. Volume 1: Attachment*. New York, NY: Basic Books.

Clear, C. (2000) *Women of the House: Women's household work in Ireland 1922–1961*. Dublin: Irish Academic Press.

Cobb, R. (2001) 'Measuring the Popliteal Heights of Women', Collaborative primary research with Lynn Jones, MA Furniture Design & Technology, September 2000–December 2001, Buckinghamshire New University.

Croney, J, (1980), *Anthropometry for Designers*. London: Batsford.

Fisher, C. (1991) *The Royal College of Midwives: Successful Breastfeeding*. London: Longman.

Fisher, C. (2000) Personal communication.

Greer, Germaine (2000) personal correspondence with Lynn Jones, 21 June.

Henry Moore Foundation (2010) Henry Moore Sculpture in the open air at Perry Green. Perry Green: Henry Moore Institute.

Inch, S. (2000) Personal communication.

Inch, S., Law, S., Wallace, L. and Hills, R. (2003) 'Confusion around Breastfeeding Terms 'Positioning' and 'Attachment'', *British Journal of Midwifery*, 11(3): 148.

Kitzinger, S. (2000) Personal communication.

Pheasant, S. and Haslegrave, C. (2006) *Bodyspace: Anthropometry, Ergonomics and the Design of Work*. London: Taylor & Francis.

Strathearn, L., Mamun, A., Najman, J. and O'Callaghan, M. (2009) 'Does Breastfeeding Protect Against Substantiated Child Abuse and Neglect? A 15-Year Cohort Study', *Pediatrics*, 123(2): 483–93.

Walker, J. and Almond, R. (2010) *Interpreting Statistical Findings: A Guide for Health Professionals and Students*. Buckingham: Open University Press.

Exploring Emotion in Midwifery Work: A First-Person Account

7

Billie Hunter

> **Key points**
>
> - Intuition can play a vital role in qualitative research
> - Undertaking 'real life' ethnographic research is both rewarding and challenging
> - Do not be afraid to question or critique the accepted view or status quo
> - Keep an open mind and attend carefully to participants' accounts – these may generate new, unexpected concepts and theories.

Introduction

This chapter uses a 'natural history' (Silverman, 2000: 236) approach to describe my personal experiences of using qualitative research to develop midwifery theory. This type of first person account is considered particularly appropriate for qualitative studies, as it affords a degree of transparency and insight into the development of the researcher's thinking, that would otherwise be invisible (Alasuutari, 1995; Silverman, 2000), and thus enhances the credibility of the study (Guba and Lincoln, 1981).

The chapter draws primarily on my doctoral research, which explored how midwives experience and manage emotion at work (Hunter, 2002). My interest in this issue stemmed from my personal midwifery experiences, particularly as a midwifery lecturer, which suggested that student midwives found their work more emotionally difficult than initially expected. This observation created an intellectual puzzle. What was it about midwifery that generated emotion? What types of emotions were experienced? How did midwives deal with these emotions?

These questions led me to the sociological theories of emotional labour and emotion work. However, although this literature generated some insights, it appeared limited in its applicability to midwifery. I also became uneasy with the lack of critical review of earlier research and what appeared to me to be a rather restricted conceptualization of 'emotional labour'. As a result, I decided to keep as open a mind as possible in my own study, avoiding the early imposition of a theoretical construct. As I describe later, this led me to adopt an ethnographic approach to exploring the issue of emotion in midwifery, collecting data from a variety of sources in order to access different perspectives. My aim was to tap into midwives' own accounts of both emotionally rewarding and emotionally difficult work. Rather than introducing concepts of emotional labour/emotion work to participants, I thought it important (and congruent to an inductive approach to theory generation) to pay proper attention to what the midwives told me.

The result was some unexpected findings regarding the sources of emotion work in midwifery that were unlikely to have become apparent had a different methodology been used. From these findings, new theories regarding the emotion work of midwives have been generated (Hunter, 2004, 2005, 2006, 2009).

My intention in writing this chapter is, therefore, to provide readers with a first-hand account of undertaking a qualitative research study, in order to provide some insights into the complexities of trying to develop new midwifery theory. In particular, I hope to show why it is important to challenge accepted wisdom, as it is only by freeing oneself from previous frames of reference and by exploring an issue with fresh eyes and an open mind that new ways of understanding can evolve.

I begin the chapter by describing how my initial interest in the subject area was sparked and then describe my 'journey' through the study. By using a first person account, my aim is to give some insights into the unpredictable and sometimes messy process of inductive theory generation. Such an account was something I would have welcomed myself as I grappled with my research apprenticeship. From conversations with experienced researchers, I realized that 'doing research' was often a very messy process, but that these (very important) experiences were rarely documented by researchers 'writing research'.

Early beginnings

My initial interest in the issue of emotions stemmed from my experiences as a midwifery lecturer in the late 1990s. My interactions with students revealed that there were many experiences in their practice that they found 'emotional', whether these were difficult or rewarding experiences. The nature of these experiences was often surprising to me. My own impression of the emotional aspects of working as a clinical midwife was frequently at odds with that described by the students. However, I did not, at the time, acknowledge the contextual differences in our experiences: the students were practising within the British National Health Service and, for much of the time, their work was institutionally based. In contrast, my own experience had been predominantly in independent midwifery practice, attending home-births. The significance of context in determining the nature of emotion in midwifery work became apparent as the study progressed, as will be seen later in this chapter.

As part of my teaching role, I was engaged in facilitating the development of the students' interpersonal and communication skills, through workshops and role play sessions. It was obviously very important to acknowledge the emotional content of midwifery work as a key aspect of these sessions. At the time, however, there was a complete absence of learning and teaching resources in this area for the students and me to draw from. Texts and resources for teaching student nurses were available but, as their focus was on ill health, these were largely inappropriate. There was also a notable absence of literature related to the emotional aspects of midwifery work; indeed, at that time, there was little published research into any aspects of midwives' personal experiences of their working lives. My early interest was, thus, triggered by a need to improve the content of my sessions to better meet the needs of students.

This primary focus on practical application locates the study firmly in the broad category of 'practitioner research', where the primary aim is 'to solve a critical problem or to develop an understanding about the nature of practice, and ultimately to contribute to the body of professional knowledge' (Reed and Procter, 1995: 11). Rather than attempting to ignore or suppress the insider knowledge and experience of the health care researcher/practitioner, Reed and Procter (1995) argue that these realities should be recognized and valued. Acknowledgement of this perspective was significant in enabling me to accept and appreciate the advantages of my own position, rather than making improbable attempts to render midwifery anthropologically strange. It was important for me to acknowledge how my own experiences, as both clinical midwife and midwifery lecturer, were influential throughout the research process, from initial planning and accessing the research setting, through to data collection and analysis. These experiences may have both positive and negative aspects. As will be seen later, however, insider research can certainly create some dilemmas for the researcher!

Choosing a research approach

Reasons for my choice of a qualitative methodology were twofold. First, qualitative methods are particularly suitable for investigating issues about which little is known, as was the case here. The aim is to develop theory inductively; that is, for theory to be developed out of the data, rather than deductively, whereby pre-existing theory is tested against the data (Morse and Field, 1996). The emphasis is on describing the phenomenon from the insider's (emic) perspective, in an attempt to understand the meaning that it holds for them (Hammersley, 1992).

Second, a qualitative approach had a much better 'fit' with the topic I was investigating. It had been apparent from my informal discussions with midwifery students that their experiences of emotion at work were both multi-faceted and profound. It was, therefore, clearly important to investigate the issue using methods that could embrace complexity and depth. A qualitative approach would enable me to view the issue holistically, and gain a more in-depth view of how emotion was experienced within a particular group of midwives. A quantitative research study would necessarily have taken the opposite approach, simplifying issues into measurable factors. That is not to say that a quantitative investigation, with the possibility of prediction of cause and effect, would not be potentially valuable in future studies of emotion in midwifery work. However, at the time, the existing state of knowledge precluded such an approach. As Hochschild (1993: xii) comments: 'Since emotion is a topic which requires subtlety of grasp, we should also refrain from counting things before we know what they are'.

Given all these points, a qualitative approach was clearly the most appropriate. The central research question became clarified as: How do midwives experience and manage emotion in their work? The broad aim of the study was to construct a picture of emotion in midwifery work from the perspective of midwives themselves, exploring how midwives make sense of emotion within the context of their occupational culture (Hammersley and Atkinson, 2007).

At this stage of the process, I can remember feeling quite ebullient: I had an interesting study, a clear research aim and question. Now, I thought, for the data collection, which I had been assured was the 'fun part'! I had reckoned at this stage without my supervisor, an experienced sociologist, who brought me back to earth by reminding me that I needed, first, to read widely about other emotions-related research, and to situate my study within this, and, second, that I needed to immerse myself in the methodological literature so that I could clarify my own ontological and epistemological positions. This was a critical part of the process that was not often reported in the research texts or papers, but was fundamental to my research apprenticeship.

Into the literature

Any foray into the literature of the sociology of emotions will very quickly lead to the influential work of Arlie Russell Hochschild (1979, 1983), who remains a central thinker in the field of emotion in the workplace. Her book *The Managed Heart: Commercialization of Human Feeling* (Hochschild, 1983) was considered ground-breaking, as it identified the significance of emotions in working life and drew attention to the work needed to manage these emotions.

This management of emotions is defined by Hochschild (1979, 1983) as 'emotion work', or 'emotional labour'. Hochschild (1983: 7) distinguishes between control of emotion in the home, which she terms 'emotion work', and 'emotional labour', which is performed in the public domain. The individual must 'work' on their emotions in order to produce the 'appropriate' emotion for the social context in which they are, thereby maintaining the social order. In Hochschild's words (1983: 7), they need: 'to induce or suppress feeling in order to sustain the outward countenance that produces the proper state of mind in others'. This work is performed according to 'feeling rules' (Hochschild, 1979: 563), the social norms that relate to feeling and display. Feeling rules relate not only to what emotions should be displayed in a given situation, but also to what an individual should feel. They are usually unspoken and generally go unnoticed until there is a disparity between what is actually felt and what an individual senses that they should feel. For example, one of the final year student midwives in my study described how sometimes she felt that 'birth was not always magical for her anymore'. She was concerned about this change, which went against the cultural norms of contemporary midwifery, which emphasize the 'specialness' of birth as a life event (Hunter, 2002).

Feeling rules are obviously present in all forms of work. For those who work in one-to-one situations with clients ('people work'), they are likely to be particularly pertinent, especially where workers are interacting with clients who are experiencing extreme emotion of some kind. In these situations, Hochschild (1983) suggests, workers will need to do more emotional labour, hiding their own feelings, however intense, in order to manage the feelings of their clients. This is clearly relevant for health care, where workers frequently engage in emotionally charged interactions (James, 1989, 1992; Smith, 1992; Froggatt, 1998; Meerabeau and Page, 1998; Bone, 2009).

The notion that managers can regulate the emotions of workers is central to Hochschild's (1983) thesis. Arguing from a perspective influenced by Marxist theory, she contends that selling emotional labour to management is likely to result in workers becoming alienated from their 'true' feelings. In this way, emotions have become commercialized and commodified in order to meet economic imperatives. In her study of American airlines (Hochschild, 1983), she observed how flight attendants were trained in techniques to enable them to control their emotions. The underpinning purpose of this was to ensure that the image conveyed by employees was congruent with the airline's corporate image of a friendly, personal service. In this way, the 'switch on smile' described by workers became part of the work contract and, thus, their emotional labour became a form of capital.

However, this emphasis on commodification may be a consequence of Hochschild's particular focus on profit-making organizations. Since her original research, a number of studies of emotions in public service work have been produced that have generated additional insights into emotion within other occupations (Steinberg and Figart, 1999a, 1999b; Fineman, 2000). As a result, we are now developing a much broader picture of the emotional labour that is carried out in a range of occupations, including medicine (Smith and Kleinman, 1989), police work (Stenross and Kleinman, 1989; Pogrebin and Poole, 1995) and nursing (James, 1989, 1992; Smith, 1992; Bolton, 2000, 2001; Bone, 2009).

Critiquing Hochschild

Given Hochschild's prominent position within the sociology of emotions, it was daunting for me as a novice researcher to critique her work. Nevertheless, there were many aspects of her book *The Managed Heart* that puzzled me, as I sensed a lack of 'fit' with my own experiences of the emotional aspects of work. First, there was an apparent assumption that workers are passive victims in the management/worker dynamic, and that they must necessarily conform to the emotional 'scripts' prescribed by management. This jarred with my own experiences, and more recent evidence also challenges this supposition. For example, Bolton's research (2000, 2001) indicates that nurses have considerable autonomy in how they display or contain their emotions, and are thus not necessarily alienated from their emotional life.

Second, Hochschild (1983) emphasizes the negative aspects of emotional labour. Again, it was far from clear to me whether this was always the case. Although there is evidence in some subsequent studies that emotional labour can lead to burn-out, exhaustion and feelings of 'inauthenticity' (James, 1989, 1992; Smith, 1992; Pogrebin and Poole, 1995), there is also a growing body of work which indicates that these negative outcomes are far from inevitable. My own study showed that, when midwives felt that they could establish a meaningful relationship with women and really 'make a difference', although they still needed to manage emotions, this was experienced positively. In the following focus group account, hospital-based midwives discuss the difference between 'positive draining', which could be interpreted as emotionally rewarding work, with work that is experienced negatively (for further discussion of these issues, please see Hunter, 2004, 2006). Emotional labour in particular was experienced negatively, especially when midwives felt that they were working primarily to meet the needs of the institution rather than the needs of the woman (Hunter, 2004):

Megan:
'I had a lovely normal delivery with a primip [primigravidae, first-time mother], had an intact perineum and I felt – even though it was draining, because it was a positive draining, you feel different about it. You feel it's okay to be drained in a positive way'. (Group agreement) 'It's back to this normal thing, it's not the same as looking after somebody with all the works and ending up in theatre, that kind of draining – then you go home and you don't know where you are.' (Focus group: hospital midwives; Hunter, 2002: 199)

Stenross and Kleinman (1989), Wharton (1993, 1999) and Bolton (2000, 2001), also provide empirical evidence that emotional labour is complex and likely to include both positive and negative emotions. Wharton's (1993, 1999) quantitative research identified a number of influencing factors, including the level of occupational autonomy, the extent of job involvement and the potential for the employee to self-monitor. When conditions are favourable, jobs that require emotional labour may bring a sense of reward, rather than burn-out, so that: 'emotion management per se may not be the problem we have assumed' (Wharton, 1999: 74).

This may be particularly true of work where there are strong elements of service and caring. Discussing the work of nurses, both Benner and Wrubel

(1989) and Bolton (2000) contend that, when emotional labour is under-pinned by a genuine sense of caring for another, there may not be negative consequences. While this may be oversimplifying matters in a different direc-tion, it certainly seems that the consequences of emotional labouring are more complex than Hochschild originally postulated.

In addition, I was increasingly perplexed by the focus of Hochschild's (1983) research on worker–client interaction as the key site of emotional labour, to the exclusion of other sources. This restricted perspective appeared to have been reiterated by most other researchers in the field, seemingly without comment, until the late 1990s (Steinberg and Figart, 1999b; Wharton, 1999). This was particularly true of the nursing-related literature, where there was an apparent assumption that emotional labour was situated solely within the nurse–patient relationship (see, for example, Smith, 1992; Smith and Gray, 2000).

This was certainly not my own experience of situations that evoked emotions and required emotion work! This is now supported by a growing literature that suggests that emotional labour is also performed within organizations as well as at the margins; for example, in interactions between colleagues, subordinates and managers (Copp, 1998; Kunda and Van Maanen, 1999; Steinberg and Figart, 1999a; Fineman, 2000; Hunter, 2004; Deery and Kirkham, 2007).

I also identified some methodological concerns related to Hochschild's study. Hochschild's work is based upon her research during the 1970s into:

- the private experience of emotion as described by American university students
- the public face of emotional labour in the labour market as experienced by American flight attendants
- a very small study into what Hochschild (1983: 16) refers to as the 'public back' (or shadow side) of emotional labour, such as that conducted by debt collectors using emotion management to induce anxiety rather than comfort in their clients.

Unusually, for qualitative research, Hochschild appears to have taken her initial conceptualization of emotional labour from the results of a question-naire. This questionnaire, used in the first study (of American undergraduate students), set two key exercises: 'describe a real situation that was important to you in which you experienced a deep emotion' and 'describe as fully and concretely as possible a real situation that was important to you in which you either changed the situation to fit your feelings or changed your feelings to fit the situation' (Hochschild, 1983: 13). The concepts derived from this study were then applied to the second study (Hochschild, 1983). This second study took an ethnographic approach to investigating the emotional labour of flight attendants, and was used to confirm and develop Hochschild's earlier theory. Imposing a theoretical framework early in ethnographic research is at odds with the inductive approach to theory generation usually associated with qual-itative research. Moreover, the questionnaire presumes that it is possible to 'work' on emotions in order to change them; that Hochschild found evidence of this is therefore hardly surprising. I was also surprised to find that no 'deviant cases' (Silverman, 1993: 44) were cited; that is, accounts that contrast with or contest the majority of accounts. This challenged my understanding of rigour in qualitative researching.

My hesitation in critiquing this seminal work was compounded by the enthusiasm of the many other researchers who followed in Hochschild's footsteps. Not only was her definition of emotional labour frequently adopted without critical reflection, but also there was no apparent questioning of her methodology. Could I be the only individual who had spotted these concerns? This seemed unlikely. It appeared that this lack of critique may have led to problems in subsequent studies.

For example, in a study of nurses, Smith and Gray (2000) presented the concept of emotional labour to participants for discussion, asking them: 'How would you define emotional labour? What does it mean to you?' (Smith and Gray (2000: 76). Although Smith and Gray (2000: 2) justified the use of this 'etic' category (that is, a category created by the researcher), claiming that it 'provides a language with which to describe and investigate what are often seen as the tacit and uncodified skills associated with care', I was concerned that giving this concept to participants would frame, and therefore restrict, their responses. It could also lead to a premature closure of the research inquiry, something that I was anxious to avoid in my own study.

Despite these reservations, however, I have no doubt about the significance of Hochschild's original work; in particular, the importance of naming this aspect of workplace behaviour. Although some aspects of the emotional life of the workplace had been described by previous sociologists (for example, Goffman, 1969; Lipsky, 1980; Hughes, 1984), Hochschild was the first to focus explicitly on this and, in doing so, capture the popular imagination in her descriptions and analysis of the phenomenon. Nevertheless, it is very important for subsequent researchers not to be afraid of critiquing established work, as it is only in this way that we can explore the social world effectively and, thus, push forward the boundaries of our understanding.

In contemporary publications, such as that of Fineman (2000), there is evidence of more open and enquiring exploration of emotion work. Fineman (2000: 13) for example, argues that a fresh approach to researching emotion is needed, if we are to gain insights that are conceptually more well-rounded and illuminating. He calls for investigative methods that: 'engage with feeling and emotion in ways traditionally proscribed by codes of "objective" social science; do so qualitatively, in a de-atomized manner; and place emotion in its wider structural and cultural contexts'.

Study design

It was with Fineman's words in mind that I decided upon an ethnographic approach to the study, using a range of data collection methods (focus groups, interviews and observation) in order to get 'the best fix on the subject matter in hand' (Denzin and Lincoln, 1994: 4).

The study was conducted in three phases:

Phase I

Phase I consisted of four focus groups undertaken with a total of 27 student midwives attending a university in Wales. Participants were from the first and the final years of both the eighteen-month programme (a 'short' course for those with prior nurse training) and the three-year programme (a 'long' or 'direct entry' course for those with no nurse training). Discussions were stimulated by the use of photographs of midwives at work; the students were asked to consider what emotions the midwife in the photo might be experiencing. This was an effective means of prompting discussion, with participants moving from the general ('how the midwife in the photo might be feeling') to the specific ('how I felt in a similar situation'). Participants were asked particularly to consider which aspects of their work they found emotionally rewarding and emotionally difficult, and how they dealt with their emotions in such situations.

Focus groups proved to be particularly suited to exploring the topic of emotions. They generated a wealth of rich data, as participants spontaneously adopted a storytelling approach to illustrate their experiences of emotion. Using a group context to explore emotion enabled me not only to gain insights into individual experiences, but also into how emotion was understood and dealt with within the culture of midwifery.

This phase of data collection occurred comparatively early on in the study, when my thinking was mainly informed by the theoretical framework of 'emotional labour' as constructed by Hochschild (1979, 1983) and subsequent authors. However, towards the end of this phase I became increasingly frustrated and dissatisfied. Although the data collection was progressing well, and the focus groups were enjoyable to conduct and were producing the rich, detailed data anticipated, I had a strong sense that I was missing something of importance. Although I was getting answers, they did not appear to be resolving the puzzle.

Two limitations within my thinking became apparent: first, the findings were restricted by the focus on student experiences. Focus group discussions were dominated by accounts of socialization into midwifery culture, rather than broader experiences of working as a midwife. Thus, while student accounts provided valuable insights, these were only part of the picture or jigsaw. Second, my initial acceptance of Hochschild's (1979, 1983) framework of emotional labour was proving to be problematic. As discussed previously, although the theoretical perspective of Hochschild and subsequent authors resonated with some aspects of the data I was obtaining, in other respects there were many disparities.

As I became aware of these limitations in my research design, I began to develop a more open-minded approach to the study. This was a significant development in my career as a novice researcher. I moved away from a conviction that there was a clearly proscribed 'way to do it' that would lead me to 'the answer', and that this would become apparent to me once I had read enough texts and talked with enough experienced researchers. Instead, I realized that, given the paucity of information related to the emotional aspects of midwifery work, it was essential to keep as truly open a mind as possible. In retrospect, I had been in danger of developing a utilitarian approach to the data, looking for examples that reflected Hochschild's framework in a manner that was antithetical to the inductive premise that is fundamental to a qualitative methodology. As Alasuutari (1995: 166) observes: 'the more open-minded you are in gathering observations, the less you exclude, the richer your material will be, and, accordingly, the better your chances of inventing new (theoretical) ideas on the basis of the material'.

Phase II: transition

My hunch was that I needed to extend my sample to include qualified midwives, and that these should represent a variety of midwifery experiences. Given my own experiences of practising as a midwife, I was well aware that the job took on very different forms in different contexts. Such inside knowledge is one of the benefits of doing practitioner research (Reed and Procter, 1995). I tested out this premise by asking an opportunistic sample of qualified midwives undertaking undergraduate studies to participate in a focus group, using the same key questions I had used with the students. These midwives represented a broad range of experiences. They worked for a variety of different NHS Trusts; were employed in both hospital, community and integrated settings; had been qualified for varying lengths of time; and were employed at different clinical grades.

My hunch appeared correct. These qualified midwives identified very different issues related to the emotional aspects of their work than had the students. Moreover, it was not only their qualified status that impacted on experiences; it was also apparent that hospital-based and community-based midwives had differing emotional issues to contend with. There were also indications that the level of clinical responsibility (as defined by clinical grade) might be of significance.

Additional evidence of the differing emotional issues confronting qualified midwives was provided by a further opportunistic sample: a chance encounter with one of the participants from Phase I, now working as a newly-qualified midwife, led to her suggesting that we reconvene the group to discuss their current experiences. While I experienced some initial hesitation, as I had not intended a longitudinal design for the study, the midwife was clearly suggesting that qualified status had brought with it a number of new and significant emotional issues, which it appeared important to explore.

The data from this group further supported my impression that student midwives and qualified midwives had differing experiences that required them to work on their emotions. Indeed, this group was particularly perceptive regarding the varied nature of these experiences, presumably as a result of their recent transition. There were also specific issues relating to their marginal position on the borders of midwifery culture – although they had successfully navigated the formal occupational boundaries, there was still considerable emotional work to be done in negotiating informal boundaries (for further exploration of this issue, see Hunter, 2006).

Phase II therefore consisted of two focus groups with 11 participants in total. By this stage in the data collection, however, I had also become aware of the limitations of focus groups as a data collection method. Focus groups were providing only one angle on the research question, as participants were 'talking midwifery' rather than 'doing midwifery'. Although participants readily identified and discussed situations that they experienced as emotionally difficult or emotionally rewarding, their accounts tended to illustrate dramatic events, rather than the more mundane, day-to-day aspects of midwifery practice. Other focus group researchers have made similar observations regarding the nature of group data (Carey, 1994; Smith, 1995). It became clear that I was in danger of missing the everyday issues that necessitate emotion management, as these taken-for-granted aspects of practice were unlikely to be elucidated.

This thinking led to Phase III, in which the research design was adapted to a multi-method approach, including periods of observation, to be undertaken with qualified midwives.

Phase III

Phase III of the study involved an in-depth substantive study of one research site over a period of eight months (November 1999–July 2000). Phases I and II had alerted me to a number of key issues related to emotion work that I was able to explore further using a mixture of focus groups, semi-participant observation and semi-structured interviews.

Purposive sampling was used to access a range of midwives with varying years of clinical experience, different levels of clinical responsibility and a range of clinical locations. In all, there were 29 participants. Of these, 17 took part in four focus groups. The remaining 12 midwives (six community-based, six hospital-based) were 'shadowed' during their working day. Field notes were made during these observations and key issues were followed up during a semi-structured interview that usually took place immediately afterwards. In this interview, I was able to compare my impressions of the emotional aspects of the midwife's day with her perceptions. This often produced some interesting differences, particularly when issues that I had identified as significant were perceived as mundane by the midwife. While this sometimes led to me re-thinking my evaluation, the opposite was also true, with midwives acknowledging, with some surprise, that aspects of their 'ordinary' daily work were actually laden with emotion.

The study differs from a traditional ethnography, as fieldwork consisted of periods of focused observation during which I watched individual midwives as they worked. Although this inevitably meant that I was also observing a number of other people, and engaging with broader aspects of the midwife's working life, this differs from the usual descriptions of ethnography as a process of 'hanging out' and participating in the day-to-day life of a particular group (Pearson, 1993). The focused nature of my observations was designed to address the unanswered questions that I had been left with at the end of Phase II. It had been evident at this stage that there were differences in the emotional experiences of hospital- and community-based midwives, and that these were influenced by a range of factors. These factors included the context in which midwives were practising, collegial relationships, relationships with women and the status of the midwife. Observations and interviews in Phase III were therefore undertaken with these issues in mind. This fieldwork generated rich and fascinating data, although this phase of the study was not without its challenges, as we will see in the next part of the chapter.

Some research dilemmas

Undertaking any type of research inevitably presents dilemmas for the researcher, and the flexible and responsive nature of ethnography makes such dilemmas even more likely. In this section, I describe two particular situations that created dilemmas for me: gaining access to the research site, and being 'behind the wallpaper'.

Gaining access

As with other aspects of qualitative research, gaining access is inevitably 'messy' and bears little relation to the straightforward process described in the research texts. Following ethical review of the study by the Local Research Ethics Committee, I negotiated access to the research site with one of the senior midwives. As agreed with the Ethics Committee, she arranged for me to be provided with names of staff and details of their clinical location, so that I could make contact. This access was relatively easy to achieve and is likely to have been facilitated by my position, at that time, as midwifery lecturer. I was not only a familiar figure, I also had a degree of professional and academic credibility. This perceived status proved to be something of a two-edged sword, as will be seen.

However, by the time recruitment to the study commenced, the original senior midwife who had given permission had left and I needed to liaise with a new senior midwife. She was very supportive and interested in the study, although it was evident that she was also somewhat anxious that my findings might be 'negative' and reflect badly on the unit. She arranged for me to attend a unit team meeting, which all midwives were expected to attend. This appeared to be an ideal opportunity to inform a large number of staff about the study and to be personally available to answer any questions. We agreed that she would briefly introduce me and then leave me to explain the project. In the event, the situation was far from what I had intended. In my research diary, I noted:

> When I arrive the room is already full. Senior midwives are sitting at the front, other midwives in rows facing them. I look for a seat amongst the main group of midwives, but am invited to sit at the front. This feels very formal and as though I am going to deliver a didactic lecture. It also aligns me with 'management' rather than 'ordinary' midwives, something that I wish to avoid. We have previously agreed that one of the senior midwives

will introduce me. She already knows about my research and is keen to be supportive to me. This becomes a much longer event than I intended. She provides many details of the study in a rather unstructured way, and includes some of the theoretical underpinning of my research, mentioning Pam Smith's work on emotional labour. From the look on most of the midwives' faces, they are totally confused. I really wish that this hadn't happened – a) because it did not present a clear picture of what the study is about, and what will be expected of participants b) because I don't want the data contaminated by the midwives being too aware of the theoretical constructs. (Research diary, 27 July 1999)

This example illustrates the power of those in 'gatekeeping' positions. As Hammersley and Atkinson (1995: 75) note: 'Even the most friendly and co-operative of gatekeepers or sponsors will shape the conduct and development of the research.' Although the senior midwife presumably acted with the best of intentions, there were potentially many negative outcomes. I was conscious of trying to redeem myself, and my study, during the more informal contact I had following this. However, it is difficult to know whether this incident affected participation rates or, indeed, the quality of the data.

Being 'behind the wallpaper'

The observational part of the data collection also challenged my theoretical understanding of 'how it should be done'. My initial intention was to be a non-participant observer but, in practice, my stance varied along a continuum of being fully participative to totally non-participative. I learnt that I had to go with the flow and adapt my role according to the midwife I was observing, the clients she was working with and the context in which we found ourselves. The textbook version, in contrast, frequently appears to imply that the researcher can adopt a consistent stance throughout. Morse and Field (1996), for example, describe four types of participant observation:

- complete participation
- participant-as-observer
- observer-as-participant
- complete observer.

The inference is that the researcher selects one of these modes prior to commencing data collection and maintains this.

My experiences were rather different. I quickly realized that sitting in the corner taking notes was perceived not only as rather peculiar behaviour, but also as intimidating. This was especially the case when I was observing the work of the community-based midwives. In family homes, it seemed particu-larly important to 'fit in', so I joined in with the social chat with the woman and her family, and generally tried to make myself appear approachable and friendly. I was very conscious that this was undertaking 'impression manage-ment' (Goffman, 1969), attempting to allay the potential fears of the midwife and the woman that I was an out-of-touch academic! The quality of my field notes, however, was in inverse proportion to my degree of participation. I quickly learnt how to multi-task, jotting down the main points while playing games with the other children and balancing a cup of tea (Hunter, 2007). The use of a Dictaphone during my car journey home proved invaluable as a memory jogger, and enabled me to record my impressions quickly, to be written up in full as soon as possible.

In hospital and clinic settings, it was somewhat easier to be 'behind the wallpaper'. The bustle of these environments appeared to afford a degree of anonymity, and I more easily became just another health worker. It was also the case that in the hospital I wore either a white coat or theatre 'greens', and this apparel appeared to act like Harry Potter's invisibility cloak and grant me instant access to any area, with no challenge. Hunt also noted the 'white coat effect' in her ethnography of a labour ward (Hunt and Symonds, 1995).

There were times, however, when I found the observer role particularly difficult to sustain. For example, when the midwives were clearly overworked and stressed, I often felt tempted to offer to help out. This tension necessitated some reflection on my part: in terms of my research, it was probable that observing midwives' emotional responses in such stressful situations would provide useful insights for my study. By offering to help – indeed, by 'going native' – I would not only contaminate the data, but also restrict my analysis. However, this research mindfulness had to be balanced against a strong desire to give something back to the midwives I was studying (and an inner voice telling me that it was the midwives who were doing real work, not I!). I discussed these dilemmas with my supervisor, an experienced ethnographer, who helped me to explore these competing pressures. My eventual compromise was to become the tea-maker whenever possible.

Similar dilemmas have been noted in other research undertaken by practitioners (Hunt and Symonds, 1995; Reed and Proctor, 1995). While shared knowledge of an occupational culture has many benefits for understanding and interpreting the data, it also brings with it many ambiguities and tensions.

A positive aspect of such difficult situations was that my empathy with the midwives was greatly increased. In the initial stages of fieldwork, I had sometimes felt disappointed with – and even critical of – the quality of communication between midwives and women, noting many closed and leading questions and missed opportunities for interaction. Increased contact with the midwives led me to see the situation through their eyes. Given the time pressures and large workloads of which I became only too aware, the midwives' communication styles could be understood not as poor practice but, rather, as strategies for managing conflicting demands. Thus, rather than clouding my view on the issues, increased empathy gave me new insights. Empathy with participants has not been widely discussed in the research literature, with Kleinman and Copp (1993) contending that this reflects a general lack of attention to the emotional aspects of undertaking fieldwork. Observational methods appear to offer particular opportunities for empathic insights, as not only does the researcher listen to the participants' accounts of difficult situations, but they may also be party to these events.

Being an observer also became difficult when interactions between midwives and clients were strained, or when serious problems arose. For example, in one situation a woman and her partner were very upset that a planned Caesarean section had been delayed. The woman was crying and her partner looked furious. In another, the midwife detected an abnormal foetal heart pattern during a routine antenatal clinic appointment. In both instances, I put my notebook away in my pocket; recording the situation no longer seemed appropriate – or indeed, important – when weighed against these real life issues. Again, it may be that my own experience as a midwife (and as a mother) heightened my sensitivity to these situations.

Despite my reservations regarding the practical and ethical difficulties of undertaking fieldwork, the advantages of this approach greatly outweighed my concerns. Watching midwives 'do' midwifery, I was able to identify many aspects of midwives' emotion work that neither the participants nor I had previously acknowledged.

Unexpected findings

So – what did I find? The study findings have been published in detail elsewhere (Hunter, 2004, 2005, 2006, 2009), so here I will provide a general overview.

In brief, the key source of emotion work for these midwives was the need to juggle conflicting ideologies of practice. Participants held a strong ideal of practising in a 'with woman' manner; that is, working in partnership with women, attending to their individual needs, promoting a normalizing approach to childbirth wherever possible. However, the demands of their day-to-day work meant that, in reality, their practice had to be 'with institution', focusing on task completion in order to 'get through the work' and meet the demands of a busy maternity service providing care for large numbers of women and their babies as they moved rapidly through the system and were discharged home. These two models of care: 'with woman' and 'with institution' were in conflict, and it was managing this tension and dissonance that created most emotion work for the study participants. In general, the midwives who were community-based were more likely to be able to work using a 'with woman' approach than their hospital-based colleagues.

My study thus provided evidence that challenged the assumption commonly found in much of the literature: that emotional labour occurred mainly within interactions between workers and clients. Although it was the case that some emotion work occurred within the midwife–woman relationship, this was far from being the key source. In fact, interactions with women were often what made the work emotionally rewarding and meaningful (for further discussion, see Hunter, 2006). Rather, it was interactions with colleagues and 'the organization' that generated most need for emotion work, and this was frequently underpinned by the conflicting ideologies (see Hunter, 2005). At the nub of such situations was a common ingredient: the dissonance felt by midwives related to ideological contradictions. Surprisingly, the need for workers to

Table 7.1 Work context, occupational identity, occupational ideology and emotion work in midwifery practice

Context	Aspects of occupational identity	Occupational Ideology	Emotion work
Hospital-based practice	– Medicalized approach – Universal provision of equitable care – Decreased autonomy – Midwives interchangeable – Decreased significance of relationships with clients – Increased sense of affiliation to colleagues and organization	'With institution'	To resolve disparity between 'with woman' ideal and 'with institution' necessity. Dominance of 'affective neutrality'.
Integrated community and hospital practice	Occupational identity = ambiguous	Ideologies incompatible ⟶	Increased emotion work
Community-based practice	– Natural approach – Individualized provision of care – Increased autonomy – Increased emphasis on use of self – Increased significance of relationships with clients – Decreased sense of affiliation to organization	'With woman'	To resolve conflicts: (a) between 'with woman ideal' and institutional demands; (b) related to sustainability of ideal. Goal = 'affective awareness'.

Source: Adapted from Hunter (2002): 227.

work on their emotions when faced with conflicting beliefs and values has rarely been identified or explored (the study by Copp (1998) is a notable exception). (See also Chapter 3, p. 77.)

The study also indicated that there were differing models relating to the management of emotion, with diverse sets of 'feeling rules' (Hochschild, 1979: 563). I suggested that an emotion management continuum existed. At one end was 'affective neutrality' (Parsons, 1951), whereby midwives suppressed emotions in order to maintain a 'professional' image. At the other end of the continuum was 'affective awareness', whereby midwives managed emotions through sharing and support. 'Affective neutrality' was more commonly described and observed within hospital midwifery, while community midwives were more likely to adopt an approach of 'affective awareness'. It was also apparent that, although some midwives might have a preference for a partic-ular emotional 'style', others moved backwards and forwards along this continuum in response to the demands of their work and their personal lives (for a more detailed discussion, see Hunter, 2009)

These differing models of emotion management are linked to the conflicting ideologies of practice described earlier. 'Affective neutrality' fits with a 'with institution' ideology aimed at minimizing the emotional content of childbirth in order to achieve institutional goals. In contrast, 'affective awareness' is linked to a 'with woman' approach, in which attention to individual psychosocial needs requires acknowledgement of the emotional elements of care.

A theoretical framework was proposed that draws together the findings of the study and identifies links between work context, occupational identity, occupational ideology and emotion management (see Table 7.1).

This study thus provides many new insights into both the sources of emotion in midwifery work, and the ways in which emotions are managed, suggesting that work context and occupational status impact significantly on the experiences of midwives. Many of the insights gained were unexpected, suggesting that emotion work occurs in situations other than those identified in the wider literature. Interestingly, there is now a growing body of literature in which authors have questioned whether the previous analysis of emotional labour had been too restricted (Dingwall and Allen, 2001; Bolton, 2005; McClure and Murphy, 2007).

The research approach that I adopted was fundamental to generating this new knowledge, and helped me to avoid reaching premature conclusions about emotion in midwifery work. The use of an ethnographic approach enabled me to obtain a well-rounded and multifaceted view of the issue, and to generate theory inductively from midwives' own accounts of emotionally rewarding and emotionally difficult work.

Conclusion

In this chapter, I have provided a natural history of a qualitative research study, telling the story of the project from my initial intuitive hunches and puzzling questions to the eventual development of new inductive theory. My aim has been to describe some of the complexities and dilemmas that are an inevitable part of undertaking a qualitative study, and the challenges of attempting to develop new midwifery theory. On the way, I hope that I have encouraged readers to keep an open mind, not to be afraid of challenging accepted wisdoms, and to be imaginative and creative in their attempts to develop new midwifery theory.

ACTIVITIES

Undergraduate

Reflect on a clinical situation in which you have left a birthing experience totally elated or totally deflated (regardless of the birth type or birth setting). Describe and discuss the range of emotions you experienced with reference to Hunter's framework described in Table 7.1.

Postgraduate

Design a research study to test Hunter's theory about 'affective neutrality' and 'affective awareness'.

References

Alasuutari, P. (1995) *Researching Culture: Qualitative Method and Cultural Studies.* Sage: London.

Benner, P. and Wrubel, J. (1989) *The Primacy of Caring: Stress and Coping in Health and Illness.* Menloe Park, CA: Addison-Wesley, Health Sciences Division.

Bolton, S.C. (2000) 'Who Cares? Offering Emotion Work as a 'Gift' in the Nursing Labour Process', *Journal of Advanced Nursing*, 32(3): 580–6.

Bolton, S.C. (2001) Changing Faces: Nurses as Emotional Jugglers. *Sociology of Health and Illness*, 23(1): 85–100.

Bolton, S.C. (2005) *Emotion Management in the Workplace.* Basingstoke: Palgrave Macmillan.

Bone, D. (2009) 'Epidurals Not Emotions: The Care Deficit in US Maternity Care', in B. Hunter and R. Deery (eds), *Emotions in Midwifery and Reproduction.* Basingstoke: Palgrave Macmillan, ch. 4: 56–72.

Carey, M.A. (1994) 'The Group Effect in Focus Groups: Planning, Implementing and Interpreting Focus Group Research', in J.M. Morse (ed.), *Critical Issues in Qualitative Research.* Thousand Oaks, CA:Sage, ch. 12: 225–41.

Copp, M. (1998) 'When Emotion Work is Doomed to Fail: Ideological and Structural Constraints of Emotion Management', *Symbolic Interaction*, 21(3): 299–328.

Deery, R. and Kirkham. M. (2007) 'Drained and Dumped On: The Generation and Accumulation of Emotional Toxic Waste in Community Midwifery', in M. Kirkham (ed.), Exploring the Dirty Side of Women's Health. Abingdon: Routledge, ch. 14: 72–83.

Denzin, N.K. and Lincoln, Y.S. (1994) 'Introduction: Entering the Field of Qualitative Research', in N.K. Denzin and Y.S. Lincoln (eds), *Handbook of Qualitative Research.* Thousand Oaks, CA: Sage, ch. 1: 1–17.

Dingwall, R. and Allen, D. (2001) 'The Implications of Healthcare Reforms for the Profession of Nursing', *Nursing Inquiry*, 8(2): 64–74.

Fineman, S. (ed.) (2000) *Emotion in Organizations*, 2nd edn. London: Sage.

Froggatt, K. (1998) 'The Place of Metaphor and Language in Exploring Nurses' Emotional Work', *Journal of Advanced Nursing*, 28(2): 332–8.

Goffman, E. (1969) *The Presentation of Self in Everyday Life*. London: Allen Lane/Penguin Press.

Guba, E.G. and Lincoln, Y.S. (1981) *Effective Evaluation*. San Francisco, CA: Jossey-Bass.

Hammersley, M. (1992) *What's Wrong with Ethnography? Methodological Explorations*. London: Routledge.

Hammersley, M. and Atkinson, P. (2007) *Ethnography: Principles and Practice*, 2nd edn. London: Routledge.

Hammersley, M. and Atkinson, P. (2007) *Ethnography: Principles and Practice*, 3rd edn. London: Routledge.

Hochschild, A.R. (1979) 'Emotion Work, Feeling Rules and Social Structure', *American Journal of Sociology*, 85(3): 551–75.

Hochschild, A.R. (1983) *The Managed Heart. Commercialization of Human Feeling*. Berkeley, CA: University of California Press.

Hochschild, A.R. (1993) 'Preface', in S. Fineman (ed.), *Emotion in Organizations*. London: Sage: p xii.

Hughes, E.C. (1984) *The Sociological Eye: Selected Papers*. New Brunswick, NJ: Transaction Books.

Hunt, S. and Symonds, A. (1995) *The Social Meaning of Midwifery*. Basingstoke: Macmillan.

Hunter, B. (2002) 'Emotion Work in Midwifery', Unpublished PhD Thesis, University of Wales, Swansea.

Hunter, B. (2004) 'Conflicting Ideologies as a Source of Emotion Work in Midwifery', *Midwifery*, 20: 261–72.

Hunter, B. (2005) 'Emotion Work and Boundary Maintenance in Hospital-Based Midwifery', *Midwifery*, 21: 253–66.

Hunter, B. (2006) 'The Importance of Reciprocity in Relationships between Community-Based Midwives and Mothers', *Midwifery*, 22(4): 308–22.

Hunter, B. (2007) 'The Art of Teacup Balancing: Reflections on Conducting Qualitative Research', *Evidence Based Midwifery*, 5(3): 76–9.

Hunter, B. (2009) 'Mixed Messages: Midwives' Experiences of Managing Emotion', in B. Hunter and R. Deery (eds), *Emotions in Midwifery and Reproduction*. Basingstoke: Palgrave Macmillan, ch. 11: 175–91.

James, N. (1989) 'Emotional Labour: Skill and Work in the Social Regulation of Feelings', *Sociological Review*, 37: 15–42.

James, N. (1992) 'Care = Organisation + Physical Labour + Emotional Labour', *Sociology of Health and Illness*, 14 (4): 489–509.

Kleinman, S. and Copp, M.A. (1993) *Emotions and Fieldwork*. London: Sage.

Kunda, G. and Van Maanen, J. (1999) 'Changing Scripts at Work: Managers and Professionals', in R.J. Steinberg and D.M. Figart (eds), *Emotional Labor in the Service Economy. The Annals of the American Academy of Political and Social Science*, 561(1): 64–81.

Lipsky, M. (1980) *Street-Level Bureaucracy: Dilemmas of the Individual in Public Services*. New York, NY: Russell Sage Foundation.

McClure, R. and Murphy, C. (2007) 'Contesting the Dominance of Emotional Labour in Professional Nursing', *Journal of Health Organisation and Management*, 21(2): 101–20.

Meerabeau, L. and Page, S. (1998) 'Getting the Job Done': Emotion Management and Cardiopulmonary Resuscitation in Nursing', in G. Bendelow and S.J. Williams (eds), *Emotions in Social Life. Critical Themes and Contemporary Issues*. London: Routledge, ch. 16: 295–312.

Morse, J.M. and Field, P.A. (1996) *Nursing Research: The Application of Qualitative Approaches*. Cheltenham: Nelson Thornes.

Parsons, T. (1951) *The Social System*. New York, NY: Free Press.

Pearson, G. (1993) 'Talking A Good Fight: Authenticity and Distance in the Ethnographer's Craft', in D. Hobbs and T. May (eds), *Interpreting the Field: Accounts of Ethnography*. Oxford: Oxford University Press. vii–xx.

Pogrebin, M.R. and Poole, E.D. (1995) 'Emotion Management: A Study of Police Response to Tragic Events', *Social Perspectives on Emotion*, 3: 149–68.

Reed, J. and Procter, S. (1995) *Practitioner Research in Health Care: The Inside Story*. London: Chapman & Hall.

Silverman, D. (1993) *Interpreting Qualitative Data: Methods for Analysing Talk, Text and Interaction*. London: Sage.

Silverman, D. (2000) *Doing Qualitative Research: A Practical Handbook*. London: Sage.

Smith, A.C. and Kleinman, S. (1989) 'Managing Emotions in Medical School: Students' Contacts with the Living and the Dead', *Social Psychology Quarterly*, 52(1): 56–69.

Smith, M.W. (1995) 'Ethics in Focus Groups: A Few Concerns', *Qualitative Health Research*, 5(4): 478–86.

Smith, P. (1992) *The Emotional Labour of Nursing*. London: Macmillan.

Smith, P. and Gray, B. (2000) 'The Emotional Labour of Nursing: How Student and Qualified Nurses Learn to Care', Report on Nurse Education, Nursing Practice and Emotional Labour in the Contemporary NHS. London: South Bank University.

Steinberg, R.J. and Figart, D.M. (1999a) 'Emotional Labor since *The Managed Heart*', in R.J. Steinberg and D.M. Figart (eds), *Emotional Labor in the Service Economy. The Annals of the American Academy of Political and Social Science*, 561(1): 8–25.

Steinberg, R.J. and Figart, D.M. (eds) (1999b) *Emotional Labor in the Service Economy. The Annals of the American Academy of Political and Social Science*, 561(1).

Stenross, B. and Kleinman, S. (1989) 'The Highs and Lows of Emotional Labor: Detectives' Encounters with Criminals and Victims', *Journal of Contemporary Ethnography*, 17(4): 435–52.

Wharton, A.S. (1993) 'The Affective Consequences Of Service Work: Managing Emotions on the Job', *Work and Occupations*, 20(2): 205–32.

Wharton, A.S. (1999) 'The Psycho-Social Consequences of Emotional Labor', in R.J. Steinberg and D.M. Figart (eds), *Emotional Labor in the Service Economy. The Annals of the American Academy of Political and Social Science*, 561(1): 158–75.

Nesting and Matrescence

8

Denis Walsh

Key points

- The birth environment is fundamental to birth experience and outcome
- Human nesting, as expressed in women's choices concerning place of birth, is sometimes premised on different dimensions of safety, such as cultural or psychosocial safety
- Women make assessments of the emotional ambience of birth settings and are drawn to nurturing, caring environments
- Matrescent (becoming mother) care is fundamental to the midwives' role in labour and is mediated through empathic relationships.

Introduction

One of the great strengths of qualitative research is not simply the illumination of a complex health care environment or the lived experience of women and midwives, but the construction of some explanatory framework (beginnings of theory generation) for what has been described. Within the variety of methods at one's disposal to undertake qualitative research, ethnography is well-suited to the task of building an explanatory framework.

Although ethnography does not require the researcher to contrive such a framework, emphasizing instead rich and detailed description, critical and institutional ethnographic approaches usually result in this (Dykes, 2005). Within maternity care, there is a rich legacy here in relation to ethnographies of birth settings such as labour wards. Kirkham's (1988) seminal study of communication in labour helped midwives 'see' the inscribing of the patient role on women, and Hunt's (Hunt and Symonds, 1995) later study of consultant labour wards exposed the stereotyping of women in these environments. Although their conclusions do not constitute theory, as such, they do give theoretical insight into a work environment and can fundamentally change the way midwives perceive these settings.

Within ethnography, the process by which explanatory frameworks through to formal theories are developed is inductive. They arise from, and are grounded, in data (Hammersley and Atkinson, 1995). This grounding is essential for credibility and transferability of theory because, once it enters the public arena through publication and presentation, researchers have no control over how it is understood and interpreted. Practitioners themselves make the judgement as to its relevance by 'seeing' whether it makes sense in their practice environment. To make this decision, they need a rich enough description of the research setting and a convincing enough argument for the researchers' interpretation to make the links. Unsubstantiated theory will be spotted quickly.

In this chapter, I will discuss the findings from an ethnographic study of a free-standing birth centre in the United Kingdom and three tentative theories developed from observations and interviews conducted there over a nine-month period (Walsh, 2004). I will then examine parallels with wider research into maternity service models in critically appraising the significance of these tentative theories.

Birth centres

Birth centres exist as integrated (attached to a consultant maternity unit) and as free-standing (some geographical distance from the host consultant maternity unit). Together, they probably support around 5 per cent of total births in the UK, and are specifically designated as midwifery-led environments (Smith and Smith, 2005). As a unique model, midwifery-led care offers a rich source of investigation for emergent midwifery theory. Free-standing birth centres offer something extra again, unencumbered as they are by a large hospital's institutional, bureaucratic and medicalised processes.

Previous qualitative research in free-standing birth centres revealed a mixed picture of empowerment for women (Esposito, 1999) and ambivalence among midwifery staff (Annandale, 1988). Women were unequivocally positive, if their experience was straight forward, but did not like the experience of transfer if complications arose during labour (Walker, 2000). If the birth centre's host unit was unsupportive, the midwives felt trapped between a model they found professionally fulfilling and a host unit hostile to their 'liberal' clinical policies. They therefore employed what Annandale (1987) terms 'ironic intervention' to reduce the transfer rates (hastening labour by routine interventions that were incompatible with their stated philosophy).

The NHS birth centre where I undertook my ethnographic study cared for about 300 women per year, and was staffed by midwives and maternity care assistants (MCAs) who provided a 24-hour service. They worked a shift system and did not practise caseload midwifery, although they did run antenatal clinics and childbirth preparation classes, which gave them opportunities to meet women antenatally who were booked with the birth centre.

I spent nine months undertaking participant observation and interviews of women and staff. Ethical approval was sought and granted and, in the following quotes, pseudonyms have been used.

Birth environment and setting

The centrality of the environment and setting for women's decision to book at the birth centre was apparent from the first interviews. Their reasons were a combination of recommendations from family, friends and work colleagues; the fact that the unit was local and easily accessible for their families and friends, and the flexibility of both when you could visit and who could visit.

The impact of the first visit to the centre was also pivotal for women in deciding to have their babies there. It is worth quoting some of their interviews:

'We went to have a look, and as soon as we walked in we thought – yep! This is the sort of place. I think it was so small and it's not like a hospital. We thought it would be a nice relaxing place to go.' (Jasmine, Transcript no. 9: 2)

Another woman said 'the birth space is somewhere you could relax'. Carmel's views also reflected this idea:

'The psychological effects of being there, it was like being at home really in terms of environment, it was very, very comfortable and calming, relaxing. It was the room itself, the way it's made up. It's got homely things in it. Most of the instruments are hidden away. They're not on display.' (Carmel, Transcript no. 21: 4)

These environmental features were repeated often as women spoke of the different pace, lack of frenetic activity and the smaller, more intimate surroundings. Some contrasted this with their previous experience of former births in hospital where they felt they were 'processed'.

In addition to environmental features, women commented on the friendliness and welcome they received from the birth centre staff. Many did not expect to be offered cups of tea and toast. Some turned up without appointments and were made welcome. One woman commented on the fact that she was greeted at the door by a staff member holding a baby. She concluded this was a baby-friendly environment.

These rationales for choosing the birth centre suggest an appraisal emanating from social (rather than clinical) criteria, and are therefore at odds with the assumption made by many maternity care professionals that evidence related to mortality and morbidity will be highly influential in the choice of where to have a baby. Women in this study commented on this latter assumption by some general practitioners (GPs), who appeared to think that all women having their first baby should give birth in a consultant unit, as the following interview reveals:

'I said why can't I go to the birth centre? ... and she said "Oh! well this is your first child, we really wouldn't advise it. There won't be any doctors present and, if anything goes wrong, they will have to take you to the hospital".' (Vivienne, Transcript no. 18: 7)

Actually, some women in the study were deterred from booking at a consultant unit by the focus on what could go wrong. One did not like a large poster on how to resuscitate a baby and the resuscitation equipment that were in the delivery room. Another expressed fear, shared by others, of the technological environment in a large hospital.

Staff focus on birth environment

The seminal influence of the birth environment for women booking at the birth centre was, unexpectedly, also reflected in the staff's priorities. There was a single-minded focus on upgrading and maintaining the décor and ambience. They had turned a traditional maternity unit into a modern birth centre by renovating and redecorating every room over a 10-year period. Most of this work had been done by the staff. To achieve this, they ran numerous fundraising events, some of which were very successful. In one three-month period, £39,000 was raised.

Another aspect of this was staff bringing in items that they no longer needed from their homes to domesticate the environment. These included crockery, cutlery, ornaments and lamps. One of the staff members had a curtain-making business and, over the years, had supplied and fitted all the curtains at no charge.

I found the freedom and discretion they exercised in addressing this aspect of the birth environment astounding. Clues as to why it was so important came in phrases the staff used from time to time. The midwives spoke of 'creating an oasis of calm', of the place 'mimicking home', of providing 'a nurturing environment', 'a quieter more relaxed ambience'. An MCA said 'a calming space and not like a hospital'.

A further aspect of this environmental focus was the attention to cleanliness, tidiness and upkeep of the facility. Although not articulated in interviews, it was an obvious priority for staff. Many of the visitors were maintenance people attending to building problems of immense variety, from replacing an ice machine to installing security cameras, from tracking down an unpleasant smell under the floor to refitting the entire kitchen. Plumbing, electrics, heating and decorating were 'bread and butter' concerns. The communications book was just as full with building-related issues as it was clinical issues, and these were handed on to the staff coming on the next shift in exactly the same way that outstanding clinical issues were.

The activities around hospitality and environment were everybody's responsibility and were no respecter of position. MCAs and midwives were completely interchangeable when any tasks related to these areas needed to be done. Midwives vacuumed floors, washed curtains, and made drinks. MCAs answered phones, conducted tours and sorted the engineering problems.

One could summarize all these activities as promoting a certain environmental ambience, and conceptualize them as environmental nurture. They were augmented by a honing of emotional ambience, which began with welcome and hospitality, and continued with one-to-one support during labour. The lead midwife at the birth centre instigated a small, but richly symbolic change when she came into post in 1993. She negotiated the withdrawal of GPs from an intrapartum surveillance role, and the admission of women's chosen birth partners. Here, she was introducing one of the most thoroughly tested and well-evaluated aspects of intrapartum care – the provision of continuous support for labouring women (Hodnett *et al.*, 2005). Anthropologists Rosenberg and Trevathan (2003) would conclude, a decade later, that childbirth has evolved over tens of thousands of years to be social because of the pain and travail that accompanies it. The role of the companions was to provide social support, not medical intervention.

The data from women's experience of labour reveal a richly nuanced account of the staff's role, oscillating between leaving alone and intense one-to-one support. The following field notes were recorded during an early shift:

'The woman was having her first baby and was obviously deep into herself, not really wanting to talk. The midwife said that she did not say a word to her until an hour had passed. This surprised me because, although women are like that in consultant units, once they get into the second stage of labour, they usually require the continuous presence of the midwife. But this woman was in the second stage of labour and still did not want the midwife in the room most of the time.' (Observation no. 4: 2)

Contrast this with a midwife's account of a labour where she was supporting her colleague:

'A teenage girl [Rachel] came in with her mother and sister. The girl became extremely distressed in the middle of the labour. She was thrashing around on the bed, so we took the bed out. Bev [the midwife] wondered whether her distress was due to the awesome responsibility of parenthood that she felt she wasn't ready for, so Bev asked her Mum and her sister to leave the room. Then she just sat with her for two hours on the floor and this girl was just sobbing into her lap, just sobbing, and then after two hours – almost as if it was out of her system – she was completely more focused and she went on and had a really good birth.' (Kerry, Transcript no. 45: 7)

Both stories illustrate the skill of promoting an appropriate emotional ambience for labour.

'Nesting' responses

All of this data emphasizes the importance of environmental, organizational and emotional ambience to women and staff in providing an appropriate setting for birth. In searching for an explanation for these behaviours and beliefs, I reprised an old-fashioned midwifery concept: nesting. Nesting was mentioned in midwifery textbooks up until the mid-1980s, when it was used to explain maternal behaviours during pregnancy (Myles, 1981). During the first 12 weeks of gestation, nesting was said to cause tiredness and lethargy that slowed women's activity during the critical embryonic phase of foetal development. Nesting behaviours returned in the weeks preceding the birth and were marked by a drive to prepare the baby's immediate environment. Decorating the nursery, purchasing the layette, cleaning and tidying the home surrounds were said to be manifestations of nesting. For reasons that are not immediately apparent, references to nesting disappeared from midwifery textbooks around the mid-1980s and only rarely appear in midwifery books today (England and Horowitz, 1996). They survive in populist magazines on new motherhood, on Internet sites; see, for example, *Nesting* (2010) and in the self-help literature around childbirth (Robertson, 1997).

Nesting links humans to the large mammalian species, where these behaviours are usually understood to be grounded in instinct – a much more problematic notion for humans because of the layers of socialization and learned behaviours that suffuse human learning and development. In reference to human behaviour, Davis-Floyd and Arvidson (1997) prefer the term 'intuition' to 'instinct', as it encompasses emotional and thinking components. Using the characteristics of an intuitive response, as identified by Bastick (1982), the women's focus on the birth environment appears strongly intuitive in nature. Bastick named these characteristics of intuition as:

- sudden, immediacy of awareness
- association of affect with insight
- non-analytical, non-rational, non-logical, gestalt nature of experience
- empathic, preverbal
- sense of certainty of the truth of insights.

The women's comments were suggestive of some or all of these features:

'... as soon as we walked in we thought – yep! This is the sort of place.' (Jasmine, Transcript no. 9: 2)

'I got stuck on it.' (Mary, Transcript no. 9: 3)

'I could picture myself there.' (Julie, Transcript no. 26: 3)

'It's really something you can't definitely put your finger on, which makes it so difficult when you're talking about it because it's so much in a woman's own mind. It's a feeling rather than an empirical value system. A woman knows immediately when it's the right atmosphere.' (Carmel, Transcript no. 21: 4)

The sense of immediacy and certainty about the birth centre being an appropriate site for birth comes through here. The final comments articulate clearly the difficulty of explaining exactly why that certainty is felt, and the visualization confirms the involvement of the non-rational, emotionally-mediated brain functions. The staff's comments reinforce this reading of the women's experience. Margaret, an MCA, told me:

'They often say "I've been to other hospitals and they're nothing like this." "This really feels like the place I would like to have my baby in." I have even had mums talking to their babies saying "This is where we want to be isn't it, in here?"' (Transcript no. 42: 4)

Gerry, a midwife, added:

'Usually people are terrified of hospitals, but they walk in and say, "It's not like a hospital is it?" I think they feel a friendly, calm atmosphere. You can see them relaxing and the look on their faces, every room they go into.' (Transcript no. 31: 6)

Clearly, the dominance of feeling seems to take precedence over a more cerebral consideration of other factors and Louise, the previous clinical leader, explicitly links what she observes in women to her understanding of animal behaviour (Transcript no. 43: 5).

Components of nesting

The intuitive 'feel' of this data reinforces the notion of nesting as an appropriate explanatory framework. Nesting activity is about preparing a safe place for offspring where, once born, they can be protected from harm. Animals and mammals, in particular, will go to extraordinary lengths to prepare such a place, and will guard it fiercely once birth has occurred (Attenborough, 1990; Cronin et al., 1996). Protection and safety may be driving women's decisions here, but applied in an alternative way that explores notions of safety beyond mortality and morbidity statistics. The possibility of seeing safety more broadly has been raised by Hirst (2004, 2005) in her review of maternity services in Queensland, Australia. In part, she was responding to a 'cultural safety' agenda regarding maternity care and indigenous groups that Ramsden (2003) had first brought to public consciousness in New Zealand. But, equally, one could speak of social and psychological safety, and these dimensions to safety are strongly hinted at in the women's accounts. Being greeted by a staff member holding a baby impressed one woman, although at one level it appears a very normal occurrence in a maternity unit. Yet, due to institutional constraints related to health and safety, this would be an unlikely occurrence in a larger hospital. In this case, the woman concluded that the birth centre was clearly a baby-friendly place where, by inference, their emotional and nurturing needs would be met. There is a sense of social safety in the request by a woman to have her teenage children present in the centre during her labour, and women's direct communication with their babies in utero as they walk around the centre suggests strong connections to an emotional comfort zone or psychological safety.

Women's nesting response appears to be unrelated to the risk discourse of childbirth safety (Bassett *et al.*, 2000; Tracey, 2006). Their thinking inverts the risk discourse's logic of protection and safety by deliberately choosing a non-medical environment for birth. Many redefined the birth centre as a hotel, 'like home', or a health farm, to disconnect it from a hospital ambience. For these women, protection and safety appeared to mean reducing the risk of iatrogenesis, associated in their minds with hospital birth. Nesting as protection and safety could also be linked to the friendliness, peace and relaxation that they experienced on visiting the centre. These qualities point to the balancing of the stress of labour, experienced internally with peaceful surrounds externally.

Women were seeking a birth ambience characterized by compassion, warmth, nurture and love. This was not just in evidence at the birth centre by the welcome, hospitality and the care they received, but also by the attention to detail that the staff had put into preparing the birth space. There is a sense in which the staff spent their working lives 'preparing for a baby'. At any moment, women may come through the door in labour and the staff's raison d'être is providing for that eventuality. Their preparing is not an idle pastime but a sustained, continuous activity as they are constantly adapting, making-over and maintaining the birth space. It is environmental nurture. There was also a spatial dimension to honing the environmental ambience – an absence of 'no-go' geographical locations within the centre. Both the women and staff interviews and the field notes recorded incidents of women, particularly during the evening and night, sitting down in the staff room and chatting with midwives and MCAs. The room was where staff went for their breaks and had a number of comfortable chairs, magazines and a television. Women and their relatives also entered the office where all the computing, telephone activity and shift handovers occurred. These actions break a strong taboo in institutions, where space is used to distribute power and to construct identities (Halford and Leonard, 2003). It contrasts with ethnographies of consultant delivery suites where there were not only prohibitions to some areas for women, but also for some ranks of staff (Hunt and Symonds, 1995; Yearley, 1999).

Human nesting instinct appears to seek out the right emotional ambience for childbearing, which is as integral to establishing a protective, safe place for birth as are the immediate physical surrounds. This marks human beings out as different from other mammals, who primarily seek solitude (Rosenberg and Trevathan, 2003). Demere *et al.* (2002) observe that, in the animal kingdom, the complexity of nesting increases as the need for parental care increases. A suitable nest is needed to continue the rearing of a newborn until it is mature enough to fend for itself: therefore, because human offspring are developmentally very immature at birth in comparison with many other mammals (Allport, 1997), women may seek out this broader range of factors when selecting an appropriate place to birth. Part of this may be making an intuitive and rapid appraisal of emotional and environmental ambience.

These findings from researching care in birth centres suggest that both women and staff will manifest nesting-like behaviours when 'freed' from the culture of hospital birth. These behaviours conceptualize safety across several domains – physical, psychological and social, emphasizing their mediation through relationships and the birth environment. The relationship focus involves a hitherto unrecognized dynamic in women's assessment of the suitability of a place of birth – its emotional ambience. Their interest in a suitable physical environment has been known about and responded to by services across the western world, as Fannon (2003) elaborates. What had been slow to be acknowledged is the potential of staff to hone environmental ambience, with consequent impact on emotional ambience, if given the remit and freedom to pursue this.

'Mother-like' care

Rachel's story described her long latent phase of labour, related earlier (p. 182), during which she was becoming very distressed. It appeared that, through a cathartic experience of emotional release, when the midwife held her in an embrace lasting two hours as she wept, Rachel reached a place of accepting her labour and the imminent birth of her baby. In this situation, the midwife could be said to have intuited an appropriate response to the girl's distress that would not be found in textbooks or within the paradigm of a biomedical model. Leap and Anderson (2004) have written that a common response of midwives to the distress of labour is treating it with a variety of pharmacological pain-relieving agents. They argue for an alternative approach, which they call 'working with pain'. This recognizes that labour pain has a physiological purpose but that it can also indicate emotional distress. The midwifery skill is in discerning these differences. Simkin and Ancheta (2005), in their book on labour progress, explore the cause of labour delay from a holistic perspective, suggesting that simply diagnosing uterine inertia is too reductionist as an explanation. In many cases of delay, a psychological component is likely to be a contributory factor, and they urge childbirth attendants to be sensitive to this possibility.

For Rachel, the 'becoming mother' journey had been a traumatic one, and the midwife's empathic care for her in labour had smoothed her path.

Another episode of care illustrated a similar dynamic. An hour after giving birth, Sarah called the midwife, complaining of abdominal pain. It was so severe that she felt cold, clammy and faint. The midwife examined her but did not feel there was any serious clinical reason for her pain. The field note continues:

'Jenny [the midwife] managed it by just sort of cradling the woman in her arms, resting her head on her lap and holding it gently and massaging her hair and scalp in a very sort of motherly, maternal way. And she did that for a long time, 20–30 minutes. Just sort of held her safe I suppose.' (Observation no. 14: 4)

During the postnatal interview, I asked Sarah about her experience of care at this point:

'She [midwife] was great afterwards because it was like having my Mum there. I remember having my head on her lap and she was just stroking the back of my head saying you will be all right. Just kind of nursing you, which was invaluable. It was like you were her daughter.' (Sarah, Transcript no. 28: 6)

Comfort and protection emanate from this incident. For Sarah, it was as a mother would care for her child.

Mothering manifested in another guise postnatally. Unlike postnatal stay times throughout the Western world, women at the birth centre frequently stayed more than three days following a normal birth. During this time, they were pampered and made to feel special. As Monica recalled:

'The next morning the tables were laid and there were lots of choices for breakfast. There were slices of melon and they had put cling film over – just lots of little things that you wouldn't expect. That evening they cooked us tea. There were only three of us so they gave us the attention there. You know when you get home, everything starts.' (Monica, Transcript no. 25: 6)

Birth centre staff seemed aware of the stresses of postnatal adjustment at home, as Nerissa states in her interview:

'They said "if you're happy to stay for the week and have that rest, then do it". And I did not kind of expect this with my second child. And they said, 'you're just as important as what he is and if you don't feel well enough to go home, you just stay with us and let us look after him a bit longer. Be spoilt for a couple of days more because when you go home, it's a twenty-four hour job and there's no switch off.' (Narissa, Transcript no. 13: 11)

Women really appreciated the little treats they received from the staff, which included ice drinks while in the jacuzzi, tea and biscuits for afternoon tea, and caring for their babies at night so the women could sleep. A staff member hand-washed a nightdress for one woman who had very few items of clothing with her.

Sharon, an MCA who worked permanent nights, told me the following story, illustrating a mothering response to the plight of staff:

'The girls here have been marvellous to me I have to say. Problems that I have had at home with elderly relatives dying of cancer. I've had a load of hassle and they have been really good. I've come in on nights and been knackered, not had any sleep and they have tucked me up in bed for a couple of hours.' (Sharon, Transcript no. 41: 6)

This anecdote borders on the subversive and, when I retold it to other midwives, some commented that sleeping on duty was a sackable offence. But here, it is an extension of the empathy shown to women and a poignant example of compassion to fellow colleagues.

There were other examples of the support the staff have received and have freely given when colleagues have been in need:

'If you come in and start your day and need a bit of counselling, they say "come on let's have a cup of tea" or "why are you so miserable today?" That's what's good about here.' (Sandra, Transcript no. 37: 14)

In all of these accounts, the midwives express a 'mothering' dimension to care.

Sketching matrescence

In the stories of Rachel (held in an embrace and consoled by the midwife as she experienced early labour) and Sarah (comforted when in pain postnatally), the midwives respond intuitively. These are non-verbal, empathic actions that spring from fairly immediate insight and awareness. There is no obvious logical or rational analysis guiding them to embrace the women in the way they did. Their actions may have been preceded by a biophysical assessment that eliminated pathology in their minds, but then the midwives appear to tap into a protective, nurturing reservoir that could be understood as 'matrescent' or 'of matrescence' (Thomas, 2001) – becoming mother. Matrescence was first coined by Raphael (1973) to emphasize that birth often 'becomes' a new mother as well as a new baby, an idea that has been echoed since by Wickham (2002) and Thomas (2001). Thomas writes of matrescence as spiritual formation, drawing analogies with the Judo-Christian tradition. Using neglected Old Testament imagery of the fecundity of God in giving birth to creation, of nurturing the people of Israel as a mother suckles her child at the breast, and of protecting the nation from harm as a hen protects its chickens, she argues for a new spiritual examination of birth as a rite-of-passage experience. It is these images of nurture and protection that can be applied to the caring by the birth attendants here. Sarah alludes to it in her extract – 'it was like having my Mum there', and Bev offers protection and nurture in place of the mother of the teenage girl. In another interview, a woman said of labour: 'you just want your Mum'.

Thomas (2001) explored another, more clearly ethical dimension to matrescence in her reflections on the physicality of pregnancy (two in one), and of childbirth (one becoming two) in the sense of selfless commitment to another. Cosslett (1994) commenting on this, notes that the concept can radically challenge the idea of the autonomous, individual subject. This connection between mother and child, although severed physically by the cutting of the cord, remains intact as the child grows, drawing selflessness and agape (Christian notion of disinterested love, as opposed to erotic love) from her. It is a kind of unconditional love that finds meaning in giving.

Matrescent care, understood in this way, incorporates an ethical disposition. It prioritizes the value of another (the baby) and responsibility to care for it. If authentic, it would manifest more broadly than in just relationships with the birth centre women. One would expect to witness its affect among staff. Sharon's experience when she was 'tucked up in bed' is one poignant example. It moved her to conclude her tale with: 'I love this place. It has been really good to me.' Sandra too, spoke of the support received from other staff at the start of a shift when you: 'need a bit of counselling'. All these actions can all be seen as matrescent in the sense of 'mothering', nurturing and protecting work colleagues. Cosslett's (1994) idea of connection to 'other' overriding the needs of the autonomous self is demonstrated by these actions.

In parallel to the metaphor of 'home' regularly spoken of by the women, so the staff used the analogy of 'family'. 'We are family here' said Sandra, an MCA, in her interview. 'It's like a family' and 'it's a family sort of thing', or 'like a second family' were other comments.

However, caution is required. Notions of home and family, idealized here as a site and environment of nurture and belonging, can be problematized. For some women and their children, home and family are places of abuse, rejection and deprivation (Mooney, 1994; Barlow and Birch, 2004). Easy elision of an optimum birth environment with the domestic setting is misleading, unless contextual meanings are made explicit. It was clear from the data that the use of this language here was intended to convey positive interpretations of home and family.

In the same way, feminist critiques of the social construction of motherhood problematize essentialist characteristics ascribed to the role (Oakley, 1993). These roles have stereotyped women as instinctive carers and home-makers, masking women's disadvantage in the private domestic sphere compared with men's position and power in the public sphere (Bordo, 1993; Upton and Han, 2003). For this reason, 'matrescence' is a better term than 'maternalism', as the latter is laden with this gender baggage. I understand matrescence as a skill in facilitating the becoming of a mother, which has generic application to either gender.

Underlying the women's gratitude for their experience of postnatal care in the birth centre may be the reality that, although becoming a mother is a major rite-of-passage event, Western cultures have all but lost its ritual-marking. Kitzinger (2000) writes, regarding indigenous cultures, of the 'sacred lying-in periods', often up to 40 days, when the woman and her baby are in a transitional, liminal stage. Other women nurture the woman into motherhood so that the mother is freed of her usual responsibilities and can 'grow with' her baby. The activity and focus of carers is to protect, to nurture and to cherish the new mother and baby.

'Care as gift'

Fox (1999) brings another lens to this analysis in his sociological critique of the professional/client relationship within the health services. He suggests that care encounters within health care are often of the 'vigil of care' variety. By this, he means that they are often surveillance-orientated and premised on a deferential relationship between client and professional. There is an expectation that the professional's expert knowledge will hold sway. His critique resonates with

Kirkham's (1996) deconstruction of 'professionalism' to reveal it as an instrument of power and coercion. It is as if the professional polices the care encounter. Fox contrasts the vigil of 'care' with 'care as gift', which he posits as a liberating alternative. 'Care as gift' is characteri\ed by trust, delight, commitment, generosity and love. It has no agenda except to encounter the other in openness and mutual respect, so that they can make health care choices with integrity.

His ideas have resonance in the maternity care context with the writings on the midwife/mother relationship. Kirkham (2000), among others, has understood this relationship as somewhat distinct from other health care professional/client alliances. This distinction has been premised on unique features such as its biologically determined longevity, its continuity through a major rite-of-passage experience, the intimate nature of its focus and the wellness status of most of the women undertaking the journey. Therefore, descriptors of the relationship have emphasized equality, partnership (Pairman, 2000), solidarity, skilled companionship (Page, 1995) and the 'professional as friend' (Walsh, 1999). Despite these descriptors, organizational methods of working have frustrated midwives' attempts to realize their potential as they struggle to establish continuity in a fragmented service and to be advocates for women within a system that makes them feel oppressed (Ball *et al.*, 2003).

The fact that labour and birth services are structured around a predominantly biomedical model has also undermined midwife/women relationships. Machin and Scamell (1997) found that women previously orientated to non-interventionist, self-directed birth submitted to an interventionist package as they encountered the 'irresistible biomedical metaphor' during labour. Midwives were the mediator of that package. Deference and paternalism marked women's response to midwives in Bluff and Holloway's study (1994) where the phrase 'they know best' was frequently used by women. Equality, partnership and authentic choice for women are a chimera within a system of professional dominance.

Midwives' own belief systems heavily influence how they relate with women and can lead to 'gently steering' women to make choices the midwives want them to make (Levy, 1999) or to agreeing to women's request for home birth but then proceed to do a 'hospital birth at home' (Edwards, 2000). All of these behaviours could be classified as having 'vigil of care' characteristics (Fox, 1998) and are a disciplining of the care relationship, hedging it round with conditions and caveats that disempower women.

Stories from the life of the birth centre stand out as different precisely because they demonstrate a reversal of this – a giving up of power by midwives and an expression of genuine agency by women as Sarah experienced. The midwife's intervention was to nurture her, holding her in a matrescent embrace, providing 'care as gift'. She is resisting an imperative 'to act' that Fox (1999) aligns with the 'vigil of care'. To embrace physically and to hold taps the relational and intuitive domains, rather than the rational and instrumental. Her care was highly appreciated by Sarah, as communicated to me during interview after the events.

Another episode of care illustrates how choices widen as 'care as gift' is enacted:

'It was the week before Christmas and I had one lady who was five centimetres when she came in. Actually, she was really more six but she was desperate to get her Christmas shopping done – you know she had this little window of time to do it and now this! So, because the labour wasn't that strong, she decided she would return to her shopping and come back afterwards. She came back and delivered a couple of hours later ... I was still here when she came back and she got her shopping done and then she went home that night after the baby was born. You have got to be flexible here.' (Gerry, midwife, Transcript no. 31: 2)

Once a woman comes into a hospital in established labour, she is kept under constant surveillance. A clinical imperative (to ensure labour is progressing at an acceptable rate (O'Driscoll and Meager, 1986)), an organizational imperative (to ensure she moves seamlessly through the hospital labour spaces (Perkins, 2004), and a professional imperative (to ensure she complies with clinician's instructions/advice (Anderson, 2004)) drive this requirement. Here, as Gerry describes, all three imperatives are subverted. The expression of agency is related to a tangential issue – the need to complete the Christmas shopping – but one that impacts on the labour because of the multiple responsibilities the woman carries. This is acknowledged by the midwife who gives her space to consider what would not normally be in the frame: returning to a supermarket in advanced labour. 'Care as gift' is realized here because the midwife demonstrates unconditional and non-reciprocal giving. She has resisted the normative professional discourse which inscribes both herself and the woman with appropriate roles for this scenario. Concomitantly, the woman sheds a normative patient subjectivity in asserting the option to leave the birth centre and return to her shopping.

One begins to glimpse Fox's attributes of 'care as gift' in this encounter: trust, confidence, generosity, admiration, allegiance. 'Care as gift' found poignant expression in a midwife's response to Jenny, who came into the birth centre in early labour and who was comforted on the floor for two hours. Here is an engagement that eschews 'doing to' for 'being with'. The 'doing to' in maternity hospitals would probably have involved administering some analgesia to relieve the pain. Such an act confirms the ordering of professional care as task-mediated, discrete and temporally-bounded. No such restrictions applied in this encounter. It was an open-ended interaction as the midwife could not have known that they would be on the floor for two hours. Her disposition is not to task but, rather, to engagement and connection: what Fox calls a 'responsibility to otherness'. She literally makes space (on the floor) for Jenny to express herself until she is ready to move on. It's as if she says: 'Here's some space for you ... go for it ... get on with it ... I trust and have confidence in you ... take my generosity of spirit' (Fox, 1998: 37)

Other attributes of 'care as gift' are in evidence in the episode where a staff member, exhausted when coming on night duty, slept for a couple of hours at the staff's invitation. Love and commitment are demonstrated in an inversion of the normal disciplining of the 'vigil of care'. Sleeping on duty would be unacceptable in most health care settings but, here, it is an outworking of compassion for a staff member going through a crisis. This demonstration of altruistic, non-reciprocal giving, directed towards the staff serves to confirm the authenticity and integrity of its expression in their relationships with the women.

Conceptualizing birth centre care as 'gift' enables some fleshing out of the characteristics of matrescent care when enacted in the professional/woman relationship.

Conclusion

Towards a synthesis of matrescence, nesting and 'care as gift'

Matrescence seems to tread a delicate path between listening, talking, showing, observing and leaving alone. A woman alluded to this when she commented in relation to her labour: 'They let me get on and find my own rhythm'. Others reflecting on their postnatal care said 'there was no fussing over you'. I have written of the difference between a 'being' disposition and a 'doing' disposition in the staff's approach to care, with the former being less time-bound (Walsh, 2009). It made space for relational and emotional work. Matrescent care requires a level of nuance-reading that is suggestive of an acute emotional intelligence (Goleman, 1996), and is sometimes recognized more easily by the absence of unhelpful behaviours (paternalism, being patronising) and attitudes (indifference and fear of intimacy). These traits are features of the 'vigil of care' paradigm.

Women recognized nurturing in care encounters when the staff response to them reminded them of their mothers. It smoothed the path of the early days of new motherhood, giving due recognition to this significant rite-of-passage experience ushered in by childbirth. Matrescence could be understood as an attitude of care as much as an attribute of care, because it permeated birth centre relationships generally.

These findings lead me to believe that midwives should seek ways to rehabilitate 'nurture' and 'love', derivative of matrescence, as familiar childbirth language and as mainstream caring activities in childbirth. These have been emasculated by the industrial model of birth, which reifies management rhetoric in labour care (Walsh, 2003), and by a professional paradigm that locates midwives and women in different planes of being (Wilkins, 2000). Matrescence as an attribute and attitude of care may also help professional birth attendants to reconnect with their empathic and intuitive self (Hunter *et al.*, 2008).

Returning to intuition completes the symmetry between matrescence and nesting. Within the childbirth carer, both seem to tap a reservoir of protection and nurture, and both could reciprocally work to enhance each other. Thus, nesting may also trigger matrescent behaviours as an extension of providing the optimum emotional ambience for birth, and matrescence inspires the refining of environmental conditions to support nesting. For the mother, nesting coaxes her towards the right space and place to give birth; matrescence, as enacted by the staff towards her, facilitates her own 'becoming mother' journey.

Both nesting and matrescence are realized and lived out through relational encounters, encounters that exhibit 'care as gift' features. Together these concepts reveal an alternative way of organizing and doing birth that should fire the imagination of all childbirth practitioners who are searching for an alternative to medically managed, industrially organized birthing provision.

ACTIVITIES

Undergraduate

How do women construct the notions of protection and safety in relation to the birth space when birth is within a hospital setting?

Postgraduate

If nesting helps explain women and staff's emphasis on the birth environment's physical and emotional ambience, then how might some of the care interactions be conceptualized and tested?

References

Allport, S. (1997) *A Natural History of Parenting*. New York, NY: Harmony.

Anderson, T. (2004) 'The Misleading Myth of Choice: The Continuing Oppression of Women in Childbirth', in M. Kirkham (ed.), *Informed Choice in Maternity Care*. Basingstoke: Palgrave MacMillan, ch. 13.

Annandale, E. (1987) 'Dimensions of Patient Control in a Free-Standing Birth Centre', *Social Science & Medicine*, 25(11): 1235–48.

Annandale, E. (1988) 'How Midwives Accomplish Natural Birth: Managing Risk and Balancing Expectations', *Social Problems*, 5(2): 95–110.

Attenborough, D. (1990) *The Trials of Life*. London: Collins.

Ball, L., Curtis, P. and Kirkham, M. (2003) *Why Do Midwives Leave?* London: Royal College of Midwives.

Barlow, J. and Birch, L. (2004) 'Midwifery Practice and Sexual Abuse', *British Journal of Midwifery*, 12(2): 72–5.

Bassett, K., Iyer, N. and Kazanjian, A. (2000) 'Defensive Medicine during Hospital Obstetric Care: A By-product of the Technological Age', *Social Science & Medicine*, 51(4): 532–7.

Bastick, T. (1982) *Intuition: How We Think and Act*. New York, NY: John Wiley.

Bluff, R. and Holloway, I. (1994) 'They Know Best': Women's Perceptions of Midwifery Care During Labour and Childbirth', *Midwifery*, 10(3): 157–64.

Bordo, S. (1993) *Unbearable Weight: Feminism, Western Culture and the Body*. London: University of California Press.

Cosslett, T. (1994) *Women Writing Childbirth: Modern Discourses on Motherhood*. Manchester: Manchester University Press.

Cronin, G., Simpson, G. and Hemsworth, P. (1996) 'The Effects of Gestation and Farrowing Environments on Sow and Piglet Behaviour and Piglet Survival and Growth in Early Lactation', *Applied Animal Behaviour Science*, 46(3–4): 175–92.

Davis-Floyd, R. and Arvidson, P. (1997) *Intuition: The Inside Story. Interdisciplinary Perspectives*. New York, NY: Routledge.

Demere, T., Hollingsworth, B. and Unitt, P. (2002) 'Nests and Nest-Building Animals', *Field Notes*, spring: 13–15.

Dykes, F. (2005) 'A Critical Ethnographic Study of Encounters between Midwives and Breast-Feeding Women in Postnatal Wards in England', *Midwifery*, 21(3): 241–52.

Edwards, N. (2000) 'Woman Planning Homebirths: Their Own Views on their Relationships with Midwives', in M. Kirkham (ed.), *The Midwife–Woman Relationship*. Basingstoke: Palgrave Macmillan, ch. 5: 55–91.

England, P. and Horowitz, R. (1996) *Birthing from Within*. Albuquerque, NM: Partera Press.

Esposito, N.W. (1999) 'Marginalised Women's Comparisons of their Hospital and Free-Standing Birth Centre Experience: A Contract of Inner City Birthing Centres', *Health Care for Women International*, 20(2): 111–26.

Fannon, M. (2003) 'Domesticating Birth in the Hospital: "Family-centred" Birth and the Emergence of "Homelike" Birthing Rooms', *Antipode*, 35(3): 513–35.

Fox, N. (1998) 'The Promise of Postmodernism for the Sociology of Health and Medicine', in G. Scambler and P. Higgs (eds), *Modernity, Medicine and Health*. London: Routledge, ch. 2: 29–44.

Fox, N. (1999) *Beyond Health: Postmodernism and Embodiment*. London: Free Association Books.

Goleman, D. (1996) *Emotional Intelligence*. London: Bloomsbury.

Halford, S. and Leonard, P. (2003) 'Space and Place in the Construction and Performance of Gendered Nursing Identities', *Journal of Advanced Nursing*, 42(2): 201–8.

Hammersley, M. and Atkinson, P. (1995) *Ethnography: Principles in Practice*. London: Routledge.

Hirst, C. (2004) Personal communication.

Hirst, C. (2005) 'Re-Birthing', Report of the Review of Maternity Services in Queensland. Brisbane: Queensland Health

Hodnett, E.D., Gates, S., Hofmeyr, G.J. and Sakala, C. (2005) 'Continuous Support for Women During Childbirth' (Cochrane Review), in the *Cochrane Library*, 1. Chichester: John Wiley.

Hunt, S. and Symonds, A. (1995) *The Social Meaning of Midwifery*. London: Macmillan.

Hunter, B., Berg, M., Lundgren, I. and Kirkham, M. (2008) 'Relationships: The Hidden Threads in the Tapestry of Maternity Care', *Midwifery*, 24(2): 132–7.

Kirkham, M. (1988) 'Midwives and Information-Giving During Labour', in S. Robinson and A. Thompson, (eds), *Midwives, Research and Childbirth, Volume 1*. London: Chapman & Hall: 117–38.

Kirkham, M. (1996) 'Professionalisation Past and Present', in D. Kroll (ed.), *Midwifery Care of the Future: Meeting the Challenge*. London: Bailliere Tindall: 164–201.

Kirkham, M. (2000) 'How Can We Relate?', in M Kirkham (ed.), *The Midwife–Woman Relationship*. Basingstoke: Palgrave Macmillan, ch. 12: 227–50.

Kitzinger, S. (2000) *Rediscovering Birth*. London: Little, Brown & Co.

Leap, N. and Anderson, T. (2004) 'The Role of Pain in Normal Birth and the Empowerment of Women', in S. Downe and C. McCourt (eds), *Normal Childbirth: Evidence and Debate*. London: Churchill Livingstone: 25–40.

Levy, V. (1999) 'Protective Steering: A Grounded Theory Study of the Processes Involved when Midwives Facilitate Informed Choice During Pregnancy', *Journal of Advanced Nursing*, 29(1): 104–12.

Machin, D. and Scamell, M. (1997) 'The Experience of Labour: Using Ethnography to Explore the Irresistible Nature of the Bio-medical Metaphor during Labour', *Midwifery*, 13(2): 78–84.

Mooney, J. (1994) *The Hidden Figure: Domestic Violence in North London*. Islington: Islington Police and Crime Prevention Unit.

Myles, M. (1981) *Myles Textbook for Midwives*. Edinburgh: Churchill Livingstone. 'Nesting' (2010) www.parents.com – accessed 24 July 2010.

Oakley, A. (1993) *Essays on Women, Medicine and Health*. Edinburgh: Edinburgh University Press.

O'Driscoll, K. and Meager, D. (1986) *Active Management of Labour: the Dublin Experience*. 2nd edn. London: Balliere Tindall.

Page, L. (1995) 'A Vision for the Future. The Challenge of Changing Childbirth', *Midwifery Educational Resource Pack No. 6*. London: English National Board.

Pairman, S. (2000) 'Women-Centred Midwifery: Partnerships or Professional Friendships?', in M. Kirkham (ed.), *The Midwife–Mother Relationship*. Basingstoke: Palgrave Macmillan, ch. 11: 207–26.

Perkins, B. (2004) *The Medical Delivery Business: Health Reform, Childbirth, and the Economic Order*. London: Rutgers University Press.

Ramsden, I. (2003) 'Cultural Safety and Nursing Education in Aotearoa and Te Waipounamu', PhD thesis. (http://culturalsafety.masey.ac.nz – accessed 24 July 2010).

Raphael, D. (1973) *The Tender Gift: Breastfeeding*. New York, NY: Schocken Books.

Robertson, A. (1997) *The Midwife Companion*. Sydney: Ace Graphics.

Rosenberg, K. and Trevathan, W. (2003) 'Birth, Obstetrics and Human Evolution', *British Journal of Obstetrics and Gynaecology*, 109(11): 1199–206.

Simkin, P. and Ancheta, R. (2005) *The Labour Progress Handbook*. Oxford: Blackwell Science.

Smith, L. and Smith, C. (2005) 'UK Childbirth Delivery Options in 2001–2002: Alternatives to Consultant Unit Booking and Delivery', *British Journal of General Practice*, 55(513): 292–7.

Thomas, T. (2001) 'Becoming a Mother: Matrescence as Spiritual Formation', *Religious Education*, 96(1): 88–105.

Tracey, S. (2006) 'Risk: Theoretical or Actual?', in L. Page and R. McCandlish (eds), *The New Midwifery: Science and Sensitivity in Practice*. London: Elsevier.

Upton, R. and Han, S. (2003) 'Maternity and its Discontents', *Journal of Contemporary Ethnography*, 32(6): 670–92.

Walker, J. (2000) 'Women's Experiences of Transfer from a Midwife-Led Unit to a Consultant-Led Maternity Unit in the UK during Late Pregnancy and Labour', *Journal of Midwifery and Women's Health*, 45(2): 161–7.

Walsh, D. (1999) 'An Ethnographic Study of Women's Experience of Partnership Caseload Midwifery Practice: The Professional as Friend', *Midwifery*, 15(3): 165–76.

Walsh, D. (2003) 'Feminism and Intrapartum Care: A Quest for Holistic Birth', in M. Stewart (ed.), *Pregnancy, Birth and Maternity Care: Feminist Perspectives*. London: Books for Midwives: 57–71.

Walsh, D. (2004) 'Becoming Mother: An Ethnography of a Free-standing Birth Centre', Unpublished PhD thesis, University of Central Lancashire, Preston.

Walsh, D. (2009) ' "Waiting on Birth": Management of Time and Place in a Birth Centre', in C. McCourt (ed.), *Childbirth, Midwifery and Concepts of Time*. Oxford: Berghahn Books, ch. 6: 126–44.

Wickham, S. (2002) 'Reclaiming Spirituality in Birth' (http://www.withwoman.co.uk/contents/info/spiritualbirth.html – accessed 24 July 2010).

Wilkins, R. (2000) 'Poor Relations: The Paucity of the Professional Paradigm', in M. Kirkham (ed.), *The Midwife–Mother Relationship*. Basingstoke: Palgrave Macmillan, ch. 4: 28–54.

Yearley, C. (1999) 'Pre-Registration Student Midwives: Fitting in', *British Journal of Midwifery*, 7(10): 627–31.

Exploring the Presence of Comfort within the Context of Childbirth

9

Kerri Durnell Schuiling, Carolyn Sampselle and Kathryn Kolcaba

---

Key points

- Comfort is common, and is commonly sought by us all: comfort is a desirable outcome of midwifery care
- Comfort is most often described in relation to experiences that deprive of us of comfort
- Comfort is a bi-dimensional concept and consists within technical senses (ease, relief and transcendence) and contexts (physical, social, psychospiritual and environmental)
- Comfort can be a strengthening experience.

Introduction

I chose to study comfort during labour because it seemed to me that much of what midwives do for birthing women is to provide comfort (KS). We assist women and support them during labour, and encourage them to use techniques that are comforting. In the United States, labour is defined within a biomedical context, and much of the care during labour is typically provided within this context. Obstetricians' education rightly focuses on how to treat pain and disease so it should come as no surprise that treating the pain of labour is common. Appreciating use of comfort measures and providing comfort during labour is undervalued in some health systems, except by health care practitioners, such as midwives, who commonly use non-pharmacologic methods to support women during labour; methods that comfort women during a very intense and painful experience.

Kathryn Kolcaba developed her theory of comfort within a framework of health. Her studies focused initially on comfort and the terminally ill, but the theory is applicable to any type of health care situation or context. In fact, more recently, comfort theory was used as a unifying framework to enhance the practice environment (Kolcaba, *et al.*, 2006) and was modified and used to direct patient care and the work of health care providers (March and McCormack, 2009). In the latter instance, the potential to facilitate greater understanding amongst disciplines and greater continuity of care for patients was realised. Dr Kolcaba assisted me in developing a Childbirth Comfort Questionnaire (CCQ), which is based on her original theory and the General Comfort Questionnaire. For further information on the theory and framework, suggestions for research and methodology for adapting the General Comfort Questionnaire for use in research, see Kolcaba (2010).

Comfort theory provided a framework that enables viewing labour and childbirth through a holistic lens; a lens that midwives use when providing care for women during labour. When care is committed to providing comfort, needs for relief, ease and/or transcendence are identified, and interventions to meet these needs can then be developed and implemented (Kolcaba and Dimarco, 2005). Comfort theory is health oriented, thus supporting the concept of normal birth. This chapter provides an overview of research undertaken by Schuiling (2003), which used comfort theory in a group of normally labouring, primiparous women. Some women were attended by midwives, others by physicians, and all received care from registered nurses. The focus of the project was to determine whether the phenomenon of comfort did actually exist during labour, and whether women could identify it as such. If comfort did exist, the next step was to explore its relationship to pain. Although the study is small (n = 64 participants, of which 53 women completed all phases of the project), it reveals new knowledge and supports the need for further studies of comfort during childbirth.

The research project

Introduction

Comfort, a holistic phenomenon and basic human need, is welcomed by most individuals because it brings about desired sensations of ease and/or relief (Schuiling and Sampselle, 1999). Seeking comfort is normal for both healthy and ill individuals. In fact, seeking comfort is one of the more common reasons people obtain health care. The concept of comfort during labour however, is a paradox to some. Interestingly though, narratives of birthing women suggest they experience sensations of both pain and comfort (Helser, 1998; Lundgren and Dahlberg, 1998) during the birthing process and that, even though the two sensations are very different, one gives meaning to the other. Additionally, those who care for birthing women would probably agree that providing comfort is an important aspect of care. Research about processes of care during labour suggests that when comforting measures are used and comfort is experienced, that comfort may be a strengthening factor during labour and may enable women to use less analgesia (Simkin, 1995).

Alleviation of pain is identified as a means of providing comfort and support to women in labour (Hodnett, 1996). Weber (1996) identifies the recognition and treatment of pain and discomfort as critical elements in the care of maternity clients. Pain adversely affects comfort, and few would argue that childbirth is not painful. However, birthing women have identified that relief of pain during labour does not necessarily result in a satisfying birth experience (Hummenick and Bugen, 1981; Green, 1993; Lundgren and Dahlberg, 1998).

Health care in North America is largely provided by practitioners educated within a biomedical model. This model is disease oriented and its goal is to 'cure'. The result is that more than 50 per cent of the two million women giving birth in the US each year receive epidural analgesia (Hawkins, *et al.*, 1999). Epidural analgesia eliminates labour pain for most women, but relieving pain and experiencing comfort address two very different needs of birthing women. Reports link epidurals with a number of adverse effects during labour, and information about additional potential side effects is uncertain (see, for example, Lieberman and O'Donoghue, 2002). Many women prefer to keep drug use to a minimum (Green, 1993) and have indicated that the experience of birthing pain, together with a perception of it as a strengthening event, gave added meaning to transitioning to motherhood (Lundgren and Dahlberg, 1998). These findings contrast sharply with the current epidemic of epidural use observed in the US. The problem addressed by this research is the assumption that pain relief meets the comfort needs of birthing women; that, if we cure the pain of birth, women will then experience comfort during the birthing process.

Marmor and Kroll (2002) explored the patterns of pain management during childbirth in the US, and addressed safe and effective methods that were available to US women. The results of their study emphasize that there is little information about what women in the US prefer, why they do so, or what influences their perception about pain management. Marmor and Kroll make it abundantly clear that US women have considerably less choice about pain control during childbirth than women in many other advanced Western industrialized democracies. The final report of the 'Listening to Mothers Survey' (Declercq, *et al.*, 2002), (the first national US survey of women's childbearing experiences) found that, even though selected comfort (non-pharmacologic) measures were often rated as highly effective by the women using them, they were used less than 8 per cent of the time. Simkin and O'Hara (2002) note further that, despite reports of the effectiveness of comfort methods, they receive little attention in the literature and are not commonly available to women in the US.

A key consideration of labour pain overlooked in the biomedical model is that labour pain is part of a physiologically normal event: childbirth. Pain – in the context of helplessness, suffering, and loss – is different from pain in the context of coping resources, comfort and a sense of accomplishment (Lowe, 2002). Labour pain can be a guide to mothers in labour; it can herald to the mother that her position needs to be changed or that progress is occurring.

Comforting interventions may enable her to interpret the nuances of pain, and provide her with the strength to continue being an active participant in the process. Focusing on comfort during labour does not negate the existence of pain but, instead, may offer birthing women expanded alternatives for pain control.

The purpose of this study was: to explore the existence of comfort during labour in a sample of healthy, primigravid women experiencing a normal labour and birth. The relationship between comfort and pain was examined, and comforting interventions that positively impacted women's level of comfort were identified.

The research questions addressed were:

- Does comfort exist during labour?
  o   If comfort exists can it be quantified?
  o   Does the level of comfort change during the course of labour?
  o   What comfort measures did the women in this study use and did they promote comfort?
  o   What is the relationship between childbirth, comfort and pain?

Study framework: Kolcaba's Theory of Holistic Comfort

Kolcaba's (2003) holistic theory of comfort encompasses process (comforting) and product (comfort), and proposes that 'comfort care' is a process of comforting actions stimulated by the individual's and care giver's perception of comfort needs. Comforting can be called such only if the product of comfort is brought into being (Kolcaba, 1995). The basic assumptions of this theory are that:

- human beings have a holistic response to complex stimuli
- comfort is a desirable outcome
- human beings strive to meet, or have met, their basic comfort needs.

Box 9.1   Kolcaba's definition of holistic comfort

Holistic Comfort
Kolcaba defines holistic comfort as the immediate experience of being strengthened by having needs for relief (the experience of having met immediate needs for comfort), ease (state of calm or contentment) and transcendence (state in which one rises above problems or pain) met in four contexts: physical (pertaining to bodily sensations and homeostatic mechanisms that may or may not be related to specific diagnoses), psychospiritual (whatever gives life meaning for an individual and entails self-esteem, self-concept, sexuality and relationship to a higher order or being), environmental (external surroundings, conditions and influences), and sociocultural (interpersonal, family and sociocultural relationships including finances, education, and support, traditions, customs and language)

Source: Kolcaba (2003).

Integral to this theory are health-seeking behaviours (Schlotfeldt, 1975) which are a wide range of subsequent activities that may be voluntary or involuntary, conscious or subconscious (Glazer and Pressler, 1989). Comfort and health-seeking behaviours have a reciprocal relationship, and the immediate outcome of comfort is a whole person response (Kolcaba, 1992).

Comfort during childbirth fits Kolcaba's (1994) theory of comfort because childbirth is a naturally occurring, usually desired, whole-person event. Consistent with the theory, 'comfort' is an umbrella term under which relief of many types of discomfort – for example, pain relief, coping and anxiety management – are subsumed.

Methods

The project consisted of four phases:

- development of the Childbirth Comfort Questionnaire (CCQ)
- assessment of internal validity of the CCQ
- assessment of effect size of comfort and adequacy of sample size
- analysis of data and answering the research questions.

Sample

Participants were selected from three regions of the US Midwest, using non-probability, convenience sampling (Polit and Beck, 2008). Births occurred at three tertiary care hospitals located in the same Midwestern state. Physicians or midwives were the primary birth attendants at each hospital. An important distinction amongst the hospitals was that one uses intrathecal analgesia, rather than epidurals, as a means of managing labour pain.

Recruitment occurred prenatally in clinicians' offices, childbirth education classes and at the time of hospital admission, if the woman was in the latent phase of labour (less than four centimetres dilated). All women at each site who met the inclusion criteria were invited to participate. Inclusion criteria were:

- 18 years of age or older
- able to speak and understand English (or have an interpreter present)
- primigravid
- anticipating a vaginal birth
- presenting in the latent phase of labour
- singleton pregnancy
- uncomplicated prenatal course.

Women who chose to use medication during labour were not excluded from the study because women living in the US commonly use medication for pain relief during labour; thus the sample reflected the general population of child-bearing women. The effect size required to detect changes in comfort during birth was unknown; therefore, initial sample size estimates using Cohen's Table of Power (Cohen, 1992; Polit and Beck, 2008; Walker and Almond, 2010) were computed using a significance level of 0.05 and a power of 0.80.

A sample size of 50 participants was deemed appropriate to detect a medium effect and to allow statistical correlation analyses. A sample size of at least 60 was set as the goal, to allow for missing data or participants dropping out during the study.

Data collection

Data collectors were nurses and midwives who had experience working with women during birth. All data collectors were trained in data collection methods. Appropriate Institutional Review Boards at each site approved the study prior to data collection. Data were collected between 2002 and 2003.

Childbirth Comfort Questionnaire

The CCQ, adapted from the General Comfort Questionnaire (Kolcaba, 1992, 2010), was used to assess women's level of comfort during labour. All aspects of the CCQ scale are interdependent; a change in one produces a change in another (Kolcaba, 1992). The CCQ consists of 14 5-point Likert scaled statements. Each statement addresses a specific sense of comfort (relief, ease or transcendence) and context (physical, environmental, psychospiritual, or social). There are an equal number of positive and negative items on the instrument, thereby decreasing the risk of response bias (Figure 9.1).

CCQ items focusing on childbirth were initially derived from labour nurses and delivery nurses, midwives, obstetricians, women who had experienced a normal labour and birth, and the extant literature. Face validity was established by a panel of experts that included midwives (n = 5), obstetricians (n = 3) and

Data Collectors please read the statement below at each data collection time point. Circle her score.

Thank-you VERY MUCH for helping in this study about the feelings women experience during labor. I am going to ask you to rate how you feel about 14 statements. Please rate each statement from 1 to 5 with '1' meaning you 'strongly disagree' and '5' meaning you 'strongly agree' at this moment.

Example:
I am glad I am being asked these questions ....1 (strongly disagree) to 5 (strongly agree).

1.	I have enough privacy.	1...2...3...4...5
2.	My pain is difficult to endure.	1...2...3...4...5
3.	I feel empowered by those around me.	1...2...3...4...5
4.	I don't think I can do this without the help of others.	1...2...3...4...5
5.	I am working well with my body.	1...2...3...4...5
6.	This chair (bed) makes me hurt.	1...2...3...4...5
7.	I can rise above my pain because it is helping me birth by baby.	1...2...3...4...5
8.	I feel confident I can birth my baby.	1...2...3...4...5
9.	This room makes me feel weak and helpless.	1...2...3...4...5
10.	The pain of the contractions motivates me to be strong.	1...2...3...4...5
11.	This is a safe place to be.	1...2...3...4...5
12.	I feel like giving up.	1...2...3...4...5
13.	I worry I will lose control.	1...2...3...4...5
14.	I need to feel better informed about my progress.	1...2...3...4...5

Figure 9.1   Childbirth Comfort Questionnaire

Note: Figure is resized for publication purposes.
Source: Schuiling (2002).

women who had experienced labour and birth (n = 5). Internal consistency reliability (Cronbach's alpha) was assessed twice: once 25 data sets were received and coded, and at the conclusion of the study. The Cronbach's alpha at both times was 0.71, which is acceptable for a new instrument (Gillis and Jackson, 2002).

Scoring the CCQ consists of adding the responses (once reverse coding is completed for negatively worded items). Possible scores range from 14–70, provided all items are answered, with higher scores indicating higher comfort levels. When data are normally distributed, the top 25 per cent of scores represent high levels of comfort and the bottom 25 per cent of scores represent low comfort.

Pain numerical rating scale

A numerical rating scale (NRS) was used to assess pain intensity. The NRS ranks pain from 0 (no pain) to 10 (worst pain imaginable). This instrument was the instrument of choice for measuring pain because each of the participating institutions typically used this instrument to assess pain, making the introduction of a second new instrument unnecessary.

Paired pain and comfort scores were obtained twice during labour:

- 1–5 centimetres of cervical dilatation   (time = T^1)
- 6–10 centimetres of cervical dilatation   (time = T^2).

Pain scores were documented prior to comfort scores. In order to keep interference with the birthing process to a minimum, the CCQ was administered between contractions. Scientifically, this was acceptable because studies about pain in labour and associated levels of endorphins indicate women rate their pain levels higher between contractions than during a contraction (Cahil, 1989).

Use of the following comfort measures (non-pharmacologic interventions used to promote comfort, including alternative and complementary methods of pain control) was documented during labour:

- aromatherapy – use of pleasing scents to assist with relaxation and comfort
- freedom of movement – being allowed or encouraged to ambulate, rock, or change position in bed at will, which enables the birthing woman to find a position of comfort
- hydrotherapy – use of water to promote comfort during labour
- imagery – use of visual imagery to promote comfort; may be guided or unguided
- massage – any type of massage of a body part that entails touch by a significant other or care provider with the intent of promoting comfort
- music – any use of music to promote relaxation and comfort
- support – one-to-one continuous support provided by a family member, significant other or care provider.

The types and number of comfort measures used at each data point were documented, as was the use and type of pain medication.

Demographic data were collected from all women in the study.

Data analysis

Demographic data were analyzed using descriptive statistics. Pearson's r was used to analyze the relationship between mean comfort and pain scores at T^1 and T^2. Mean comfort and pain scores were analyzed using analysis of variance (ANOVA) and covered women who used:

- no pain medication
- pain medication other than an epidural
- only epidural analgesia for pain relief.

Data on independent variables considered 'standard care' were collected, and bivariate analysis was used to test the difference between the means of two independent groups; for example, comfort scores and number of comfort measures. When three or more independent group means were available, an ANOVA was used. Appropriate F statistics and degrees of freedom are reported for all ANOVAs and *post hoc* testing using a Scheffé was done when indicated.

Results

Preliminary analysis of 25 data sets revealed that:

- comfort scores were highly correlated between T^1 and T^2 (Pearson's r = 0.73)
- there was no significant change in the comfort scores, as indicated by a paired t-test (t = −1.2, df = 26, p = 0.231).

These findings reflect stability of the data and, therefore, a minimum sample size of 50 was determined likely to be sufficient to allow correlation analyses.

Sixty-four primiparous women, ranging in age from 18 to 40 years, participated in the study. Most were Caucasian, high school or college graduates, married, and employed with an average annual family income of US$50,000 or more (Table 9.1). A majority of the women planned their pregnancies (59.4 per cent) and most attended childbirth preparation classes (64.1 per cent). Physicians attended the majority of the births (65 per cent), although 38.2 per cent of the women indicated they had a midwife birth attendant (some had both a physician and a midwife birth attendant). Most women were admitted to the labour unit when they were between two cms and three cms dilated. The average length of labour was 19.5 hours, which is within normal limits for primiparous women (Varney, *et al.*, 2003). The majority (71 per cent) received pitocin either to augment or to induce their labour, and 84 per cent had continuous electronic foetal monitoring. Baby outcomes were excellent: 100 per cent of the births were live and full-term, and all of the infants had Apgar scores ranging between 7 and 10 at five minutes.

Scores on the CCQ at T^1 ranged from 33 to 67 (M—54.48), and at T^2 from 32 to 69 (M—55.68). The highest subscale scores at T^1 were observed when women reported a sense of ease occurring in an environmental (4.79/5.00) or

Table 9.1   Demographic characteristics of participants

Characteristic	Number (valid %)		Mean	Standard Deviation	Range
Age (years)			26.25	± 5.12	18–40
Race					
Euro/Caucasian	58.9	(90.6)			
African Am.	2	(3.1)			
Hispanic/Latino	1	(1.6)			
Native Am.	1	(1.6)			
Asian/Pacific Islander	0				
Middle Eastern	1	(1.6)			
Other	1	(1.6)			
Education (highest level completed)					
Elementary	4	(6.3)			
High School	27	(42.2)			
College	27	(42.2)			
Graduate School	6	(9.4)			
Employment					
Yes	46	(74.2)			
No	16	(25.8)			
Marital Status					
Married	42	(65.6)			
Single	8	(12.5)			
Divorced	0				
Separated	12	(18.8)			
Widowed	0				
Live with S/O	2	(3.1)			
Family Income (U.S. dollars)					
Less than $10,000	6	(9.5)			
$10,000–$19,999	7	(11.1)			
$20,000–$29,999	6	(9.5)			
$30,000–$39,999	8	(12.7)			
$40,000–$49,00 0	10	(15.9)			
$50,000 or more	26	(41.3)			

social context (4.78/5.00). The lowest subscale scores at T^1 were observed when women reported a sense of relief occurring in a psychospiritual (1.58/5.0) or physical context (3.29/5.00) (see Table 9.2 and Box 9.1).

At T^2, highest subscale scores are observed when women reported a sense of ease occurring in an environmental (4.92/5.00) and/or social context (4.74/5.00). However, the sense of transcendence received high scores when experienced within environment (4.58/5.00), social (4.36/5.00), or psychospiritual (4.35/5.00) contexts (see Table 9.2).

Table 9.2   Childbirth comfort questionnaire subscale scores at $Time^1$ and $Time^2$

	Relief			Ease			Transcendence		
	T^1	T^2	% Change	T^1	T^2	% Change	T^1	T^2	% Change
Physical	3.29	3.09	−7%	3.85	4.19	+8%	3.49*	3.66*	+5%
Psychospiritual	1.58	1.66	+5%	3.82	3.72	−3%	4.34**	4.35**	+1%
Social	4.16	4.30	+3%	4.78	4.74	−1%	4.16	4.36	+5%
Environmental	3.55	3.83	+7%	4.79	4.92	+3%	4.58	4.58	0

Note: *Scores averaged for questions 7 & 10. **Scores averaged for questions 8 & 12.

Table 9.3   Statistical findings of comfort and pain scores at $Time^1$ and $Time^2$

	Pain T^1	Pain T^2	Comfort T^1	Comfort T^2
Pain T^1	1.00			
	r = .275			
Pain T^2	p = .06	1.00		
	r = −.283*	r = −.107		
Comfort T^1	p = .03	p = .46	1.00	
	r = −.047	r = −.545**	r = .577**	
Comfort T^2	p = .74	p = < .001	p < .001	1.00
Mean Score	4.78	4.13	54.48	55.68
S.D. ±	2.9	3.6	6.63	7.7

*p ≤ 0.05; **p ≤ .001.

The women in this study maintained their level of comfort throughout their labour. Total CCQ scores at T^1 significantly correlated with CCQ scores at T^2 (r = 0.577, p < .001) regardless of comfort or pain measures used. A small change in pain scores occurred between T^1 (M—4.78) and T^2 (M—4.13), but this finding did not reach significance (r = 0.275, p = 0.06) – see Table 9.3.

Pearson's r revealed that comfort and pain were significantly correlated in a negative direction at T^1 (r = −0.283, p = 0.03) and at T^2 (r = −0.545, p < 0.001) (see Table 9.3). Pain scores at T^1 ranged from 0 to 10, with a mean score of 4.78 (S.D. 2.9 [n = 62]). Pain scores at T^2 again ranged from 0 to 10, with a mean score of 4.13 [S.D. 3.6 [n = 53]). Initially, these results seemed to suggest that, as pain scores rise, comfort scores would fall (or the converse). However, further analysis revealed that this assumption is incorrect. Although pain scores fell in response to epidural analgesia, the total comfort scores remained the same or nearly the same as observed during T^1.

Women receiving epidurals noted an increase in comfort within the physical context, but not necessarily within the other contexts of comfort. Comfort

Table 9.4   Comparison of comfort and pain scores of women who did not use pain medication with women who used any type of pain medication

No Pain Medication (n @ T^1 = 36; n @ T^2 = 10)			Used Pain Medication (n @ T^1 = 24; n @ T^2 = 40)				
Scores	Mean	SD	Mean	SD	t	df	
Comfort T^1	54.97	7.52	53.71	4.97	.729	60	
Pain T^1	4.94	2.37	4.54	3.71	.515"	58	
Comfort T^2	55.50	7.65	55.72	7.85	−.08	51	
Pain T^2	5.55	3.32	3.78	3.66	1.39	48	

Note: Comfort scores were not significantly different between T^1 and T^2. Pain scores are significantly correlated between T^1 and T^2. *$p < .05$.

scores of women who chose not to use pain medication versus those who used any type of pain medication (including epidural analgesia) were not significantly different between groups at either T^1 ($t = 0.729$, df = 60, p = 0.09) or T^2 ($t = 0.081$, df = 51, p = 0.99). However, there was a statistically significant difference in mean pain scores between the two groups at T^1 ($t = 0.515$, df = 58, p< 0.001), with women using pain medication reporting lower scores although not at T^2 ($t = 1.39$, df = 48, p = 0.139) (see Table 9.4).

An ANOVA was computed to assess the differences between the mean comfort and pain scores at T^1 and T^2 among:

- women who used no pain medication
- women who used pain medication other than an epidural
- women who used epidural analgesia.

The group's mean comfort scores were not significantly different from one another at either T^1 or T^2 (see Table 9.5). Mean pain scores amongst the three groups varied significantly at T^1 (F = 12.92, df2, 50, p < .001) and at T^2 (F = 13.61, df = 2, 40, p < 0.001). A Scheffé *post hoc* test revealed that, at both T^1 and T^2, women using epidural analgesia had significantly lower mean pain scores than women who used medication other than an epidural (see Table 9.5).

Women in this study used an average of two or three comfort measures during their labour; the most common measures were:

- one-to-one continuous support (T^1 n = 47; T^2 n = 46)
- freedom of movement (T^1 n = 43; T^2 n = 22)
- massage (T^1 n = 25; T^2 n = 23).

T-tests on comfort scores between women who used a comfort measure at T^1 and those not using comfort measures at T^1 were not significantly different. However, women who had freedom of movement at T^1 had significantly higher comfort scores at T^2 ($t = −3.43$, df = 51, p < 0.001), and women who

Table 9.5   ANOVA summary for effect of medication on pain and comfort scores at Time^1 and Time^2

Variable and Source	df	SS	MS	F	p
Comfort T^1					
Between groups	2	39.64	19.82	0.519	0.598
Within groups	52	1987.56	38.22		
Comfort T^2					
Between groups	2	183.65	91.82	1.303	0.282
Within groups	43	3029.83	70.46		
Pain T^1					
Between groups	2	149.71	74.86	12.92*	0.000*
Within groups	50	289.61	5.79		
Pain T^2					
Between groups	2	239.79	119.89	13.606*	0.000*
Within groups	40	352.46	8.81		

*p ≤ .05.

Table 9.6   Difference in comfort scores at Time^2 for women using a comfort measure at Time^1

	Used Comfort Measure at T^1		Did Not Use Comfort Measure at T^1			
Measure	Mean Scores	S.D.	Mean Scores	S.D.	t	df
Free Movement	57.76	6.72	50.40	7.83	−3.43**	51
1:1 Support	57.19	7.55	49.91	5.58	−2.98**	51

Note: Only significant findings presented. **p ≤ .001.

had one-to-one support at T^1 had significantly higher comfort scores if one-to-one support were also used at T^2 (t = −2.98, df = 51, p = 0.004) (see Table 9.6). Bivariate analysis of the mean comfort scores of women who used comfort measures at T^2 and those who did not revealed that women who used massage had significantly higher comfort scores than those who did not use massage (t = −2.29, df = 51, p < .05).

T-tests on mean pain scores of women using comfort measures at T^1 and those who did not revealed that women who had one-to-one support had significantly higher pain scores than women who did not have one-to-one support (t = −2.05, df = 58, p = 0.04). Women who had freedom of movement at T^2 had significantly higher pain scores at T^2 (t = −2.26, df = 48, p = 0.03), even though the mean comfort scores of this group were also higher (see Table 9.7).

Table 9.7   Pain score differences between women who used comfort measures and women who did not

T^1 (n = 60) and T^2 (n = 50)						
Used Comfort Measure T^1			Did Not Use Comfort Measure T^1			
Measure	Mean	S.D.	Mean	S.D.	t	df
Massage	5.24	3.27	4.46	2.70	−1.01	58
Hydrotherapy	4.67	2.89	4.83	3.01	.199	58
Music	3.43	2.88	4.96	2.94	1.30	58
Imagery	4.43	3.31	4.83	2.93	.336	58
1:1 Support	5.19	2.95	3.31	2.56	−2.05*	58
Ambulation	4.76	3.04	4.83	2.83	.085	58
Used Comfort Measure T^2			Did Not Use Comfort Measure T^2			
Measure	Mean	S.D.	Mean	S.D.	t	df
Massage	3.70	3.57	4.64	3.66	1.17	48
Hydrotherapy	3.70	3.74	4.31	3.63	.544	48
Music	4.50	3.70	4.00	3.70	.210	48
Imagery	3.43	3.60	4.24	3.67	.547	48
1:1 Support	4.38	3.82	3.00	2.50	−1.03	48
Freedom of movement	5.55	3.36	3.26	3.57	−2.26*	48

* $p < .001$.
Note: Women who had 1:1 support had significantly higher pain scores than women not using 1:1 support at T^1. However, women who had 1:1 support at T^2 had significantly higher comfort scores at T^2 (t = −2.98, df = 51, p = .004). Women who had freedom of movement at T^2 had significantly higher pain scores than women who did not have freedom of movement.

Discussion

The findings of this study suggest that women experience comfort as a state of being that is distinct from pain during childbirth, and that relief of pain during labour is not sufficient to ensure that a labouring woman will experience comfort. That is, pain management and the experience of comfort are not synonymous: pain relief does not assure comfort. The higher comfort scores observed at T^1 and T^2 occurring when a sense of ease was experienced within an environment or social context supports theories of the importance of the childbirth environment and human presence. Green et al. (1990) comment that little attention is paid to a woman's relationship with her care givers, but that this relationship may well have relevance to subsequent psychological states during childbirth. The higher CCQ scores found at these intersects may be women's voices telling us that the birth environment and the relationship the woman forms with her birth attendant is of considerable importance, particularly in enabling her to feel a sense of comfort.

Mean comfort scores at T^1 positively correlated with those at T^2; most women in this study maintained a moderate level of comfort throughout their labour. The lack of significant differences between comfort scores may be due to the healthy population of women participating in this study. It is very likely these women actively sought to maintain their level of comfort. If labour is viewed through a lens that frames the process as normal, then it makes sense that healthy women would actively seek to maintain their comfort. They would ask for a back-rub, or change their position to one of greater comfort, or ask for medication. All of these activities would have been well within the locus of control of the women participating in this study. Additionally, the majority of women in this study had one-to-one support, and women who had one-to-one support had higher comfort levels at T^2, which may have offset the increasing pain of contractions. However, women who had one-to-one support at T^1 also had significantly higher pain scores at T^1, even though the comfort score remained the same. It is difficult to discern the nuances of this finding, although it may simply mean that women who received one-to-one support were experiencing greater pain and their clinician and family responded by providing one-to-one support.

Although the use of comfort measures and comfort scores at T^1 was not significantly correlated, it is interesting that women who used freedom of movement at T^1 had significantly higher comfort scores at T^2 and also had significantly higher pain scores at T^2. Women who have freedom of movement may feel more in control of the birthing process, and therefore have a higher level of comfort. Many studies document that control is important to women during labour (Lowe, 1987; Green, 1993; Halldorsdottir and Karlsdottir, 1996; Hodnett, 2002; Green and Baston, 2003). However, with ambulation comes gravity's pull. Some studies suggest that when women labour in upright positions, they may experience a shorter phase of maximum slope (Andrews and Chrzanowski, 1990; Gupta and Hofmeyr, 2004). Although the upright position may cause contractions to be more frequent and more intense, studies suggest that the cervix tends to dilate faster and the descent of the foetus is more rapid, resulting in a shorter phase of maximum slope and a shorter labour. It makes sense that freedom of movement could positively impact comfort and negatively impact pain levels. Some women may choose to tolerate an increase in pain intensity, if they know their labour may be shorter and they feel in control. It is noteworthy that, in a study of the effects of women walking during labour, the women who walked did not have shorter labours, but 99 per cent said they would like to walk again during labour (Bloom *et al.*, 1998). A test of the speculated relationship between labouring upright and length of labour is beyond the scope of this investigation, but warrants further study.

Women using massage at T^2 had significantly higher comfort scores. Massage takes many forms and, in theory, it stimulates a variety of sensory receptors in the skin and deeper tissues, bringing about inhibition of pain awareness. A controlled study of touch during active labour compared women's behaviour and vital signs, and found that women in the massage group had improved coping abilities, greater comfort and lowered systolic blood pressure and pulses than the no-massage group (Simkin, 1995). These findings about touch support those of the current study.

Pain scores at T^1 and T^2 were positively correlated. There are two possible explanations for this finding. Many of the women in the study controlled their pain by using epidural analgesia. At T^1, 12 out of 53 women were using epidural relief and at T^2, 27 out of 53 were receiving epidural analgesia. This suggests that, as women's pain increased, they sought out methods to assist them in controlling their pain and the most popular method was pharmacologic. It is unknown whether or not the method of pain control used by each woman was her choice or her clinician's. It is also unknown whether comfort measures were offered as pain increased.

It is noteworthy that pain scores of women who used no medication were not significantly different from those who used medication, other than an epidural. In fact, the group using pain medication other than an epidural had slightly higher (though not significantly higher) pain scores than the unmedicated group. A possible explanation for the stability of pain scores in this group is physiologic. A study of a labouring women's level of plasma beta-endorphins (the body's natural analgesic) suggests that beta-endorphins have a positive effect on pain perception during labour, blunting the pain but not obliterating it (Lowe, 2002). A significant correlation has been demonstrated between plasma concentrations of beta-endorphins and labour pain; the level of beta-endorphins rose as labour pain increased (Bacigalupo et al., 1990; Chan et al., 1993).

Comfort and pain scores were negatively correlated at both T^1 and T^2. This appears to be a logical finding, but further analysis revealed that women who received epidural analgesia had significantly lower pain scores compared with women who did not. However, at the same time, the comfort scores did not vary significantly between these two groups. Therefore, it seems that the dramatic decrease in the pain scores of women using epidurals caused a statistically significant negative correlation between comfort and pain scores. It was probably more a reflection of the dramatic change in the pain scores than change in the total comfort score that produced the negative correlation. In fact, this finding suggests that that the relationship between comfort and pain is not entirely reciprocal, and that the experience of comfort during labour requires more than pain management. Additionally, the finding that pain relief does not necessarily provide comfort is reflected in studies of childbirth satisfaction that demonstrate pain relief does not automatically mean the childbirth experience was satisfying (Hodnett, 2002).

A limitation of this study is the non-experimental design, which does not allow for causal inference or explanation. Using a larger sample size decreases this limitation, but cannot eliminate it. Additionally, convenience sampling carries inherent bias with it, as those willing to participate may not be typical of the population with regard to the phenomenon of interest. This limitation was decreased because the sample was drawn from three different sites in different geographic regions. Also, trend bias was avoided because data collection took place over the span of 18 months.

Conclusion

This study begins to describe the complex comfort needs women have during childbirth. The findings suggest that comfort during childbirth occurs in different contexts and senses of experience, and that comfort is complex, requiring care giver expertise in assessment, evaluation and management. Clinical observations and birth narratives describing comfort and pain relief as different aspects of the experience of labour and birth have been quantified with the use of the CCQ. This preliminary work provides a foundation upon which to build the state of the science about providing pain relief and comfort during childbirth, in an effort to increase options for both women and their clinicians.

ACTIVITIES

Undergraduate

Undertake a concept analysis of 'comfort in labour' and identify how you would confirm the defining attributes of this concept.

Postgraduate

As stated above (p. 211):

> A study of a labouring women's level of plasma beta-endorphins (the body's natural analgesic) suggests that beta-endorphins have a positive effect on pain perception during labour, blunting the pain but not obliterating it. (Lowe, 2002)

> A significant correlation has been demonstrated between plasma concentrations of beta-endorphins and labour pain; the level of beta-endorphins rose as labour pain increased. (Bacigalupo, et al., 1990; Chan et al., 1993)

Design a research trial to test these assumptions.

References

Andrews, C. and Chrzanowski, M. (1990) 'Maternal Position, Labor and Comfort', *Applied Nursing Research*, 3(1): 7–13.

Bacigalupo, G., Riese, S., Rosendahl, H., and Saling, E. (1990) 'Quantitative Relationships between Pain Intensities during Labor and Beta-Endorphin and Cortisol Concentrations in Plasma: Decline of the Hormone Concentration in the Early Postpartum Period', *Journal of Perinatal Medicine*, 18(4): 289–96.

Bloom, S.L., McIntire, D.D., Kelly, M.A., Beimer, H.L., Burpo, R.H., Garcia, M.A. and Leveno, K.J. (1998) 'Lack of Effect of Walking', *New England Journal of Medicine*, 339(2): 117–18.

Cahil, C. (1989) 'Beta-Endorphin Levels during Pregacy and Labor: A Role in Pain Modulation?', *Nursing Research*, 38(4): 200–3.

Chan, E., Smith, R., Lewis, T., Brinsmead, M., Zhang, H., Cubis, J., Thornton, K. and Hurt, D. (1993) 'Plasma Corticotropin-Releasing Hormone, Beta-Endorphin and

Cortisol Inter-Relationship during Human Pregnancy', *Acat Endocrinologica*, 128(4): 339–44.

Cohen, J. (1992) 'A Power Primer', *Psychological Bulletin*, 112(1): 155–9.

Declercq, E., Sakala, C., Corry, M., Applebaum, S. and Risher, P. (2002) 'Listening To Mothers: Report of the First National US Survey of Women's Childbearing Experiences'. New York, NY: Maternity Center Association.

Gillis, A., and Jackson, W. (2002) *Research for Nurses: Methods and Interpretations*. Philadelphia, PA: F.A. Davis.

Glazer, G., and Pressler, J. (1989) 'Schlotfeldt's Health Seeking Nursing Model', in J. Fitzpatrick and A. Whall (eds) *Conceptual Models of Nursing Practice*, 2nd edn. Englewood Cliffs, NJ: Prentice-Hall.

Green, J.M. (1993) 'Expectations and Experiences of Pain in Labor: Findings from a Large Prospective Study', *Birth*, 20(2): 65–72.

Green, J.M. and Baston, H. (2003) 'Feeling in Control during Labor: Concepts, Correlates and Consequences', *Birth*, 30(4): 235–47.

Green, J.M., Coupland, V., and Kitzenger, J. (1990) 'Expectations, Experiences and Psychological Outcomes of Childbirth: A Prospective Study of 825 Women', *Birth*, 17(1): 15–24.

Gupta, J.K., and Hofmeyr, G.J. (2004) 'Position for Women during Second Stage of Labour', *Cochrane Library (Intervention Review)* (CD002006) (www.mrw.inter-science.wiley.com/cochrane – accessed 24 March 2008; 4 August 2010: edited, no changes to conclusions, Issue 4 2009).

Halldorsdottir, S. and Karlsdottir, S. (1996) 'Journeying through Labor and Delivery: Perceptions of Women who Have Given Birth', *Midwifery*, 12(2): 48–61.

Hawkins, J., Beaty, B., and Gibbs, C. (1999) 'Update on Anesthesia Practices in the US', Society for Anesthesia and Perinatology, *Abstracts*, A53.

Helser, D. (1998) 'Women's Experiences of Comfort and Discomfort in Childbirth as Expressed in Published Birth Narratives', Paper presented at the meeting of the American College of Nurse-Midwives Annual Meeting, San Francisco.

Hodnett, E. (1996) 'Nursing Support of the Laboring Women', *Journal of Obstetrical, Gynecologic & Neonatal Nursing*, 25(3): 257–64.

Hodnett, E. (2002) 'Pain and Women's Satisfaction with the Experience of Birth: A Systematic Review', *American Journal of Obstetrics and Gynecology*, 186(5), Suppl. S160–S172.

Hummenick, S., and Bugen, I. (1981) 'Mastery: The Key to Childbirth Satisfaction? A Study', *Birth and the Family Journal*, 8: 84–90.

Kolcaba, K. (1992) 'Holistic Comfort: Operationalizing the Construct as a Nurse-sensitive Outcome', *Advances in Nursing Science*, 15(1): 1–10.

Kolcaba, K. (1994) 'A Theory of Holistic Comfort for Nursing', *Journal of Advanced Nursing*, 19(6): 1178–84.

Kolcaba, K. (1995) 'Comfort as Process and Product, Merged in Holistic-Nursing Art', *Journal of Holistic Nursing*, 13(2): 117–31.

Kolcaba, K. (2003) *Comfort Theory and Practice: A Vision for Holistic Health Care and Research*. New York, NY: Springer.

Kolcaba, K. (2010) 'The Comfort Line' (http://www.thecomfortline.com – accessed 4 August 2010).

Kolcaba, K. and Dimarco, M. (2005) 'Comfort Theory and its Application to Pediatric Nursing', *Pediatric Nursing*, 31(3): 187–94.

Kolcaba, K., Tilton, C. and Drouin, C. (2006) 'Comfort Theory: A Unifying Framework to Enhance the Practice Environment', *Journal of Nursing Administration*, 36(11): 538–44.

Lieberman, E., and O'Donoghue, C. (2002) 'Unintended Effects of Epidural Analgesia during Labor: A Systematic Review', *American Journal of Obstetrics and Gynecology*, 186(5), Suppl. S31–S68.

Lowe, N. (1987) 'Parity and Pain during Parturition', *Journal of Obstetrics, Gynecology & Neonatal Nursing*, 16(5): 340–6.

Lowe, N. (2002) 'The Nature of Labor Pain', *American Journal of Obstetrics and Gynecology*, 186(5), Suppl. S16–S24.

Lundgren, I., and Dahlberg, K. (1998) 'Women's Experiences of Pain during Childbirth', *Midwifery*, 14(2): 105–10.

March, A. and McCormack, D. (2009) 'Modifying Kolcaba's Comfort Theory as an Institution-Wide Approach', *Journal of Holistic Nursing*, 27(2): 75–80.

Marmor, T. and Kroll, D. (2002) 'Labor Pain Management in the United States: Understanding Patterns and the Issue of Choice', *American Journal of Obstetrics and Gynecology*, 186(5), Suppl. S173–S180.

Polit, D. and Beck, C. (2008) *Nursing Research: Generating and Assessing Evidence for Nursing Practice*. Philadelphia, PA: Wolters/Lippincott Williams & Wilkins.

Schlotfeldt, R. (1975) 'The Need for a Conceptual Framework', in P. Verhonic (ed.), *Nursing Research*. Boston, MA: Little, Brown: 241–53.

Schuiling, K.D. (2003) 'Exploring the Concept of Comfort within the Context of Childbirth', Unpublished PhD thesis, University of Michigan.

Schuiling, K. D. and Sampselle, C. (1999) 'Comfort in Labor and Midwifery Art', *Image: Journal of Nursing Scholarship*, 31(1): 77–81.

Simkin, P. (1995) 'Reducing Pain and Enhancing Progress in Labor: A Guide to Nonpharmacologic Methods for Maternity Caregivers', *Birth*, 22(3): 161–71.

Simkin, P. and O'Hara, M. (2002) 'Nonpharmacologic Relief of Pain during Labor: Systematic Reviews of Five Methods', *American Journal of Obstetrics and Gynecology*, 186(5), Suppl. S131–S159.

Varney, H., Kriebs, J. and Gegor, C. (eds) (2003) *Varney's Midwifery*, 4th edn. Boston, MA: Jones & Bartlett.

Walker, J. and Almond, P. (2010) *Interpreting Statistical Findings: A Guide for Health Professionals and Students*. Buckingham: Open University Press

Weber, S. (1996) 'Cultural Aspects of Pain in Childbearing', *Journal of Obstetric, Gynecologic & Neonatal Nursing*, 25(1): 67–72.

Birth Territory: A Theory for Midwifery Practice

10

Kathleen Fahy, Jenny Parratt, Maralyn Foureur and Carolyn Hastie

---

Key points

- Birth Territory Theory can be used to describe, explain and predict how the 'birth territory' affects women and babies at all stages of childbearing, in particular during labour and birth
- The theory shows how to restructure the 'birth territory' to create a 'sanctum' rather than a 'surveillance environment'
- One factor that has a large impact on a woman's well-being as an embodied self is whether 'integrative power' or 'disintegrative power' is used by the woman herself and/or by others in the 'birth territory'
- We hypothesize that, when 'integrative power' is used within a 'sanctum', the woman is most likely to experience a 'genius birth': a 'genius birth' is one where a woman feels good about herself, however the baby is born.

Introduction

The physical environment is known to impact cognition, problem solving, pain tolerance and mood (Sternberg and Wilson, 2006). The importance of the environment to birth is often assumed in midwifery literature but, until recently, there has been little theory and research to justify this claim. Denis Walsh (2000; see Chapter 8) wrote about the negative impact of a 'bed birth' and argues for mobility in labour, removing the bed from centre stage. Gould (2002) alleged the standard hospital birth suite acts subliminally to medicalize birth in the mind of the woman and midwife. Women in a National Childbirth Trust (United Kingdom) survey identified that being able to move around and having a less clinical looking room, as well as access to an en suite toilet and birth pool, were important aspects of the birth environment (Newburn and Singh, 2005). However, the key environmental factors identified by the women were overwhelmingly related to the relationship the woman experienced with the midwife and also the woman's sense of control. Even though midwives recognize the importance of the environment in women's birthing experience and why it matters, the midwives' role within that environment has needed to be systematically conceptualized.

Our work has been to theorize what constitutes an optimal birth environment. Knowing what an optimal birth environment is allows midwives and women to create each individual's appropriate space. Our approach is an extension of the salutogenic (health promoting) model applied to birth (see Chapter 3). The expected outcome of creating and maintaining optimal birth territories is salutogenic, in that the majority of women will have physiologically normal births. We agree with Downe and McCourt (2004) that a flexible definition of normality is required in recognition of the 'unique normality' of each woman.

This chapter develops the ideas that were first presented in earlier works (Fahy, 1995; Rowley (Foureur), 1998; Parratt, 2000, 2002; Parratt and Fahy, 2004; Foureur and Hunter, 2006; Foureur, 2007; Hastie and Fahy, 2009). These ideas were first organized and developed as theoretical concepts by Fahy and Parratt (2006). The synthesis of Birth Territory Theory also stems from current post-structural research about the factors that impact upon women's changing embodied self during childbearing (Parratt and Fahy, 2008; Parratt, 2010). The chapter also draws on, condenses and refines information that is included in our book: *Birth Territory and Midwifery Guardianship* (Fahy *et al.*, 2008), in which there is a full exploration of our theory, supporting examples and research evidence.

Birth Territory Theory is applicable in any setting at any stage of the childbearing experience: peri-conception, antenatal, intrapartum and postpartum. This theory can be used to describe, explain and predict how the 'birth territory' affects women, babies, and midwives in terms of both process and outcomes. Birth Territory Theory in some ways stands in contrast to the obstetric paradigm that is most commonly used to describe, explain and predict pregnancy, labour and birth. Obstetrical thinking posits that birthing can be understood, and improved upon, by the application of a reductionistic, disembodied and mechanistic model (see Chapter 2).

Birth Territory Theory takes a 'both/and' approach to valuing both reductive theory and holism. For example, we value holism and inductive thinking when we consider the multiple and complex factors that interact to make up 'birth territory'. Equally, we value the reductionist science of physiology, which provides a scientific, theoretical evidence base that explains how the environment can impact upon reproductive physiology right down to the level of gene expression and hormone release. But, if the only lens one uses to consider childbearing is reductionistic, then much of importance is left out. Our theory is the first to examine the impact of environment on childbearing in a way that is experientially grounded, theoretically integrated and supported by physiological evidence.

Overview of Birth Territory Theory

The theory derives from reflections upon our empirical experiences as midwives, researchers and childbearing women. Collectively, we have extensive clinical experience in a variety of service models, predominately continuity of care models that include attendance at homebirths, birth centre births and births in standard hospital environments. All four authors are active in research and theory development. All four are reflective practitioners who engage with each other in critical conversations. 'Birth territory' has been inductively developed, primarily by synthesis of new ideas based on analysis of existing and new research data, as well as our own experiences as women, mothers and midwives. This inductive method is a recognized strategic approach to theory development (Peterson and Bredow, 2004; Walker and Avant, 2004). Our midwifery theory draws from and contributes to biological, architectural, psychological, sociological, post-structural and feminist theory. In the realm of psychoanalytic, post-structural and feminist theory, important theorists that have influenced this work are Liz Grosz (1994, 1995, 2004), Luce Irigaray (1993, 2001, 2003), Julia Kristeva (1982), Iris Marion Young (2005) and Jacques Lacan (1977a, 1977b). Our power-related concepts build upon some of the ideas of Michel Foucault (1979, 1980, 1982).

In this section, we present an overview of the whole theory. The overarching concepts are introduced with details about the individual concepts presented in the sections that follow. A glossary of concepts and brief definitions is given in Table 10.1 (at the end of the chapter). Within Birth Territory Theory, 'birth' is defined as that period extending from peri-conception up to and including early parenting. 'Birth territory' is defined as the environment that is external to the woman/baby. The concept of 'birth territory' includes the physical features of the environment (the 'terrain') and the use of power by people within the environment ('jurisdiction'). 'Birth territory' deals with the space for birth. This space can be conceptualized at a number of levels. First, using a particular conceptual lens, 'birth territory' can be seen as the micro-level of the individual birth space (here, we also mean antenatal and postnatal spaces as well). Using a wider conceptual lens, 'birth territory' can be seen as the birth space within the broader environment. For most birth rooms, this means conceptualising 'birth territory' as the delivery suite, maternity unit and the health service, which operates as an integrated social system. Opening the conceptual lens even further, 'birth territory' encompasses all of the above, plus the historical, regulatory, legal, professional and political frameworks that direct, limit and control what is possible at the micro-level. This totality, the macro- and the micro-environment for birth, is termed 'birth territory' (Fahy et al., 2008). Most midwives work with women in the 'birth territory' at the micro-level, the primary focus of our theory. Labour and birth are the times of women's greatest vulnerability and greatest personal growth/change, and therefore this chapter focuses mostly on the territory for birth, although the theory is equally relevant to antenatal and postnatal territories.

The aim of Birth Territory Theory is: to explain how a woman can be supported to have a 'genius birth'. A 'genius birth' is defined as one where a woman responds to labour challenges by drawing from usually hidden capacities deep within her embodied self (see concepts on power and spirituality, pp. 222–5). In actualizing her inner power, she combines it with her conscious intention to experience a physiologically normal birth. A 'genius birth' is not contrived but, rather, is conscious and effortful even if, in taking account of her holistic well-being at that particular moment of her life, medical interventions are accepted (Parratt, 2008, 2010). The effort involved in achieving 'genius birth' means a woman will feel not only a degree of joy and relief in the presence of her baby, but also in her own achievement; she may even feel like a genius (Parratt, 2010). What is critical to a 'genius birth' is that the woman stays fully empowered throughout, and that as much normality as possible is maintained (Parratt, 2010). This normality is maintained through 'jurisdiction' and 'midwifery guardianship' discussed on pp. 222, 225–7.

A 'forced birth' is defined as one where power is used to try to force a particular type of birth. A 'forced birth' involves cutting off from one's own inner power. There are two types of 'forced birth'. One type is an outcome of the woman's collapse into powerlessness and victim-hood creating the need for a 'medically forced birth'. The other type is a 'maternal forced birth', which occurs because a woman responds to labour challenges by forcefully directing her egoic power to achieve the kind of birth she wants. This use of egoic power ignores capacities hidden within a woman's embodied self. Egoic power limits the woman's powers to her existing beliefs about what she can accomplish. If, however, she can let go of her pre-conceived views of what is possible, then she will find that she is capable of much more than she realizes. Neither a medical nor maternal 'forced birth' is likely to be optimally suited to a woman's holistic well-being (Parratt, 2008, 2010). Following 'forced birth', a woman's feelings of self-appreciation will be limited and she is likely to focus her joy and relief on the presence of her baby (Parratt, 2010). A 'forced birth' divides the power available to a woman for birthing and, thus, undermines her physiology and that of the baby. We hypothesize that, compared with women who have a 'forced birth', women who experience a 'genius birth' have a more positive sense of self and a more positive attachment to their babies, regardless of whether or not the birth was 'normal'.

In order to appreciate fully the importance of an optimal environment for birth, what is needed is an understanding of the neurophysiology of conception, pregnancy, labour, birth and the post-birth period. Unfortunately, few current text books provide us with the detailed descriptions that are required for this understanding to evolve. Therefore, we either have to locate a myriad of research material and assimilate it ourselves, or we have to rely on already collected and reconstructed accounts of what is important to consider. Here, we provide a brief summary of what we understand to be fundamental to integrating 'Birth Territory Theory' into the way care is provided to childbearing women (Fahy et al., 2008).

The physiology of undisturbed birth

At a physiological level, each person can be considered as an entire neuro-hormonally regulated, dynamic, physical system that interacts with, and is constantly altered by, whatever is encountered in the actual or perceived environment. The encounter happens from moment to moment through our senses of smell, sight, hearing, touch and taste. The brain processes what the senses encounter. Through the brain, we perceive the world as safe or unsafe through the emotional encoding and expression of these 'encounters'. Emotions are translated into neuro-hormones (brain chemicals) that instantly and constantly manipulate physiology by altering and regulating every body system (Pert, 1997; Foureur, 2008). For example, neuro-hormones influence breathing, blood pressure and rate of blood flow throughout the body, as well as temperature and immune functioning (to name just a few). Importantly, because neuro-hormones are brain chemicals, they also alter behaviour with the intent of increasing the individual's sense of safety – and, therefore, their well-being. All of these processes happen without conscious awareness as a result of the powerful effects of either the parasympathetic or sympathetic nervous systems.

For 'genius birth' to occur, the woman/baby dyad needs to exist in a protected and undisturbed space. In such a space, the woman/baby will perceive the environment as safe and birth physiology will be optimized (Foureur, 2008). It is important to recognize that what is considered to be 'safe' may differ for each woman (Parratt and Fahy, 2004; Parratt, 2010). Some will only feel safe at home with known and trusted care givers. Others may only feel safe in an environment that is highly medicalized and technologically sophisticated. These two 'safe spaces' are part of a continuum, and women will position themselves somewhere along it. Birth Territory Theory reveals the many aspects of environment that will influence perceptions of safety, and the following section demonstrates how these may alter birth physiology. When women feel unsafe, they feel fear – and that has negative consequences for birth physiology (Rowley (Foureur)), 1998; Foureur and Hunter, 2006; Foureur, 2008).

The fear cascade

Decades of research supports the role of the sympathetic nervous system in an automatic, innate response to acutely stressful events. A surge of catecholamines (such as adrenaline and nor-adrenaline) is secreted in response to acute stress, initiating what is known as the 'fright, flight or fight response' (Stable and Rankin, 2005). Adrenaline constricts blood vessels causing blood pressure and heart rate to rise as blood is diverted from non-essential organs to the brain, to aid clear thinking, and to the muscles of the legs and arms, ready to run or fight. The Fear Cascade hypothesises that, during labour and birth, the perception of an 'unsafe' environment may similarly trigger the sympathetic nervous system to initiate a flood of neuro-hormones that will impact both maternal and foetal physiology (Inch, 1984; Rowley (Foureur),

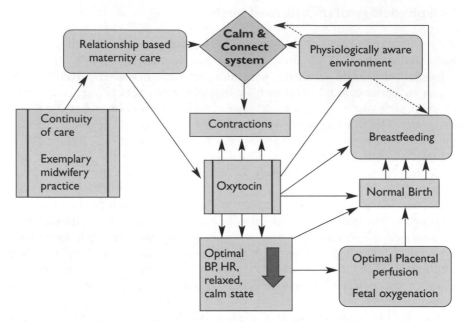

Figure 10.1   The optimising birth spiral – the integrating role of oxytocin

Source: Foureur (2007).

1998; Foureur, 2008; Hastie, 2008a). Adrenaline can disrupt the secretion of oxytocin, which may result in changes to the nature of labour contractions. Contractions may become irregular, slow down or stop altogether. In addition, the vasoconstrictive effect of adrenaline in diverting blood away from the abdomen means that there is less blood available for placental perfusion and, therefore, foetal oxygenation. This may lead to foetal distress. The Fear Cascade provides a biologically plausible theory as to why there are two main reasons for all intervention in childbirth (once labour has begun). The corollary is that providing an environment that women perceive as supportive, protected and safe enables optimal physiological functioning.

There is also now a greater understanding of the physiology of a positive and supportive birth environment. Part of that understanding is presented in Figure 10.1, which includes the key elements of an optimal birth space and is discussed more fully in Fahy *et al.* (2008).

Optimizing birth physiology

In essence, Figure 10.1 provides a model of the physiological consequences of a safe birth environment. The parasympathetic nervous system is triggered by the perception of safety and security. The neuro-hormone that orchestrates this system is oxytocin. Oxytocin is integral to the functions of what is termed, by some researchers, as the 'calm and connect system' (Uvnas-Moberg, 2003). Oxytocin initiates a range of behaviours that:

- enhance attachment of the pregnant woman to those who will help her in childbirth and early parenting
- enhances attachment of the woman to her unborn and then newly-born baby
- decreases stress
- increases pain threshold
- enhances labour contractions, leading to normal birth
- helps the mother to relax, by lowering blood pressure and heart rate, particularly during breastfeeding
- is essential for breastfeeding to occur and, in turn, enhances the attachment of the baby to the mother.

In this section, we have argued that women need to be protected, so that they can have an undisturbed birth. Being protected is critical to the woman's feeling safe. Feeling safe is critical for the birth physiology of the woman/baby dyad to function optimally. Optimal physiological functioning is also necessary for optimizing mother–infant attachment and breastfeeding. In the following section, we give more detail about Birth Territory Theory including the 'terrain', 'jurisdiction', power, spirituality and 'midwifery guardianship'.

The terrain of Birth Territory Theory

In Birth Territory Theory, 'terrain' denotes the physical features and geographical area of the individual birth space, including the furniture and accessories that the woman and her support people use for labour and birth (see Chapter 6). Two sub-concepts – 'surveillance environment' and 'sanctum' – lie at opposite ends along this continuum called 'terrain'.

Environment as a sanctum

'Sanctum' is defined as a homely environment designed to optimize the privacy, ease, control and comfort of the woman; there is easy access to a toilet, a deep bath and the outdoors. Provision of a door that can close meets the woman's need for privacy and safety. The more comfortable and familiar the environment is for the woman, the safer and more confident she will feel. An experience of 'sanctum' protects and potentially enhances the woman's embodied sense of self; this is reflected in optimal physiological function and emotional well-being.

The surveillance environment

'Surveillance environment' is the other sub-concept of 'terrain'. It denotes a clinical environment designed to facilitate surveillance of the woman and to optimize the ease and comfort of the staff. This is relevant to the concept of 'jurisdiction' (discussed on p. 222). A 'surveillance environment' is a clinical-looking room where equipment the staff may need is on display and the bed dominates. It has a doorway but no closed door, or the door has a viewing window. The woman has no easy access to a bath, a toilet or the outdoors.

Our theory hypothesizes that the more a 'birth territory' deviates from a 'sanctum', the more likely it is that the woman will feel fear. This deviation from the 'sanctum' will, in turn, reduce her embodied sense of self; it will be reflected in inhibited physiological functioning, reduced emotional well-being and possibly overt emotional distress. As we argue later, a woman's sense of safety is paramount for her to be able stay on a trajectory towards 'genius birth'. A greater level of surveillance is therefore appropriate, if that is what the individual woman needs in order to feel safe.

Jurisdiction in 'birth territory'

'Jurisdiction' means having the power to do as one wants within the birth environment. Within the broad concept of 'jurisdiction', there is a continuum of 'integrative power' and 'disintegrative power'. Two concepts are directly derived from 'integrative power' and 'disintegrative power': namely 'midwifery guardianship' and 'midwifery domination'. First, the underlying concepts of power, spirit and the self that are essential to understanding all the concepts associated with 'jurisdiction' are discussed (see Table 10.2 at end of the chapter).

Power

'Power' is an energy that enables one to be able to do or obtain what one wants (Northrup, 1998). Power is essential for living; without it we would not move at all. We see power as ethically neutral. This is consistent with Foucault's notion of power – which he argued was productive, not necessarily oppressive (Foucault, 1980). Power can be used to get others to submit to one's own wishes. Health professionals who want women to submit to their authority (to be docile) normally use a subtle form of coercive power that Foucault called 'disciplinary power' (Foucault, 1979, 1980, 1982).

Power and spirituality

We recognize the inherent contradictions in trying to put conceptual boundaries on spiritual ideas, and yet we need to do so in order to be able to communicate. Birth Territory Theory is holistic and based on the assumption that universal energy (power) is everywhere and always operating. Universal energy is everywhere within the environment; it contains both *yin* and *yang*, good and bad, light and dark, being and non-being (Jung, 1960; Grof, 1985, 1988, 1993; Leder, 1990; Kovel, 1991; Kornfield, 2002). Universal energy is the power that energizes atoms, cells, organs, people, the world and the cosmos. This concept is more familiar within Eastern, rather than Western, philosophy (Jung, 1960; Kovel, 1991; Grof, 1993; Irigaray and Pluhacek, 2002; Kornfield, 2002; Barrett, 2006). The concept of Universal energy is, however, compatible with Western physics, most particularly quantum physics. Albert Einstein famously wrote $E = mc^2$ (meaning energy and matter are interchangeable within the universe), which is another way of saying that energy is universal (Einstein, 1987).

Universal energy is an organizing power that can be conceptualized as promoting increasing levels of organization and complexity (Barrett, 2006). The human spirit is an indivisible part of universal energy. Spirit is non-rational, which is not the same as 'irrational' (Parratt and Fahy, 2008). Spirit is ever-moving and acts, sometimes, in idiosyncratic ways that promote the person's psychophysiological organization towards maximum health and well-being. Spirit, unlike ego, is free of what is rationalized by people to be either possible or impossible; thus, spirit can achieve the seemingly impossible (Kovel, 1991). An extended discussion of spirituality and spiritual power is beyond the scope of this chapter – and, indeed, this theory. The theory does, however, acknowledge that the power of spirit may be felt as sacred, mysterious or wondrous. It may be experienced as a passive yielding or surrendering. Spirit may also be experienced as energy or enthusiasm, as an intuitive gift, or simply as the life-giving force of the breath (Kovel, 1991).

Power and the embodied self

The embodied self is an integrated, whole body/soul/mind who is continually changing according to the internal and external powers with which it is relating. Within the embodied self, the interaction of these powers is complex. In order to simplify the internal powers, we consider them in two contrasting ways. 'Egoic power' arises from the 'ego', and 'inner power' is derived from what we call the 'inner self'.

The ego and egoic power

'Ego' is a learned part of the personality structure that is powerful, verbal, rational and conceptual. Development of the ego enables a person to know how to behave in the external, social environment (Lacan, 1977a, 1977b; Grof, 1985; Peck, 1993; Grosz, 1994, 1995). The relationship between the person's external environment and their inner self creates egoic power. Egoic power is a self-protective force that enables a person to compare and assess their relative safety (Lacan, 1977a, 1977b). The ego assesses safety by perceiving divisions within the inner and outer environments. Egoic power is, therefore, valuable and necessary to the embodied self. In addition, egoic power can prioritize, judge and be biased, thereby giving a person the capacity to take a self-protective stance, should threats be perceived. But these defensive capacities may also mean that a person is self-aggrandizing through the use of arrogance and aggression, or self-sacrificing through the use of diminutive or submissive behaviours. While these behaviours may seem self-protective to the biased ego, they can also damage a person's sense of self as an embodied whole. This is because, unless egoic power is used mindfully, it dominates, hides and ignores the softer 'inner self'.

The inner self and inner power

The 'inner self' is 'spirit', uniquely manifested within each person as their 'soul' (Grof, 1985; Kovel, 1991; Peck, 1993). As the 'inner self' is non-verbal and non-rational, it communicates symbolically and emotionally (Grof, 1985; Kovel, 1991; Peck, 1993). The 'inner self' is subtle, creative, intuitive, and powerful. 'Inner power' moves the self to take action in ways that are sensed to be in the higher interests of the whole embodied self (Grof, 1985; Peck, 1993; Taylor, 1994). 'Inner power' is usually 'integrative' of body, mind and soul. It prompts the self towards more of everything that life has to offer. 'Inner power' is accessed rather than exercised. Accessing inner power can occur in different ways. One way is for a person to get the mind and ego out of the way, such as through some form of meditative practice. Another way to access inner power is to mindfully surrender egoic attempts at control; for example, through the mindful release of egoic desires to dominate or submit to a situation. However, even if egoic power has attempted to repress the inner self, the non-rational spontaneity of inner power will still be experienced. A person's ego may then feel this repressed inner power as a confusing, even terrifying, threat to the ego.

Integrative power

'Integrative power' integrates all forms of power within the environment towards a shared higher goal – in this case, 'genius birth'. Using 'integrative power' promotes mind–body integration for the woman and all other people in the environment. This mind–body integration is essential for the woman, so that she feels able to respond spontaneously and expressively to her bodily sensations and intuitions. We use the word 'intuitive' in a way that is similar to, but also different from, the common understanding of 'instinctive'. The idea of 'instinctive' behaviour is based on a version of evolutionary theory, which claims that human evolution has made such characteristics as social hierarchy, gender inequality and violence inevitable features of all societies (Gasper, 2004). Sigmund Freud (1856–1939) claimed that 'anatomy [read biology] is destiny'; that is, one's sex determines one's personality and, there-fore, desires and behaviours (Thurschwell, 2009). Leading feminist scholars such as Karen Horney (1939), Betty Friedan (1963) and Kate Millett (1969) disagreed; they argued, instead, that cultural programming is the major deter-minant of women's personalities. If a woman feels inferior to a man, Horney contended, it is not due to some universal process such as Freud's concept of 'penis envy'. Rather, she wrote:

> the wish to be a man ... may be the expression of a wish for all those qual-ities or privileges which in our culture are regarded as masculine, such as strength, courage, independence, success, sexual freedom, the right to choose a partner. (Horney, 1939: 108)

The belief that all women are the same and biologically programmed by their 'instincts' has limited, and is used to limit, the roles that women play in society to those of wives, mothers, daughters and sisters. So, distancing ourselves from these common meanings, we consciously take our meaning of women's intuitions and instincts from Liz Grosz's analysis (2004). Thus, 'instinct' is a non-rational (but not irrational) bodily response that occurs relative to the moment and the unique body who is experiencing the sensation (Parratt, 2010). 'Intuition' is an integrated reflection on both the non-rational responses of instinct and the rationally mediated desires of the ego (Parratt, 2010). Women are often disconnected from their bodily instincts and use their higher brains to ignore and over-ride the intuitive messages coming from their embodied selves.

When the woman needs to make decisions about her care options, then the use of 'integrative power' harnesses the power of all participants in the birth environment, so that power is focused on the woman's enhanced mind–body integration. As such, the focus of power within the birth space is on the woman's self-expression and confidence in being the one who is making the ultimate choice about what happens. This integrative use of power then enables the woman to actualize her own power according to her lived experiences at that time (Parratt, 2008, 2010). Importantly, the use of 'integrative power' supports the woman in feeling good about her embodied self, even if the birth outcome is not as she had wished.

Midwifery guardianship

'Midwifery guardianship' is a form of 'integrative power' that involves guarding the woman and her birth 'terrain'. Guarding the 'birth territory' allows the woman to labour undisturbed. 'Midwifery guardianship' also entails nurturing the woman's sense of safety through the respect of her attitudes, values and beliefs. It involves ensuring, as far as possible, that those who enter the boundaries of the birth 'terrain' are committed to using 'integrative power'. 'Midwifery guardianship' promotes and respects the woman's own intrinsic capacity, by which we mean her internal, 'integrative power', enabling the woman to find her own way to birth. The idea being that women can birth their own babies and that the power to do so comes from within (England and Horowitz, 1998). Integrating her inner powers means harnessing the power of her body, mind and soul towards her ultimate aim: 'genius birth'. Note that integrating inner power needs work to be done by the woman: she cannot be passively anaesthetized and integrate all her powers. We are arguing that feeling safe, being undisturbed and activating her own inner power is critical for the woman to optimize her labour and birth.

A brief clinical story from Jenny Parratt's research gives an example of both forms of 'integrative power'; with the midwife and within the woman (Parratt, 2009; 2010) (Box 10.1).

We have discussed the concept of 'midwifery guardianship' back and forth between ourselves because we know that some midwives act like guardians while others are dominating. Similarly, some doctors act like guardians while others are dominating. We thought about changing the concept to 'birth guardian', but that took the focus off the woman – which, we think, is wrong. So, we returned to the roots of the word 'midwife', and it means 'with woman'. We interpret the meaning of 'with woman' as being in a particular relationship to the woman that, in a way, integrates the professional's power

---

Box 10.1   Emily's story of integrative power

Emily was 38 years old in her first pregnancy. She had planned to give birth at a birth centre. She found it challenging that labour didn't start until 42 weeks. She was transferred to the labour ward due to meconium liquor. Emily explained that she felt trapped in the system; she became 'quite defensive' and felt unable to trust the labour ward midwife (Parratt, 2009: 333). Emily agreed to have labour augmented but she also negotiated to have a birth centre midwife whom she felt she could trust. Emily made steady progress through the labour, in part, she said, because of the trusting relationship with the midwife; that relationship enabled her to feel more secure and less trapped. Shoulder dystocia complicated the birth. Emily continues the story in her own words:

> It was like my body interpreted what it meant to have shoulder dystocia at birth, I never went through the 'what ifs' of possible damage or disablement; I wasn't even focused on making her safe ... my body was totally focused on opening up ... My power at birth overrode any sense of vulnerability ... They put her onto my stomach, Graeme and I were crying, he said 'it's a girl' ... My feelings weren't about being a mother; they were about how excited I felt. She was beautiful but I felt more of a sense of relief because I had done it and she was OK. (Parratt, 2009: 342; 356)

Emily's postpartum experience was marred by her mother's death and a rift with her family; this created stress that impacted on other areas such as her return to work. Antidepressants temporarily provided an added sense of security and self-trust while Emily sorted through her changing sense of self. Emily remembered the power of birth as an extension of trust beyond the physical realm. She was aware of a similar power associated with breastfeeding and recognized that awareness of this power is a 'huge strength' that will get her 'through life' (Parratt, 2009: 357).

---

with the woman's power. Since not only midwives can take the role of being truly 'with woman', we have decided that the role of 'midwifery guardianship' is open to doctors as well as midwives (Smellie, 1785; Hastie, 2008b). Note that we are using the word 'midwifery' as derived from the verb 'to midwife', rather than from the noun describing what a person is. We are talking of an action that may or may not be happening from one moment to the next. We are not trying to label whether a person is a 'midwifery guardian' or not. We have, thus, de-personalized the concept 'midwifery guardianship', because a person's actions may change; the same person may act as a guardian and then not act as one. Thus, being a midwife does not necessarily make someone a 'midwifery guardian', and undertaking 'midwifery guardianship' does not assume that the person is a professional midwife.

Disintegrative power

'Disintegrative power' is an ego-centred use of power that disintegrates other forms of power within the environment and imposes the user's self-serving goal. The use of 'disintegrative power' in the 'birth territory' diminishes a woman's capacity for 'genius birth'. 'Disintegrative power' may be used by the woman, the midwife and/or any other person in the territory. When it is used by the woman, it is an ego-based determination to have a particular experience or outcome that is a 'forced birth' (Parratt, 2008). Regardless of who uses it, 'disintegrative power' leads to the disintegration of the woman's mind–body unity and, thus, separates her from her embodied power to birth instinctively (Parratt, 2010). 'Disintegrative power', when used by professionals, undermines the woman as the decision-maker in her own care and leads to a 'forced birth' (Parratt, 2010). The use of 'disintegrative power' by maternity clinicians diminishes the woman's sense of self, regardless of the physical birth outcome. The negative effects of the use of 'disintegrative power' within the 'birth territory' can be inferred from research showing that women's perceptions of low levels of support coupled with surgical births are most related to their experiences of postnatal distress, depression and problems with maternal–infant bonding (Smellie, 1785; Creedy *et al.*, 2000; Davis-Floyd, 2003; Boarders, 2006; Cigoli *et al.*, 2006; Hastie, 2008b).

Midwifery domination

'Midwifery domination' is a form of 'disintegrative power' that is based on the use of disciplinary power. Disciplinary power is a subtle and manipulative form of power that is usually not able to be detected until the subject of power offers resistance (Foucault, 1979, 1980). 'Midwifery domination' is disturbing, because it interferes with the woman's labouring process by inducing the woman to become either docile or aggressive in response (Fahy, 2002). Being docile requires the woman to follow the midwife's guidance and, therefore, give up her own embodied knowledge and power. A woman may respond to 'midwifery domination' by using her own 'disintegrative power', where she attempts to dominate the midwife and may even become aggressive toward her care givers. In a situation of 'midwifery domination', the woman is cut off from her inner power. When a woman is cut off from her inner power, it is very hard for her, or the midwife, to trust that the woman is perceiving and responding to her intuitive bodily sensations. In contrast, when a woman is consistently exposed to 'midwifery guardianship' and uses 'integrative power', midwives can more easily 'trust' a woman's expressions of power and her 'intuitions'.

The clinical stories

Birth Territory Theory is next applied to two birth stories, those of Tara and Niki. These births occured in hospital but, in other respects, they are different. It is this contrast that allows us to exemplify the concepts and illustrate the significance of the Theory. As Birth Territory Theory falls within critical post-structural feminism, this is reflected when the theory is applied to the stories. We are aware that the honesty of the critical stance can create unpalatable reactions, and we acknowledge that others may have different perspectives on the stories. While other people may have other perspectives, in our opinion critical feminism is preferable in this situation, because it can take into account more of the available data than other methodologies. These stories are discussed in greater detail in two chapters – Fahy (2008) and Fahy and Hastie (2008) – in Fahy *et al.* (2008).

Application to Tara's birth in a 'surveillance environment'

Kathleen observed the following episode as a researcher (Fahy, 1995). Although this episode occurred some years ago, it was observed and analyzed as part of a research study. The other stories available for our current theoretical analysis were anecdotal or part of a woman's or midwifes' narrative and were thus not as detailed as these two stories. The birthing rooms and the ways that maternity staff relate have not changed substantially, in our view. Our interpretive comments linking this story to the theoretical concepts are presented as bullet points at the end of each relevant section.

Tara (not her real name) was aged 19 years, having her first baby and well-known to me as a research participant. With my help, Tara had devised a birth plan that included that she would have an epidural if she felt she couldn't cope with the pain.

Here is the scene that I encountered on arriving to be with Tara in late first-stage labour. The delivery suite where Tara was labouring was on the third floor of the hospital. There was no door to Tara's room, just a pink curtain partly covering the entrance. Tara was in a large, modern, clinical-looking room. All the furniture was made of metal. It had two windows, but the view was of another building. The room was air-conditioned, but not cold. The lighting was by artificial recessed fluorescent tubes. There was a large, mobile operating theatre light (turned off) hanging over the bed. There was oxygen and suction on the wall. A baby resuscitation trolley was partially 'hidden' behind a pink screen. The bed was in the centre of the room; its end was facing the curtained doorway. Tara was lying on her side on the bed, covered by a sheet. Her mother sat quietly beside her. Tara was awake and apparently relaxed. She had a working epidural, and an electronic foetal monitor was attached.

- This is a 'surveillance environment', and there is no evidence that Tara has any 'jurisdiction'.

Shortly after I arrived, the epidural wore off and Tara wanted it topped up. Her request was refused by the midwives, who explained that, as her cervix was fully dilated, she wouldn't feel the urge to push and have a normal birth if she had a working epidural. Tara said she didn't care about a normal birth, she just wanted the epidural topped up, but the midwives would not do what she wanted.

- This is 'disintegrative power' and 'midwifery domination'. It is possible that a different midwife with a different approach may have been able to gain Tara's commitment to a normal birth.

After the midwife's refusal, Tara became passive and sullen. She continued to want the epidural topped up, but she was not assertive in making this clear.

- Evidence of submission and docility is accompanied by reduced emotional well-being.

I urged her to speak up for herself, which she did, saying 'I want the epidural topped up please'. This was met with silence and the midwife left the room. Shortly afterwards, the senior medical registrar (whom Tara had never seen) came in and stood at the end of the bed and said, with a degree of anger, 'We will top you up but you will probably need forceps now and that can damage the baby's head. You are a selfish girl who is putting her baby at risk.' Not waiting for a response, he walked out and was never seen again.

- This is 'disintegrative power' and medical domination.

Tara turned her face away and, without talking, she cried softly. Except for crying, she was essentially silent for the rest of the labour. Throughout the rest of the labour, Tara was passive and sullenly compliant.

- This is evidence of serious emotional distress and submission. The theory, through the concept of 'disintegrative power', predicts that Tara will not be able to birth independently because of this emotional distress and disempowerment.

The epidural was finally topped up but only worked on one side, so Tara continued to feel the pain fully on one side. After the episode with the doctor, Tara's contractions became less frequent and much shorter. On medical orders, the midwives began a Syntocinon infusion. She had six hours in a painful second stage with no progress.

- This is evidence of sub-optimal physiological functioning related to the use of 'disintegrative power'.

Finally, a junior doctor decided to do a vacuum delivery and an episiotomy.

- For Tara, the negative 'birth territory' was a medical and midwifery 'forced birth': it was experienced by Tara as a disempowering and painful ordeal.

We recognize that the 'birth territory' alone cannot, in any simple way, be 'blamed' for the negative outcomes of mother and baby. We are claiming, though, that these experiences did contribute to her emotional distress and postnatal depression. We are also claiming that a positive experience of 'birth territory' is likely to have had a very different outcome.

Application to Niki's birth in a 'sanctum'

Kathleen and Carolyn were the midwives at this birth and recorded this as part of Kathleen's professional journaling. The story has been approved for publication by the woman and the other participants at the birth. All names have been changed. Once again, our interpretive comments that link to the theoretical concepts are presented as bullet points at the end of each section.

Niki was having her first baby and labour had progressed well. She stayed in the deep birth pool for eight hours, using meditation techniques to cope with the pain. Gavin (Niki's partner) was a quiet, loving and supportive presence. Carolyn and I were quiet and unobtrusive; however, in line with medical protocols we recorded Niki's blood pressure and pulse hourly, and assessed the baby's heart rate at 15-minute intervals.

- The 'jurisdiction' of the space is Niki's, and the midwives are acting as midwifery guardians.

Labour had begun with the baby's head in an occipito-transverse position, but we assumed that the head would rotate naturally. All went well until transition, which continued for about three hours. During the first part of this time, Niki wanted to get out of the bath and change positions, and we encouraged her to follow this inner instinct.

- 'Integrative power' is being used by Niki and the midwives.

As the time progressed and we saw no signs of second stage activity, Carolyn suggested that Niki move her hips in particular ways to assist with pelvic opening. With great strength, courage and endurance Niki followed Carolyn's advice and squatted, walked, tried the hands-and-knees position and tried the birth stool – all to no avail.

- This is a use of 'integrative power'; it brings midwifery power/knowledge to the situation and integrates with the power of the woman and her body.

We discussed with Niki and Gavin that, on palpation, the baby's head was still in the occipito-transverse position. A vaginal examination confirmed that the head may, indeed, be a bit stuck at the ischial spines. As the cervix was not yet fully dilated, the obstetrician (Jonathan), whom they knew a little, suggested to Niki that she may want to have her contractions strengthened by the use of a Syntocinon infusion.

- Jonathan's use of power/knowledge is integrative, as it leaves the choice of having Syntocinon up to Niki.

These words had an almost immediate effect on Niki. She turned on her side, went physically limp as if giving up, and cried. She said, 'I don't want Syntocinon'. Up until this point, Niki had been strong and active; suddenly, she appeared weak and passive.

- Niki's ego-based determination to have a particular experience has created 'disintegrative power' that has undermined her embodied sense of self, causing a loss of power illustrated by her passivity.

Carolyn spoke firmly to her. 'No, Niki, you don't have to have Syntocinon. There are midwifery strategies that we can try, you can still have a normal birth, but we need you to *be here* and fully present. You need to come back here right now and you need to be strong and courageous. I want you to get up and start moving. Gavin', she directed, 'I want you to come and help Niki. Jonathan', she said, and turned to him, 'can you give us 40 minutes and come back then'. Jonathan agreed and quietly left the room.

- This is the midwife using 'integrative power'. Carolyn moves to reverse Niki's use of 'disintegrative power'; she uses 'integrative power' to call for Niki's fully embodied presence.

The effect of Carolyn's powerful intervention was amazing. Niki regained her strength and confidence. With fortitude and grace, Niki got up and started moving as Carolyn instructed. She began stepping sideways up the steps of the birth pool with Gavin providing physical and psychological support. After a time, Carolyn advised squatting for a few contractions and Niki did this; again, with Gavin's loving support. This movement went on for the next 40 minutes of labour, with all of us actively involved in supporting Niki and listening to the baby's heart sounds every 15 minutes.

- This is 'integrative power' in action.

During this time, Niki's facial expressions showed she was in pain, but she didn't complain or cry out; she was too busy putting all her energy into helping her pelvis to open and the baby to turn.

- This is evidence of her greater mind–body integration and enhanced embodied sense of self.

After talking quietly together, Carolyn and I agreed that there were three options if the head did not rotate within the 40 minutes allocated. We discussed them with Niki and Gavin before Jonathan returned.

- This is 'midwifery guardianship'.

When Jonathan got back, he examined Niki and found her fully dilated, but the head was still in the occipito-transverse position. At this point, all five of us discussed the three options for moving forward. Niki chose a manual rotation. Jonathan said it might be too painful, but he was willing to try if Niki was. With Niki sitting on the birth stool, Jonathan performed a manual rotation when Niki had a contraction. The head moved easily into the correct position and baby Declan was born normally about two hours later.

- This is the use of 'integrative power', and the outcome is a 'genius birth'.

Immediately after birth, Niki, Gavin and baby Declan were bonding beautifully; nearly two hours later, Niki birthed the placenta with minimal blood loss and they went home after four hours. Niki and Gavin described amazing feelings of being overwhelmed with love for Declan. Niki was proud of herself and very pleased with Gavin's support in labour. Gavin was proud of Niki and himself; they were both thrilled with the outcome. Niki and Declan proceeded to have a positive postnatal and breastfeeding experience.

Niki, Gavin and I discussed the birth about a week afterwards. They were convinced that the respectful and positive care that they received prevented a caesarean section. When asked how she felt about Carolyn's forceful intervention asking her to be strong, get moving and not give up, Niki said 'I thought she was great because she made me feel that what I wanted (a normal birth) was possible, that I didn't have to give up. Someone else who really knew about birth believed in me and in my dream, and I was able to trust myself again and to keep on going'.

- Evidence of how 'midwifery guardianship' and 'integrative power' can harness the woman's own power while using midwifery and medical interventions only as they are specifically needed.

We acknowledge that the 'birth territory' was not the only factor that was involved in creating the positive outcomes for Niki and her family. Niki had experienced continuity of carer with her midwives and knew us both well. In addition, she had personal characteristics that were central to her outcomes: she had read widely, had discussed birthing options fully with her midwives, and she was committed to natural birth. This story and Niki's own words demonstrate, however, that Niki would have been most unlikely to have given birth normally had she been cared for in a 'surveillance environment' without 'midwifery guardianship'.

Tara experienced negative 'birth territory' in all aspects of 'terrain' and 'jurisdiction'; she had no 'jurisdiction' over her room. 'Midwifery guardianship' was absent and 'disintegrative power', both medical and midwifery, was used. Labour and birth were an ordeal for Tara, who experienced a 'forced birth' that was a source of anger and shame for her. As the theory of 'birth territory' predicts, Tara had a very negative postnatal period and difficulty bonding with her baby.

By comparison, Niki experienced almost ideal conditions for birth and had a joyful, 'genius birth' outcome. She had a 'sanctum' to labour in and she experienced 'jurisdiction' over the territory. She used her own 'integrative power', and she was the beneficiary of the use of 'integrative power' by the midwives and the obstetrician. For Niki, the 'birth territory' was experienced as nurturing, so that labour, even though painful, did not involve anguish. As the theory predicts, she had an easy and positive postnatal transition, capably bonding with her baby and breastfeeding successfully.

Conclusion

Birth Territory Theory can be used to describe, explain and predict how the 'birth territory' affects women and babies at all stages of childbearing, in particular during labour and birth. Birth Territory Theory is a practical, evidence-based theory that can be used to guide midwives and administrators in practice. The theory shows how to restructure the 'birth territory' to maximize a woman's 'integrative power' so that she is able to have a physiologically normal pregnancy, labour and birth.

One factor that has a large impact on a woman's well-being as an embodied self is whether 'integrative power' or 'disintegrative power' is used by the woman herself and/or by others in the 'birth territory' (Parratt, 2010). We hypothesize that, when 'integrative power' is used within a 'sanctum', the woman is then most likely to experience a 'genius birth'. The role of the midwife – to provide 'midwifery guardianship' in the 'birth territory' – seems to be paramount in promoting the use of 'integrative power' by the woman and others within the territory. The central proposition of the theory of 'birth territory' is that, when midwives create and maintain an ideal 'birth territory', maximum support is provided to the woman and foetus in labour and birth which results in an increased likelihood that the woman will experience a 'genius birth' – which, in most cases, will also be a physiologically normal birth. We have argued that when the woman has a 'genius birth', whether or not it ends up being physiologically 'normal', she is more likely to be satisfied with the experience, feel good about her embodied self and adapt with greater ease in the post-birth period.

We believe our theory meets the accepted professional criteria to be considered a formal theory for midwifery (Fawcett, 2000; Peterson and Bredow, 2004; Walker and Avant, 2004). The limitations of the theory include the fact that the theoretical and empirical links between how women feel and how they function physiologically needs further development. The theory currently does not describe the mechanism that creates the broader and longer-term benefits that we are predicting as the outcomes. Research is also needed to strengthen the evidence for our proposition: that providing an ideal 'birth territory' will result in the majority of women actually experiencing physiologically normal birth. Finally, the theory is currently focused on the individual birth room, but it would benefit from being developed at the social level, so that theory could guide public practice about the desired location, structure and function of maternity services.

The strengths of Birth Territory Theory include that the theoretical concepts and propositions were originally derived from reflections on the practice of four senior midwifery clinicians and researchers. The concepts are well-defined and the propositions are clearly stated. The theory displays internal validity, in that the concepts and propositions are logically structured in relation to each other. Since we have been developing this theory, we have constantly tested it against our previous and current practice and find it has good explanatory and predictive power. This demonstrates that the theory has face validity (Fawcett, 2000). We believe that the theory is sufficiently well developed to be evaluated, critiqued and tested in both practice and further research.

ACTIVITIES

Undergraduate

Consider, discuss and explore the meaning of the following statements from the chapter:

... a woman's sense of safety is paramount for her to be able stay on a trajectory towards 'genius birth' ...

Some will only feel safe at home with known and trusted care givers. Others may only feel safe in an environment that is highly medicalized and technologically sophisticated.

Postgraduate

The central proposition of the theory of 'birth territory' is that, when midwives create and maintain an ideal 'birth territory', maximum support is provided to the woman and foetus in labour and birth, which results in an increased likelihood that the woman will experience a 'genius birth'.

Design a clinical research study to test this proposition.

Table 10.1   Glossary of key Birth Territory concepts

Birth	Birth is defined as that period extending from peri-conception up to and including early parenting.
Birth territory	'Birth territory' is defined as the environment that is external to the woman/baby. The concept of 'birth territory' includes the physical features of the environment (the 'terrain') and the use of power by people within the environment ('jurisdiction').
Disintegrative power	'Disintegrative power' is an ego-centred use of power that disintegrates other forms of power within the environment and imposes the user's self-serving goal. 'Disintegrative power' may be used by the woman, the midwife and/or any other person in the territory. The use of 'disintegrative power' by anyone in the birth room may create mind–body disintegration and undermine the woman and baby in their ability to have a 'genius birth'.
Forced birth	A 'forced birth' is defined as one where power is used to try to force a particular type of birth. A 'forced birth' involves cutting off from one's own inner power. There are two types: medically forced and maternally forced. Neither medical nor maternal 'forced births' are likely to be optimally suited to a woman's holistic wellbeing at that particular moment of her life. Following a 'forced birth', a woman's feelings of self-appreciation will be limited, and she is likely to focus her joy and relief on the presence of her baby.

Table 10.1 *continued*

Genius birth	A 'genius birth' is defined as one where a woman responds to labour challenges by drawing from usually hidden capacities deep within her embodied self. In actualizing her inner power, she combines it with her conscious intention to experience a physiologically normal birth. A 'genius birth' is not contrived but, rather, is conscious and effortful even if, in taking account of her holistic wellbeing at that particular moment of her life, medical interventions are accepted.
Integrative power	'Integrative power' integrates all forms of power within the environment towards a shared higher goal, in this case; 'genius birth'. Using 'integrative power' promotes mind–body integration for the woman and all other people in the environment. This mind–body integration is essential for the woman so that she feels able to respond spontaneously and expressively to her bodily sensations and intuitions.
Jurisdiction	'Jurisdiction' means having the power to do as one wants in the birth environment. Within the broad concept of 'jurisdiction' there is a continuum of 'integrative power' to 'disintegrative power'. Two concepts are directly derived from integrative and 'disintegrative power'; namely 'midwifery guardianship' and 'midwifery domination'.
Midwifery guardianship	'Midwifery guardianship' is a form of 'integrative power' that involves guarding the woman and her birth 'terrain'. Guarding the 'birth territory' allows the women to labour undisturbed. 'Midwifery guardianship' also entails nurturing the woman's sense of safety through the respect of her attitudes, values and beliefs. Here, we use the term 'midwife', not in the professional sense but in the active sense, meaning the actions undertaken by any birth attendant to 'be with' a woman integratively.
Terrain	'Terrain' denotes the physical features and geographical area of the individual birth space, including the furniture and accessories that the woman and her support people use for labour and birth. Two sub-concepts, 'surveillance environment' and 'sanctum', lie at opposite ends along this continuum called 'terrain'.

Table 10.2   Glossary of key power terms

Ego	'Ego' is a learned part of the personality structure. Ego is powerful, verbal, rational and conceptual. Ego is formed to enable the person to know how to behave in the external, social environment. Ego can easily dominate the 'inner self'.
Egoic power	'Egoic power' is a self-protective force arising from the ego. It compares and assesses perceived divisions within inner and outer environments in order to determine relative safety. But egoic power is divisive and dominating, so it also hides and ignores 'inner self' and 'inner power'.
Inner power	'Inner power' is an energy that moves the self to take action that is sensed to be in the higher interests of the whole self. 'Inner power' is 'integrative' of body/soul/mind. 'Inner power' prompts the self towards more of everything that life has to offer. 'Inner power' is accessed rather than exercised. It can only be accessed by surrendering egoic attempts to control the situation. An experience of inner power may be confusing, even terrifying, to the person's ego.
Inner self	The 'inner self' is 'spirit' uniquely manifested within each person as their 'soul'. The 'inner self' is non-verbal and non-rational, it communicates symbolically and emotionally. The 'inner self' is subtle, creative, intuitive and powerful.
Spirituality	Humans long to feel whole or connected with the sacred dimensions of life. Sometimes this quest is towards something bigger and more powerful than us, and sometimes the quest is inwards towards knowing our inner self more fully. This quest for wholeness and connection is termed 'spirituality'
Universal energy	'Universal energy' is the power that energizes the world and the cosmos. This concept is more familiar within Eastern, rather than Western, philosophy. As Einstein noted, energy is everywhere within the environment and within all living and non-living people and things; in this way, energy is universal. Universal energy contains yin and yang, good and bad, light and dark, being and non-being. Human beings are animated by universal energy, which is sometimes referred to as 'spirit'. In our theory, we see a person's spirit as non-rational, ever-moving and acting, sometimes, in unexpected and idiosyncratic ways. Spirit may be suppressed or liberated by egoic power.

References

Barrett, R. (2006) *Taijiquan: Through the Western Gate*. Berkley, CA: Blue Snake Books.

Boarders, N. (2006) 'After the Afterbirth: A Critical Review of Postpartum Health Relative to Method of Delivery', *Journal of Midwifery and Women's Health*, 51(4): 242–8.

Cigoli, V., Gilli, G. and Saita, E. (2006) 'Relational Factors in Psychopathological Responses to Childbirth', *Journal of Psychosomatic Obstetrics and Gynaecology*, 27(2): 91–7.

Creedy, D.K., Shochet, I.M. and Horsfall, J. (2000) 'Childbirth and the Development of Acute Trauma Symptoms: Incidence and Contributing Factors', *Birth*, 27(2): 104–11.

Davis-Floyd, R. (2003) *Birth as an American Rite of Passage*, 2nd edn. Berkley, CA: University of California Press.

Downe, S. and McCourt, C. (2004) 'From Being to Becoming: Reconstructing Childbirth Knowledges', in S. Downe (ed.), *Normal Childbirth: Evidence and Debate*. London: Churchill Livingston, ch. 1: 3–24.

Einstein, A. (1987) *The Collected Papers of Albert Einstein 1905–1920*, (A. Beck, trans.) Princeton, NJ: Princeton University Press.

England, P. and Horowitz, R. (1998) *Birthing from Within: An Extra-Ordinary Guide to Childbirth Preparation*. Albuquerque, NM: Partera Press.

Fahy, K. (1995) 'Marginalised Mothers: Teenage Transition to Motherhood and the Experience of Disciplinary Power', Unpublished PhD, University of Queensland, Brisbane.

Fahy, K. (2002) 'Reflecting on Practice to Theorise Empowerment for Women: Using Foucault's concepts', *Australian Journal of Midwifery*, 15(1): 5–13.

Fahy, K. (2008) 'Theorising Birth Territory', in K. Fahy, M. Foureur and C. Hastie (eds), *Birth Territory and Midwifery Guardianship*. Edinburgh: Elsevier, ch. 2: 11–19.

Fahy, K., Foureur, M. and Hastie, C. (eds) (2008) *Birth Territory and Midwifery Guardianship*. Edinburgh: Elsevier.

Fahy, K. and Hastie, C. (2008) 'Midwifery Guardianship: Reclaiming the Sacred in Birth', in K. Fahy, M. Foureur and C. Hastie (eds), *Birth Territory and Midwifery Guardianship*. Edinburgh: Elsevier, ch. 3: 21–37.

Fahy, K. and Parratt, J. (2006) 'Birth Territory: A Theory for Midwifery Practice', *Women and Birth*, 19(2): 45–50.

Fawcett, J. (2000) *Analysis and Evaluation of Contemporary Nursing Knowledge: Nursing Models and Theories*. Philadelphia, PA: F.A. Davis.

Foucault, M. (1979) *Discipline and Punish: The Birth of the Prison*. (A. Sheridan, trans.) New York, NY: Vintage Books.

Foucault, M. (1980) *Power/Knowledge: Selected Interviews*, (C. Gordon, L. Marshall, J. Mepham and K. Soper, trans.). New York, NY: Pantheon Books.

Foucault, M. (1982) 'The Subject and Power', afterword in H. Dreyfus and P. Rabinow (eds) *Michel Foucault: Beyond Structuralism and Hermeneutics*. New York, NY: Harvester Wheatsheaf: 208–26.

Foureur, M. (2007) 'Establishing the Principles for Creating Positive Birth Space', Keynote Address, Australian College of Midwives State Conference, Queensland, July 2007.

Foureur, M. (2008) 'Creating Birth Space to enable Undisturbed Birth', in: K. Fahy, M. Foureur and C. Hastie (eds), *Birth Territory and Midwifery Guardianship*. Edinburgh: Elsevier, ch. 5: 57–77.

Foureur, M. and Hunter, M. (2006) 'The Place of Birth', in S. Pairman, J. Pincombe, C. Thorogood and S. Tracey (eds), *The Midwifery Textbook*. Sydney: Elsevier.

Friedan, B. (1963) *The Feminist Mystique*. New York, NY: W. Norton.

Gasper, P. (2004) 'Is Biology Destiny?', *International Socialist Review*, (38). Online journal available at: http://www.isreview.org/issues/38/genes.shtml – accessed 15 August 2010.

Gould, D. (2002) 'Birthwrite: Subliminal Medicalisation', *British Journal of Midwifery*, 10(7): 418.

Grof, C. (1993) *The Thirst for Wholeness: Attachment, Addiction and the Spiritual Path*. San Francisco, CA: Harper Collins.

Grof, S. (1985) *Beyond the Brain: Birth, Death and Transcendence in Psychotherapy*. New York, NY: State University of New York Press.

Grof, S. (1988) *The Adventure of Self-Discovery*. New York, NY: State University of New York Press.

Grosz, E. (1994) *Volitile Bodies*. Sydney: Allen & Unwin.

Grosz, E. (1995) *Space, Time and Perversion: The Politics of Bodies*. Sydney: Allen & Unwin.

Grosz, E. (2004) *The Nick of Time. Politics, Evolution and the Untimely*. Sydney: Allen & Unwin.

Hastie, C. (2008a) 'The Spiritual and Emotional Territory of the Unborn and Newborn Baby', in K. Fahy, M. Foureur and C. Hastie (eds), *Birth Territory and Midwifery Guardianship*, Edinburgh: Elsevier, ch. 6: 79–94.

Hastie, C. (2008b) 'Putting Women First: Interprofessional Integrative Power', Unpublished Master's Dissertation, University of Newcastle: Newcastle.

Hastie, C. and Fahy, K. (2009) 'Optimising Psychophysiology in Third Stage of Labour: Theory Applied to Practice', *Women and Birth*, 22(3): 89–96.

Horney, K. (1939) *New Ways in Psychoanalysis*. New York: Norton.

Inch, S. (1984) *Birthrights: What Every Parent Should Know about Childbirth in Hospitals*. New York, NY: Pantheon Books.

Irigaray, L. (1993) *An Ethics of Sexual Difference*, (C. Burke and G.C. Gill, trans.) London: Athlone.

Irigaray, L. (2001) *To Be Two*, (M. Monoc and M. Rhodes, trans.) New York, NY: Routledge.

Irigaray, L. (2003) *The Way of Love*, (H. Bostic and S. Pluhacek, trans.) New York, NY: Continuum International Publishing Group.

Irigaray, L., and Pluhacek, S. (2002). *Between East and West* (European Perspectives; A Series in Social Thought and Cultural Criticism). New York, NY: Columbia University Press.

Jung, C.G. (1960) 'On the Nature of the Psyche', in *Collected Works, Volume 8*, (R. Hull, trans.). Princeton, NJ: Princeton University Press.

Kornfield, J. (2002) *A Path with Heart: The Classic Guide through the Perils and Promises of Spiritual Life*. London: Random House.

Kovel, J. (1991) *History and Spirit: An Inquiry into the Philosophy of Liberation*. Boston, MA: Beacon Press.

Kristeva, J. (1982) *Powers of Horror: An Essay on Abjection*, (L. S. Roudiez, trans.) New York, NY: Columbia University Press.

Lacan, J. (1977a) *Ecrits: A Selection*, (A. Sheridan, trans.) London: Tavistock.

Lacan, J. (1977b) *The Four Fundamental Concepts of Psycho-Analysis*. Book XI of seminar series (A. Sheridan, trans.) Harmondsworth: Penguin.

Leder, D. (1990) *The Absent Body*. Chicago, IL: Chicago University Press.

Millett, K. (1969) *Sexual Politics*. Chicago, IL: Chicago University Press.

Newburn, M. and Singh, D. (2005) *Are Women getting the Birth Environment They Need?: Report of a National Survey of Women's Experiences*, London: National Childbirth Trust.

Northrup, C. (1998) *Women's Bodies, Women's Wisdom*. Bath: Piatkus.

Parratt, J. (2000) 'Trusting Enough to be Out Of Control: The Impact of Childbirth Experiences on Women's Sense of Self', Unpublished Master's Dissertation, University of Southern Queensland, Toowoomba.

Parratt, J. (2002) 'The Impact of Childbirth Experiences on Women's Sense of Self', *Australian Journal of Midwifery*, 15(4): 10–16.

Parratt, J. (2008) 'Territories of the Self and Spiritual Practices during Childbirth', in K. Fahy, M. Foureur and C. Hastie (eds), *Birth Territory and Midwifery Guardianship*. Edinburgh: Elsevier, ch. 4: 39–54.

Parratt, J. (2009) 'Feelings of Change: Stories of Having a Baby'. Lulu.com: Raleigh. (http://www.lulu.com/content/paperback-book/feelings-of-change-stories-of-having-a-baby/7846284 – accessed 15 August 2010).

Parratt, J. (2010) 'Feeling Like a Genius: Enhancing Women's Changing Embodied Self during First Childbearing', Unpublished PhD, University of Newcastle, Newcastle.

Parratt, J. and Fahy, K. (2004) 'Creating a "Safe" Place for Birth: An Empirically Grounded Theory', *New Zealand College of Midwives Journal*, 30(1): 11–14.

Parratt, J. and Fahy, K. (2008) 'Including the Nonrational is Sensible Midwifery', *Women and Birth*, 21(2): 37–42.

Peck, M.S. (1993) *The Road Less Travelled: A New Psychology of Love, Traditional Values and Spiritual Growth*. London: Hutchinson.

Pert, C. (1997) *The Molecules of Emotion: The Science behind Mind–Body Medicine*. New York, NY: Scriber.

Peterson, S.J. and Bredow, T.S. (2004) *Middle Range Theories: Application to Nursing Research*. Philadelphia, PA: Lippincott Williams & Wilkins.

Rowley, M. (Foureur, M.) (1998) 'Evaluation of Team Midwifery Care in Pregnancy and Childbirth: A Randomised Controlled Trial', Unpublished PhD, University of Newcastle, Newcastle.

Smellie, W. (1785) *A Set of Anatomical Tables with Explanations and an Abridgment of the Practice of Midwifery*. Edinburgh: Charles Elliott.

Stable, D. and Rankin, J. (2005) *Physiology in Childbearing with Anatomy and Related Bioscience*, 2nd edn. Edinburgh: Elsevier.

Sternberg, E.M. and Wilson, M.A. (2006) 'Neuroscience and Architecture: Seeking Common Ground', *Cell*, 127(2): 239–42.

Taylor, K. (1994) *The Breathwork Experience: Exploration and Healing in Nonordinary States of Consciousness*. Santa Cruz, CA: Hanford Mead.

Thurschwell, Pamela (2009) *Sigmund Freud*. London: Routledge. (Retrieved from Taylor and Francis e-library, www.ebookstore.tandf.co.uk – accessed 15 August 2010).

Uvnas-Moberg, K. (2003) *The Oxytocin Factor: Tapping the Hormone of Calm, Love, and Healing*. Cambridge, MA: Merloyd Lawrence Books.

Walker, L. and Avant, K. (2004) *Strategies for Theory Development in Nursing*. Norwalk, CT: Appleton & Lange.

Walsh, D. (2000) 'Part Five: Why We Should Reject the 'Bed Birth' Myth', *British Journal of Midwifery*, 8(9): 554–8.

Young, I.M. (2005) *On Female Body Experience: Throwing Like a Girl and Other Essays*. Oxford: Oxford University Press.

Developing a Model of Birth Technology Competence using Concept Development

11

Kenda Crozier, Marlene Sinclair, George Kernohan and Sam Porter

---

Key points

- Application of the Hybrid Method of Concept Development in midwifery practice
- Outline of a stepwise approach to Concept Development
- Demonstration of the existence of birth technology in midwifery practice
- Further development of the Concept Development process by introducing another step to validate the concept.

Introduction

As health care has changed through the advance of science and technology, this has had an impact on pregnancy for women with medical conditions. According to Lee (2004), more women are embarking on high-risk pregnancies complicated by medical conditions because science and technology have developed to support them in their aim of achieving motherhood. These women need to be cared for by midwives who are competent in the use of high technology.

Polemical issues in midwifery

There is debate within the midwifery profession about the continuing drive towards more technologically mediated birth (Rothwell, 1995; Kirkham and Stapleton, 2000; Walsh, 2009). Cowie and Floyd (1998) expressed concern that midwives were becoming distracted from the real work of midwifery by the technological machines that they use in practice. Their implication, that midwives are becoming dependent on machines in practice, is refuted by the work of Sinclair (2001), who found that midwives disagreed with any suggestion that they might be dependent on the technology. Nevertheless, Sinclair (2000) argued that midwives do need to develop skills in use of technology, including key skills in information technology, to ensure the health and safety of women and their unborn and newly born infants (Sinclair, 2000).

The reasons for the use of technology in midwifery practice are many and complex. Consumer demand, changing societal acceptance of everyday technology, and the inextricable link between advances in medicine and technology are some of the driving forces (Henley-Einion, 2003).

In describing midwifery work, many authors compare and contrast approaches to pregnancy and birth taken by the medical and midwifery professions in order to highlight that midwifery philosophies and knowledge are separate from those defined within the medical specialty of obstetrics (Chalmers *et al.*, 1980; Oakley, 1987; Bryar, 1995; Davis-Floyd, 2003). In response to the current debate within midwifery about the return to normality, it was important in this study to develop an understanding of midwives' competence in the use of technology and the place that technology holds in midwifery practice (Crozier, 2005). Before any change can take place, there needs to be an understanding of the current status quo.

Aim of the study

The aim of the research was to identify birth technology competencies used by midwives to support women during the birthing process. The key questions were:

1. What is birth technology competence?
2. What are the key skills required by midwives to enable them to function competently and effectively in their technological role?

Deciding on the use of a concept development method

The purpose of the research study was theory-building, in that it sought to explain a dimension of the role of the midwife, in relation to technology, that had not previously been explored in this manner. There was a need to examine midwives' use and competence in the use of technology in a hospital setting. The majority of technologies are used as a matter of routine in delivery suites, although technologies are also used in antenatal wards, day assessment units and postnatal wards. Birth technology competence is a concept that has not previously been defined; therefore, it was important to use a method that would suit the exploratory nature of the investigation. The method needed to include a means of developing the concept beyond a discourse analysis, and contextualizing it within the real world of midwifery. The starting point was defining the concept of birth technology through a process of concept analysis leading to identification of attributes, a model case, and a definition. To ensure the concept analysis was 'real', or could be

Table 11.1   Three phases of the Hybrid Model of Concept Development

PHASE I *Theoretical*	PHASE II *Fieldwork*	PHASE III *Final analysis*
Selecting a concept	Setting the stage	Weighing findings
Searching the literature	Negotiating entry	Working out
Dealing with meaning and measurement	Selecting cases	Writing-up findings
Choosing a working definition	Collecting and analyzing data	

confirmed as clinically meaningful, further refinement of the concept had to be explored through fieldwork. Bringing together the theoretical components and their clinical application through the use of ethnography facilitated the development of a model of midwifery competence in the use of birth technology.

The Swartz-Barcott and Kim (2000) Hybrid Model of Concept Development utilizes a three-phase approach incorporating:

1. a theoretical phase, which examines the literature and discourse surrounding the phenomenon under question – in other words 'concept analysis';
2. a fieldwork phase, which serves to illuminate the concept in action; and
3. an analytical phase, which utilizes the combined information from the first two phases in order further to refine the concept.

A modified approach – consisting of both the Chinn and Kramer (1999) framework for concept analysis in the theoretical phase and the Hybrid Model of Concept Development (Swartz-Barcott and Kim, 2000) – was used in this work to analyse and develop the concept of birth technology competence. The hybrid approach has been used to examine, among others, concepts such as family-centred care (Hutchfield, 1999) and the professional identity of the nurse (Ohlen and Segesten, 1998). The major components of each of the phases in the Hybrid Model of Concept Development are set out in Table 11.1.

Figure 11.1 illustrates a semi-formal audit trail outlining the methods used throughout the process of concept development as a guide to the process followed in this work.

Phase I: theoretical phase

Technology in use

Having established that technology in the birthing process is far from unusual, it was necessary to ascertain the type of technologies used by midwives. Sinclair (1999) created detailed inventories of technology used in midwifery work. These were adapted using information from literature to identify the type of technology that might be encountered in the observation phase of the

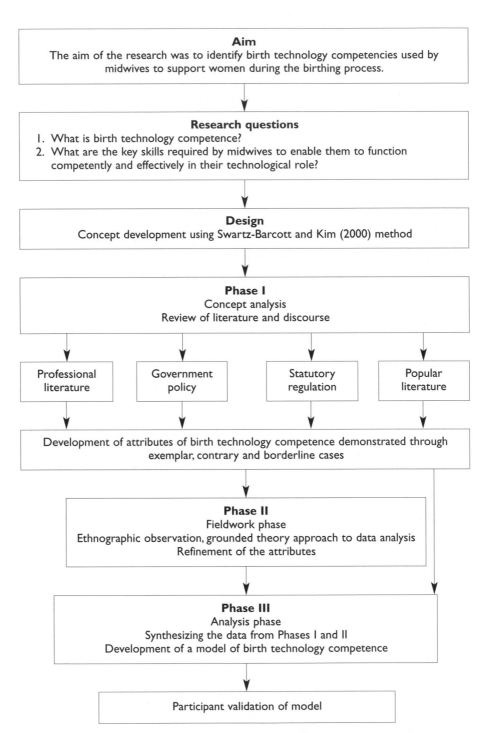

Figure 11.1   Audit trail outlining the methodology

study. Sinclair's inventories have been adapted and subdivided into five main categories:

1. monitoring the mother and foetus;
2. controlling labour;
3. pain relief;
4. resuscitation; and
5. bureaucracy.

The categories were used to identify the types of machines used in the field-work phase of the study (see Table 11.2).

These categories encompass a large part of the work of a midwife on labour wards. The technical skills required to incorporate these activities into practice and to maintain the woman as the focus of care have, perhaps, led to the divergence of the role of the midwife in technological and normal birth.

Defining competence

Eraut (1994) asserts that, in general usage, the term 'competent' is associated with a person who is regularly engaged in a task or range of tasks, and who has attained a level of skill through the regular performance of the work. It is accepted that competence is seen as specific to a particular set of circumstances.

Competence in clinical practice

Defining competence in relation to clinical practice is essential because it is one of the attributes that define a profession. To a certain extent, competencies are defined by the professional bodies that govern practice – for example, the Nursing and Midwifery Council in the UK. The general public, therefore, expect that a doctor, nurse or midwife has undergone a statutory period of training and education, and has qualified with the requisite knowledge and skills to practise safely.

Competence in relation to midwifery practice in the UK and Ireland includes not only knowledge of how to conduct practical tasks, but also the application of theory in practice. It incorporates knowing how to conduct the tasks in the context of a wider worldview. It is a synthesis of theoretical knowledge and practical skill, the ability to make decisions based on evidence, sound judgement and experience. It also includes the ability to interact with women on a personal and professional level – in other words, caring. Fraser *et al.* (1998: 28) sum this up by stating that: 'The public needs to be reassured that those about to become midwife practitioners have developed the right knowledge, skills and attitudes to become competent'. Norman (1985) developed a model defining clinical competence based on five areas that could reasonably be assessed. These would seem to be applicable to an assessment of midwifery competence in the use of birth technology. The competencies he described are: clinical skills; knowledge and understanding; interpersonal attributes; problem-solving and clinical judgement, and technical skills.

Table 11.2 Types of technology

Category	High technology	Low technology	Uses in practice
Monitoring the mother and foetus	CTG machine (with or without foetal ECG)		Monitoring contractions and foetal heart responses to contractions. Uses ultrasound wave technology.
	Handheld Doppler device		Used to monitor foetal heart rate in antenatal period and during labour; allows woman to hear heartbeat. Uses ultrasound wave technology.
		Pinard stethoscope	Low technology means to enable the midwife to hear foetal heart without use of ultrasound wave technology.
	Electronic blood pressure monitor		This device has the functions of blood pressure recording, mean arterial pressure reading, pulse, temperature, oxygen saturation and cardiac monitor. The device can be programmed to make regular recordings and store them in the electronic memory. It also produces a printout of the recordings.
		Sphygmomanometer	This low technology device is used to measure blood pressure. The midwife has to pump up the cuff manually and listen to hear the Karotkoff sounds to determine blood pressure.
	Digital thermometer		This electronic device measures temperature, which is displayed on a digital display
	Oxygen saturation monitor		This device can be attached to a finger and will take measurements of saturation levels of perfused oxygen and carbon dioxide.
	Cardiac monitor		This device is used in women with underlying cardiac conditions, and is most likely to be used post-operatively, as women with pre-existing cardiac conditions are usually advised to have a Caesarean section.
	Glucose meter		For women who are diabetic, the control of blood sugar and insulin administration during labour is vital.

Controlling labour	Amnihook	This device is used for rupturing membranes.
	Electronic infusion pump/syringe drivers	This is used to deliver intravenous fluids. Drugs may be added to the infusion in order either to stimulate or to suppress uterine contractions. The rate at which the fluid and drug are delivered is controlled by the pump in order to reduce the risk of side effects or complications. Syringe drivers may also be used for the administration of drugs for controlling diabetes and pre-eclampsia, among other conditions.
Pain relief	Syringe pump/driver	Epidural analgesia may, in some cases, be administered by a syringe pump or driver. Syringe pumps may also be used for patient controlled analgesia systems, which are normally set up by an anaesthetist.
	Entonox	This inhalation analgesia is self-administered by the woman under the guidance of the midwife. The midwife needs to be skilled in coaching the woman in how to use the apparatus.
	Transcutaneous Electrical Nerve Stimulation (TENS)	This machinery can be sited by the midwife or the woman's partner and is controlled by the woman.
Resuscitation	Resuscitaire table	With equipment including oxygen, suction, and intubation equipment. All the equipment on the Resuscitaire should be checked by the midwife to ensure that it is available and in working order so that it may be readily used in an emergency.
	Drugs	The drugs commonly used in resuscitation of the newborn should be checked to ensure that they have not expired.
	Resuscitation trolley	Contains drugs and equipment needed in the event of maternal collapse, and should be checked on a daily basis to ensure it is fully stocked and all drugs are in date.
Bureaucracy	Computers	Used to record patient admission details, used for recording care episodes and delivery details. Birth records and NHS numbers for newborn babies are generated by computer.

The use of exemplar cases

An exemplar case can illustrate the attributes of the concept – providing, here, a means of showing what is meant by the concept of 'birth technology competence'. A literature search was undertaken using key words including 'midwifery', 'competence', 'birth technology' and 'technological competence'. The cases were constructed from the experience of the authors and from the process of reviewing the literature, and seek to illustrate how the authors view the concept after the examination of the literature. The development of the cases also acts as a means of clarifying meaning and drawing out criteria of relevance to the concept. The criteria generated were used to inform the observations in the fieldwork stage.

Exemplar case to illustrate the concept of birth technology competence

In the context of the labour ward, a midwife should be able to admit a woman to the labour ward, carry out a physical examination, take a history, and perform an assessment including general and vaginal examinations (Nursing and Midwifery Council, 2009). She should be able to:

- communicate effectively with the woman to elicit sufficient detail for an assessment of risk
- use the machinery with dexterity, whilst explaining its purpose to the woman
- demonstrate a caring approach, enabling the woman to take decisions about her care
- provide privacy for the woman and her partner during assessment, examination, and discussion
- interpret information obtained using all these tools and construct, with the woman, a plan of midwifery care to meet her individual needs
- explain the findings to the woman and write a detailed account in the midwifery record.

This process should be the basis of producing a plan of care for the labour in partnership with the woman.

The midwife should be able to interpret the findings, assess progress and make decisions about whether to increase the rate of infusion. She must communicate with the woman throughout, having established a relationship of trust with her. She also has a statutory professional obligation to record, contemporaneously, the events of the labour and delivery. The technology used in this case is the intravenous infusion and pump, the electronic blood pressure monitoring machine and the cardiotocograph machine.

Attributes of birth technology competence

According to Chinn and Kramer (1999), creating conceptual meaning produces tentative criteria for determining whether the concept under investigation exists in a given situation. The various sources from which the meaning is drawn create layers of meaning. In adapting Norman's (1985) five areas of clinical competence, it is possible to collapse them into three defined areas

Table 11.3   The five areas of competence

Norman's competences	Domains of midwifery competence
Interpersonal attributes	Interpersonal skills
Knowledge and understanding	Professional knowledge
Clinical skills	
Problem-solving and clinical judgement	Clinical proficiency
Technical skills	

Source: Adapted from Norman (1985).

for midwifery competence in birth technology: interpersonal skills, professional knowledge and clinical proficiency (see Table 11.3).

The attributes identified in the theoretical phase of the study provided a basis for the fieldwork observations (see Table 11.4). Having recognized birth technology competence as a concept and identified attributes associated with the concept, it was important to test the existence of the concept in midwifery practice. The strength of the Hybrid Model of Concept Development (Swartz-Barcott and Kim, 2000) is that it links theory and practice. Therefore, the fieldwork phase aimed to explore whether the concept could be confirmed and, if so, how well the theoretical aspects fitted into the world of everyday midwifery practice.

Phase II: fieldwork phase

Setting

The fieldwork took place in the labour wards, antenatal assessment units, and postnatal wards in two consultant maternity units in England. Both units had a mixture of consultant-led and midwifery-led care, although one managed 5,000 births per year and the other 2,000. One is described as the 'central unit', and the other as the 'peripheral unit'.

Sample

Six midwives in the central unit and ten in the peripheral unit consented to being observed in their everyday practice. As the process moved forward, the observations became more focused on situations where technology was used, and observations continued until data saturation was achieved (Spradley, 1980; Strauss and Corbin, 1998).

Selection criteria

The managers were approached about the midwives who would be deemed competent in technology use. The managers agreed that newly qualified midwives could not be considered technologically competent, which mirrors

Table 11.4 Tentative attributes of birth technology competence from the theoretical phase

Domain	Element	Attribute
Interpersonal skills	Caring Touch	The ability to demonstrate a caring approach to the woman and her family
		The use of touch to examine women and babies
		The use of touch to calm and relax women in pain
		The use of touch involved in palpation of contractions during labour to identify length, strength, and frequency
	Communication	The ability to communicate with women and their families to share information
		The ability to communicate between the machinery and the woman, to interpret the findings so that she can understand
		The ability to communicate with other health professionals involved in the care of the woman
		The ability to communicate by recording episodes of care, both in written and electronic form
	Woman-centred care	The ability to provide individualized care, taking into account the needs and wishes of the woman
		Demonstrating respect for the individual rights of women in making choices about their care
Professional knowledge	Midwifery subject knowledge	Knowledge of the normal mechanism of labour, and ability to identify when deviations occur
		Ability to identify risk
		Understanding how interventions impact on normal labour progress
		Knowledge of sound evidence on which practice is based
		Knowledge of the unit policies and guidelines
	Professional accountability and responsibility of the midwife	Knowledge of how practice is governed by legislation and unit protocols
		Sphere of practice
		Knowledge of when it is appropriate to refer, and to whom
		Record-keeping, both written and electronic

Clinical proficiency	Skills in using the machinery	Ability to switch on the machine and understand that it is working correctly
		Ability to identify and report faults in the machinery
		Dexterity in programming the machinery, making changes to the programme during care including:
		• increasing dosage rate for a pump or syringe driver
		• changing the fluid bag in a pump
		• changing the syringe in a driver
		• changing the paper in a CTG machine
		• changing the date and time on a CTG machine
		• programming an electronic blood pressure monitor to take readings at regular intervals.
		Making the connection between woman and machine
		Understanding where to find information concerning hazard warnings
	Decision-making	The ability to understand the technological products of the machines and to make decisions based on these.
		To refer to appropriate personnel when deviations from the norm are detected
	Traditional midwifery skills	The ability to demonstrate traditional midwifery skills used in diagnosis, planning and implementing care including:
		• palpation of the abdomen
		• vaginal examination
		• auscultation of the foetal heart.

Table 11.5   Inclusion and exclusion criteria for midwifery participants

Inclusion criteria	Exclusion criteria
Midwives who have personal responsibility for caring for or managing individual women in labour or on wards.	Midwives with overall responsibility for running of labour ward during a shift (and who would, therefore, not have responsibility for individual women)
Midwives who have been qualified for more than six months (and have finished their period of preceptorship)	Midwives who have been qualified for less than six months
Midwives who have worked on a labour ward, or the ward where the observation is being carried out, in their particular unit for more than six months (and are, therefore, are fully orientated to the environment, and familiar with policies and guidelines for practice in that area)	Midwives who have been working on a labour ward, or the ward on which the observation is taking place, for less than six months and are, therefore, orientating to the environment
Midwives considered by managers and peers to be technologically competent	Midwives who are undergoing a period of supervised practice Midwives in a period of preceptorship

findings from other studies (Fraser *et al.*, 1998; Sinclair, 1999). Table 11.5 demonstrates the inclusion and exclusion criteria agreed for both units.

Ethnographic observation schedule

The lead researcher (KC) informed the unit in question of the dates when observations would take place. The researcher would usually arrive on the unit at the beginning of a shift and would be present for the shift handover. A midwife who had previously consented to be observed would be approached and asked again for permission to shadow her during the shift. The midwife would seek permission from the woman/women for the researcher to be present, and the observation would take place over the period of a shift. The researcher made written notes during the observation.

Research ethics

Ethical approval for the study was granted by the local research ethics committee, which covered both units. Each hospital had a separate research governance committee that also approved the study.

Involvement of women

The researcher approached women to explain that she was shadowing the midwife as part of a research study into midwifery work. Women were asked for consent to allow the researcher to observe midwives caring for them in labour. It was explained to the women that the researcher was a midwife and, therefore, bound by the same rules of confidentiality and code of conduct as those caring for them. Women were assured that their names would not be used in the research. An information sheet provided further written details about the researcher and the study.

Analysis of data

Field notes were transcribed as soon as possible after the observation, and initial coding of the data was made using the software QSR NVivo. The transcripts were check coded for consistency. Data were analyzed using a grounded theory approach so that each observation informed the next (Charmaz, 2006). Therefore, the researcher began with a wide focus and this gradually became more refined with each observation session. The transcribed data were coded before the next observation event so that the observation could inform the data to be collected at the next episode. Coding consisted of reading the transcripts and assigning codes as they arose using the broad conceptual framework from the literature. The researcher assigned codes to themes emerging (open coding); this process involved assigning attributes to the codes so that, when a recurrence was found, it was possible to check that it met the criteria previously assigned. Observations continued until data saturation was reached and themes were found to be recurring with no new themes emerging. Categorising of the data enabled connections to be made between the coded concepts.

This development of axial coding led to the advance of a framework of technological competence. The relationships between categories were tested by constant referral to the data to ensure that the conceptual links were sound. Theoretical validation involved the process of constant referral to the raw data and was repeated often throughout the stages of coding, categorizing, and developing the model. The synthesis of the fieldwork phase and the concept development phase also ensured that the theoretical validity could be constantly tested to ensure the reliability of confirmation.

Phase III: analytical phase

In this phase, the researcher synthesized the data from fieldwork with the results of the concept analysis. This involved the comparison of findings from the concept analysis with the findings from the fieldwork phase in order to generate deeper meaning for the concept of birth technology competence in midwifery. An in-depth analysis of the competing paradigms in midwifery and the concepts that impinge upon birth technology competence in midwifery took place during this phase. The model of birth technology competence in midwifery emerged from this process.

The final phase in the research involved validating the model by means of respondent validation (Silverman, 2001). This is not part of the process recommended by Swartz-Barcott and Kim (2000). However, as a means of ensuring that the model was grounded in midwifery practice, and as a tool for validating the method of concept development, it was deemed appropriate. The model was presented to a focus group of eight midwives from the field of study. The midwives were asked to comment on the model and its applicability within midwifery practice.

Findings from the fieldwork phase

Themes

The initial themes used for coding were the attributes from the concept analysis but, as the study progressed, new concepts began to emerge in the field. The voices and actions of the participants gave increased strength to concepts that could not have been ascertained from the concept analysis data. As the study evolved, the observations became more focused, and new themes began to emerge during coding. This meant that earlier observations needed to be re-examined and recoded with the new themes. Miles and Huberman (1994) recommend this approach as an ongoing form of data management and analysis.

The ethnographic fieldwork confirmed the appropriateness of the attributes identified in the first stage of concept analysis as being an integral part of the concept in the clinical context and included two new attributes:

1. the ability to use evidence and clinical judgment in conjunction to inform practice decisions; and
2. the ability to demonstrate appropriate use of technology (see Table 11.6).

The use of the concept of birth technology competence in the field is not straightforward, and is altered in some ways according to individual midwifery practice. A closer examination of birth technology competence reveals that other concepts impinge on it. Therefore, although the attributes of birth technology are supported in the empirical observations, the perception of the way the concept is operationalized has been altered by the empirical observations in the field. The relationships between categories in the empirical data point to competing paradigms in midwifery practice, which impinge on the operation of birth technology competence.

In the final analytical phase of the Swartz-Barcott and Kim (2000) Hybrid Model of Concept Development, the synthesis of theoretical work and fieldwork takes place. The researcher takes a step back from the field and re-examines the findings in light of the initial focus of the study. Swartz-Barcott

Table 11.6 Altered attributes of birth technology competence

Domain	Element	Attribute
Interpersonal skills	Caring Touch	The ability to demonstrate a caring approach to the woman and her family
		The use of touch to examine women and babies
		The use of touch to calm and relax women in pain
		The use of touch involved in palpation of contractions during labour to identify length, strength and frequency
	Communication	The ability to communicate with women and their families to share information
		The ability to communicate between the machinery and the woman, to interpret the findings so that she can understand
		The ability to communicate with other health professionals involved in the care of the woman
		The ability to communicate by recording episodes of care, both in written and electronic form
	Woman-centred care	The ability to provide individualized care, taking into account the needs and wishes of the woman
		Demonstrating respect for the individual rights of women in making choices about their care
Underpinning theoretical knowledge	Midwifery subject knowledge	Underpinning theory for midwifery practice
		Knowledge of the normal mechanism of labour, and ability to identify when deviations occur
		Ability to identify risk
Professional knowledge	Professional accountability and responsibility of the midwife	Understanding of how interventions can impact on normal progress of labour
		Knowledge of sound evidence to inform practice
		Knowledge of how practice is governed by legislation
		An understanding of the development of local policies, guidelines, and protocols
		Understanding of the role of policies and guidelines
		Sphere of practice
		Knowledge of when it is appropriate to refer, and to whom
		Record keeping, both written and electronic

continued overleaf

Table 11.6 *continued*

Domain	*Element*	*Attribute*
Clinical proficiency	Skills in using the machinery	Ability to switch on the machine and understand that it is working correctly Ability to identify and report faults in the machinery Dexterity in programming the machinery, making changes to the programme during care including: • increasing dosage rate for a pump or syringe driver • changing the fluid bag in a pump • changing the syringe in a driver • changing the paper in a CTG machine • changing the date and time on a CTG machine • programming an electronic blood pressure monitor to take readings at regular intervals Making the connection between woman and machine Understanding where to find information concerning hazard warnings **Appropriate use of technology**
	Decision-making	The ability to understand the technological products of the machines and to make decisions based on these. To make appropriate referrals when deviations from the norm occur **Ability to use evidence to inform practice in conjunction with the skill of clinical decision-making** **Demonstration of involvement of women in decisions surrounding technology use**
	Traditional midwifery skills	The ability to demonstrate traditional midwifery skills used in diagnosis, planning, and implementing care including: • palpation of the abdomen • vaginal examination • auscultation of the foetal heart

Note: The additional attributes, identified in the fieldwork phase are highlighted in bold text.

and Kim (2000: 147) advocate the use of three questions to guide this process.

1. To what degree is the concept applicable and important to nursing [in this case midwifery]?
2. Does the initial selection of the concept seem justified?
3. To what extent do the review of literature, theoretical analysis, and empirical findings support the presence and frequency of this concept within the population selected for empirical study?

In this case, the fieldwork phase has confirmed the frequency of the use of technology in midwifery practice and, therefore, the importance of birth technology competence to midwifery practice, which justifies the initial selection of the concept.

The process of the final analytical phase took place after the fieldwork data had been analyzed. Once initial categories had been identified within the fieldwork data and relationships were made, it was necessary to go back to the literature and the concept analysis. Figure 11.2 illustrates the process involved.

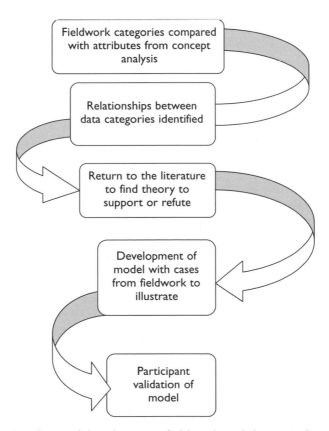

Figure 11.2   Synthesis of data between fieldwork and theoretical work in the final analytical phase

A model of birth technology competence

The comparative analysis led to the development of a model of midwifery competence in birth technology that has three identifiable strands depending on the knowledge, skills, and attitudes of the midwife. In an ideal world, it would be possible to identify one type of technology competence in midwifery. Yet, because birth is a process with constantly changing situations and a range of different women with different needs, midwifery is not static. Therefore, not one but three typologies of midwifery birth technology competence emerged: Bureaucratic, Classical and New Professional.

Table 11.7 identifies the traits of each of the typologies. These reflect different paradigms of midwifery competence in the use of birth technology.

Table 11.7   Model of midwifery competence in birth technology

	Bureaucratic competence	*Classical professional competence*	*New professional competence*
Decision-making	Decisions made on the basis of policies	Decisions made by the professional	*Involves women in decision-making*
Belief in the physiological processes	Tends not to trust the physiological processes	Believes in the efficacy of natural physiological processes	Believes in the efficacy of natural physiological processes
Traditional midwifery skills	Tends not to trust the traditional skills, preferring technology	Exercises traditional midwifery skills	Exercises traditional midwifery skills
Individual clinical judgement	More likely to seek medical opinion than act on own judgement	*Makes judgements based on own expertise/ experience*	Acts on the basis of individual clinical judgement
Belief in efficacy of technology	Believes in the efficacy of technology	To some extent, believes in the efficacy of technology	To some extent, believes in the efficacy of technology
Role of policy and guidelines in decisions	*Governed by guidelines and policy*	To some extent, is governed by guidelines and policy	To some extent, is governed by guidelines and policy

Note: The defining attributes of each of the typologies are *italicized*.

These also appear to represent, to some extent, the culture in which midwives work.

Validation of the model

The validity of the model was tested by a process of respondent validation (Silverman 2001), where the model was presented to a focus group of midwives who had participated in the study. The process of theory-building work has suffered criticism for being removed from the reality of practice, according to Rodgers and Knafl (2000). The purpose of using a research design that allowed for ethnographic fieldwork was to enable the link to be made between theory and practice in relation to birth technology competence. The final phase of participant validation also tested whether the model had meaning for midwives in practice.

The focus group participants regarded the model as a hierarchical one in which midwives would progress through the bureaucratic stage to classical professional and, finally, to new professional competence. In their opinion, the ideal typology was that of New Professional Competence, with the emphasis on woman-centred care. They clearly identified the Bureaucratic typology as that of a novice practitioner who used the policies and guidelines to inform their decisions. The consultation of other midwives and doctors to aid decision-making was also regarded as a trait of the novice. The reliance on technology, and lack of appreciation of the efficacy of the physiological processes, were seen as consequences of inexperience.

The focus group saw the New Professional Competence as the ideal to which to aspire because of the involvement of women in the decision-making process. The participants regarded this as a hallmark of an experienced and confident midwife who was able to hand over control to the woman. In reflecting on their own practice, they seemed to regard themselves as 'veering towards New Professional Competence' (Midwife FG 3) or 'wavering somewhere between Classical and New' [Professional] (Midwife FG 5), although one midwife firmly stated that she regarded herself as working within the framework of Classical Professional Competence.

Although midwives see the value of New Professional Competence, it is the least prevalent type of competence demonstrated in the empirical work. Bureaucratic Competence was the most prevalent type of competence displayed in practice; to a certain extent, the focus group midwives, although professing to practice in a manner that they felt veered between Classical Professional and New Professional Competence, actually displayed attributes of Bureaucratic Competence in their discussion. Their concerns with the avoidance of litigation, the importance they placed upon guidelines and protocols, and their use of doctors to cover their decisions, were clear indications of the Bureaucratic approach.

The confirmation of the focus group gives strength to the model; the midwives agreed the typologies, although it was remarkable that they all saw themselves as either fitting the Classical Professional or New Professional typologies. They did, however, recognize the prevalence of Bureaucratic

Competence. In validating the model, the group also validated the method that was used to produce the result. The occurrence of birth technology competence as a concept in midwifery work was confirmed.

Conclusion

In terms of a contribution to midwifery theory, this research offers evidence of a robust and transparent approach to developing, testing and confirming a specific theory for clinical midwifery practice. It is important to midwifery as a profession to develop the necessary competence and confidence required to build theories that will become pillars of midwifery knowledge: 'The end result of sound theoretically-based research is filtration and absorption of knowledge that trickles and merges into the thought processes and senses of clinicians. If midwifery research is to be efficacious and effective, its contribution must be made visible – better research, underpinned by sound theory and leading to demonstrable effects on practice' Sinclair (2007: 39).

ACTIVITIES

Clinical observation

Review the tentative theoretical attributes defined in Table 11.4. Familiarize yourself with these and begin critical observation of clinical situations in which birthing technologies are commonly used to confirm or refute the visibility of these theoretically-defined attributes.

Postgraduate

The model provided by Crozier et al. as a result of this study requires further development and testing. Design a research proposal that will build new midwifery knowledge using this model.

References

Bryar, R.M. (1995) *Theory for Midwifery Practice*, 1st edn. London: Macmillan.

Chalmers, I., Oakley, A. and Macfarlane, A. (1980) 'Perinatal Health Services: An Immodest Proposal', *British Medical Journal*, 280(6217): 842–5.

Charmaz, K. (2006) *Constructing Grounded Theory: A Practical Guide Through Qualitative Analysis*. London: Sage.

Chinn, P.L. and Kramer, M.K. (1999) *Theory and Nursing: Integrated Knowledge Development*. London: Mosby.

Cowie, J.L. and Floyd, S.R. (1998) 'The Art of Midwifery: Lost to Technology?', *Australian College of Midwives Journal*, 11(3): 20–4.

Crozier, K. (2005) 'The Development of a Concept of Birth Technology Competence in Midwifery', Unpublished PhD thesis, University of Ulster, Belfast.

Davies-Floyd, R.E. (2003) *Birth as an American Rite of Passage*, 2nd edn. Berkeley, CA: University of California Press.

Eraut, M. (1994) *Developing Professional Knowledge and Competence*. London: Falmer Press.

Fraser, D., Murphy, R. and Worth–Butler, M. (1998) *Preparing Effective Midwives: An Outcome Evaluation of Pre-registration Programmes of Midwifery Education*. London: English National Board.

Henley–Einion, A. (2003) 'The Medicalisation of Childbirth', in C. Squire (ed.) *The Social Context of Birth*. Abingdon: Radcliffe Medical Press.

Hutchfield, K. (1999) 'Family-centred Care: A Concept Analysis', *Journal of Advanced Nursing*, 29(5):1178–87.

Kirkham, M. and Stapleton, H. (2000) 'Midwives' Support Needs as Childbirth Changes', *Journal of Advanced Nursing*, 32(2): 465–72.

Lee, B. (2004) 'Ill Mothers and Critical Care: The Challenge in the 21st Century', *Midwives*, 7(2): 522–4.

Miles, M.B. and Huberman, A.M. (1994) *Qualitative Data Analysis*, 2nd edn. Thousand Oaks, CA: Sage.

Norman, G.R. (1985) 'Objective Measurement of Clinical Performance', *Medical Education*, 19(1): 43–7.

Nursing and Midwifery Council (2009) *Standards for Pre-registration Midwifery Education*. London: NMC.

Oakley, A. (1987) 'From Walking Womb to Test-tube Babies', in M. Stanworth (ed.) *Reproductive Technologies. Gender Motherhood and Medicine*. Cambridge: Polity.

Ohlen, J. and Segesten, K.P. (1998) 'The Professional Identity of the Nurse', *Journal of Advanced Nursing*, 28(4): 720–7.

Rodgers, B.L. and Knafl, K.A. (2000) (eds) *Concept Development in Nursing: Foundations, Techniques and Applications*, 2nd edn. Philadelphia, PA: W.B. Saunders.

Rothwell, H. (1995) 'Medicalisation of Childbearing', *British Journal of Midwifery*, 3: 318–31.

Silverman, D. (2001) *Interpreting Qualitative Data: Methods for Analysing Talk, Text and Interaction*, 2nd edn. London: Sage.

Sinclair, M. (1999) 'Midwives' Readiness to Use Technology on the Labour Ward', Unpublished PhD thesis, Queens University, Belfast.

Sinclair, M. (2000) 'Birth Technology: Observations of High Usage in the Labour Ward', *All Ireland Journal of Nursing and Midwifery*, 1– (3): 83–8.

Sinclair, M. (2001) 'Midwives' Attitudes to the Use of the Cardiotocograph Machine', *Journal of Advanced Nursing*, 35(4): 599–606.

Sinclair, M. (2007) 'A Guide to Understanding Theoretical and Conceptual Frameworks', *Evidence Based Midwifery*, 5(2): 39.

Spradley, J.P. (1980) *Participant Observation*. London: Harcourt Brace.

Strauss, A. and Corbin, J. (1998) *Basics of Qualitative Research: Techniques and Procedures for Developing Grounded Theory*, 2nd edn. Thousand Oaks, CA: Sage.

Swartz-Barcott, D. and Kim, H.S. (2000) 'An Expansion and Elaboration of the Hybrid Model of Concept Development', in B.L. Rogers and K.A. Knafl (eds), *Concept Development in Nursing*. Philadelphia, PA: W.B. Saunders.

Walsh, D. (2009) 'Pain and Epidural Use on Normal Childbirth', *EBM*, 7(3). Accessed 21 July 2010 at http://www.rcm.org.uk/ebm/ebm-2009/september-2009/pain-and-epidural-use-in-normal-childbirth/.

Contemporary Caesarean Section Theory: Risk, Uncertainty and Fear

12

Michelle Kealy and Pranee Liamputtong

Key points

- Caesarean section is a birth technology employed in childbirth in a range of circumstances (life-saving, situations of clinical uncertainty, and in the absence of clinical indications)
- Care givers and women adopt different approaches to decision-making (paternalistic, shared, informed choice) depending on individual circumstances
- Social theories including risk, uncertainty and trust in authorities help to explain why the caesarean section rate is rising steadily in highly-industrialized countries.
- A new theoretical framework of three zones of clinical practice is described.

Introduction

In this chapter, we discuss several theoretical concepts relevant to an explanation of the contemporary use of caesarean section. We contend that, in order to provide safe and appropriate maternity care, midwives need to understand the multiple factors that influence the increasing use of caesarean birth by care givers and women.

To begin, the prominent discourses of the competing ideologies of childbirth and the general changes to maternity care practices that have occurred over time are discussed. We then describe three 'zones of clinical practice' that help us to understand traditional and contemporary reasons for caesarean section, as described in the scientific literature. From there, we critique three commonly reported approaches to decision-making in health care and suggest the limitations of these approaches in relation to decision-making for interventions, such as caesarean section. The theoretical framework developed, encompassing three zones of clinical practice and three decision-making styles draws on findings from an interview study of women's experiences of caesarean section (Kealy, 2007). With increasing use of technologies such as caesarean section, discourses of risk, fear, uncertainty, trust and confidence are shown to influence decision-making in childbirth.

In contemporary life, the pursuit and practice of health is closely linked to biomedicine (Crawford, 2006). It requires extensive social resources and permeates all levels of institutions, creating a need for increasing goods, services and knowledge in professional and commercial settings. According to Crawford (2006), health is a goal to which to aspire, and a source of anxiety; it shapes identity and requires constant assessment and reassessment. From birth to death, the physical, mental and social aspects of a healthy life are mediated by medicine, an agency of surveillance and intervention. This medicalization of health; the dominant role of the obstetric profession; and heightened community-sensitivity to risk, fear and uncertainty has changed the cultural and social norms of childbirth for women in high- and middle-income countries in the past one hundred years (Lane, 1995; Possamai-Inesedy, 2006). Today, we live in a globalized world, where notions of consumerism, individualism and informed choice are politically and economically encouraged by a market-driven health care system, with quick-fix solutions readily available. Arguably, caesarean section has become a purchasable commodity (Beckett, 2005; Elliot and Lemert, 2006).

The increasing use of caesarean section has been a public health concern since the 1980s, when the rate escalated in many high- and middle-income countries (WHO, 1985). Sociologists such as Oakley and Richards (1990) highlighted a lack of research on women's health and well-being in association with the rapidly rising rate of caesarean births. Others argued that the increasing use of caesarean section was an issue of gender in male-dominated medicine (LoCicero, 1993); was socio-economically determined (Hurst and Summey, 1984; Sakala, 1993; Leone et al., 2008); or related to financial incentives in some countries (Rocha et al., 1985; Barros et al., 1986). Since then, new evidence on what this and other high-technology and interventionist maternity care practices might mean to childbearing women has contributed to a more contemporary understanding of some of the issues (Beckett, 2005; Liamputtong, 2005; McCallum, 2005), yet consensus on an optimal rate of caesarean section (Cyr, 2006) or factors that might succeed in reducing the rate, remain elusive (Chaillet and Dumont, 2007). In addition, and possibly most importantly, while maternal morbidity and mortality related directly to caesarean birth remains difficult to measure (Waterstone et al., 2001), the international consensus favours vaginal birth in the absence of complications, albeit without evidence from randomized clinical trials (Kingdon et al., 2006; Federation of International Gynecologists and Obstetricians, 2007; Miesnik and Reale, 2007).

Natural childbirth or technological birth: competing ideologies

What exactly is natural childbirth, and is it different to normal childbirth in existing discourses? Natural childbirth, according to Treichler (1990: 129), can mean 'birth without the panoply of hospital procedures' or 'birth with Lamaze and/or without anaesthetic', outside of hospital, or vaginal birth instead of caesarean section, or not artificial (as in *in vitro* fertilization). Normal/natural birth will be used here to mean a spontaneous vaginal birth but, following the lead of Frost *et al.* (2006: 301), the term 'normal' will be avoided for its connotation in Western societies with the 'normalcy of intervention'. Frost and colleagues also refer to 'interventionist birth' as oppositional to the discourses of 'natural' birth.

Natural childbirth discourses have been largely driven by Western, white, middle-class women (Nelson, 1983; Lazarus, 1994; Zadoroznyj, 1999). Lupton (2003) argues that middle-class women in high-income countries value personal control, and therefore cannot relax and relinquish control of their own bodies in childbirth. In contrast, Lupton suggests, working-class women are not so concerned about having control of childbirth, and have fewer difficulties with the notion of not having control (see also Lazarus, 1994; Liamputtong, 2005, 2007). Natural childbirth, emphasizing the natural or biological experience of giving birth untainted by drugs, places extra pressure on women and is seen as problematic. Mansfield (2008: 1094) takes this debate further. She states:

> natural childbirth is not just a worldview or set of cultural ideas, but is instead a set of practices: things women, their caregivers, and their wider social networks do to make birth a normal, physiological – not risky, pathological – experience.

Mansfield also suggests that the role of nature and society, in facilitating natural childbirth, requires social and active engagement – it is not a passive process; and argues that this is an area of research that warrants additional investigation.

Childbirth in high-income countries now takes place in a highly technological environment. Davis-Floyd (1996: 156) calls this a 'technocratic model of birth'. By this, she means a hegemonic model where technology is highly valued in an autocratic and bureaucratic society, which organizes itself around the technology. In a technocratic paradigm, women's bodies are considered deficient, unable to give birth safely without technological intervention. Davis-Floyd (1996) contests that, in this environment, medical knowledge is the only knowledge that has value, is authoritative, in contrast to women's intuitive or inner knowledge, which is devalued by medicine. She asserts, however, that women who believe in natural childbirth, or a holistic approach to birth, place greater value on the authoritative knowledge of women than, for example, laboratory results obtained by scientific means. The technocratic model views the woman separately from her baby, considers her body to be distinct from her mind, and assesses childbirth within a risky mechanical framework that is in need of monitoring and control. Further, the management of pregnancy and labour is conducted increasingly with the interests of the foetus rather than the woman paramount.

For decades, women have had a negative view of the use of technology in childbirth (Oakley, 1980). The more technology employed, the less likely women were to feel satisfied with their birth experience, and the more likely to feel depressed with maladjusted feelings towards the baby in the early post-partum. In addition, women's perspectives on pregnancy as a normal life-event were shown to conflict ideologically with the views of medical practitioners, who were likely to view each pregnancy as an isolated episode of care (Graham and Oakley, 1981). Interestingly, in the United Kingdom, women appear to be less negative and more accepting of interventions with the increasingly routine use of technology in 'normal' birth (Sinclair and Gardner, 2002; Green and Baston, 2007).

Beckett (2005) and Lupton (2003) argue that the natural birth movement promoted limited choices for women in childbirth. The ideology of natural childbirth does not adequately consider the needs of women for whom medical interventions such as caesarean section are essential. Such women may feel they have failed, or feel excluded and cheated within the natural birth discourse. In contrast, contemporary hospital birth places women, at the most vulnerable time of their lives, in positions of compliance in a process that is geared more to efficiency than meeting women's social and emotional needs. Hospital-based birth emphasizes that health care professionals are the experts, and pregnancy and childbirth are illness states to be managed with constant surveillance. Since the normalization of hospital-based, physician attended childbirth (in some countries), some argue that the only real alternative birth model is non-hospital-based and non-physician attended. This strict interpretation of natural birth is not common in most high-income countries (Frost *et al.*, 2006).

Women's attitudes to technology in childbirth, especially in light of the rising caesarean section rate, have been increasingly explored over the last 25 years (Sandelowski and Bustamante, 1986; Oakley and Richards, 1990; Kornelsen, 2005; Liamputtong, 2005, 2007; Liamputtong and Watson, 2006). Some have suggested that a broadening of the natural versus technological birth dichotomy may better encapsulate women's complex understandings of technology and use of different types of intervention (Beckett, 2005; Frost *et al.*, 2006).

Caesarean section: three zones of clinical practice

A Finnish sociologist, Alasuutari (1995), describes how qualitative researchers may seek to explain human behaviour by organizing interview data into various types or groups. The process begins with the two most extreme cases, cases that 'differ from each other as much as possible', and then the researcher thinks about the special or distinguishing features that makes these two cases different. Then, writes Alasuutari (1995: 49), the researcher works to categorize all the other cases into these two extreme groups, or, if they do not match, other features or dimensions would be sought to classify cases until there is a 'typology in which every case fits in a box'. This classification system helps to explain why people behave the way they do, but it is only the beginning of analysis, not the final product.

Table 12.1 Theoretical framework

Zones of clinical practice	Description of the zone of clinical practice	Model or style of decision-making used in maternity care	Examples in clinical practice
Central zone	Life-saving caesarean section. No doubt that the benefits vastly overwhelm the potential harm; mother and or baby in grave danger of loss of life or serious morbidity	Paternalistic style; decision to intervene made by physician, usually alone, due to urgency of situation. Woman readily consents to surgery in presence of real danger	Cord prolapse, fulminating pre-eclampsia, massive antepartum haemorrhage, obstructed labour with malpresentation
Grey zone	Caesarean section undertaken in times of clinical doubt about the best course of action. Uncertain benefit–harm ratio	Usually shared decision-making style; between doctor and woman (and/or partner). May occasionally be paternalistic (doctor decides unilaterally) to intervene; women unhesitatingly accept medical authority	Maternal fatigue, foetal distress measured on CTG alone, suspected 'small' or 'large' baby
Peripheral zone	Caesarean section undertaken for non-clinical reasons. The potential harm associated with major abdominal surgery is likely to outweigh the potential benefit	Women convince their decision-making care giver (usually physician) that they want a caesarean (either during pregnancy or after labour has commenced)	Caesarean on maternal request (previous negative birth experience, fear of labour pain, fear for foetal wellbeing during labour, fear of failure to give birth vaginally)

In addition to the vast literature on the reasons for caesarean section, Kealy (2007) used women's explanations of the reasons for their first caesarean to develop a theoretical framework. Thematic analysis of the interview data supported classification of three different experiences of women. The main reason women gave for their first caesarean section was used to classify their accounts into three groups:

- life-saving caesarean section – central zone
- caesarean section undertaken in uncertain clinical situations – grey zone
- caesarean section performed in the apparent absence of medical reasons – peripheral zone.

This framework is built, in part, on the concept of the 'grey zone', posited by Naylor (1995: 840), who noted: 'evidence-based medicine offers little help in the many grey zones of practice, where the evidence about risk–benefit ratios of competing clinical options is incomplete or contradictory'. Both before and since the Naylor paper, authors have alluded to 'grey areas' or doubt about the benefits of the increasing use of caesarean section, in Australia and abroad (Francome and Savage, 1993; Sakala, 1993; Shearer, 1993; Renwick, 1991; Robson and Ellwood, 2003; Kalish *et al.*, 2004). It seemed appropriate to develop a theoretical framework that extended the concept of the grey zone to take account of all the reasons for caesarean section in contemporary practice.

In addition to the grey zone are those caesarean sections undertaken in other circumstances; that is, those that are clearly life-saving and those that are clearly performed for non-clinical reasons. The 'central' zone applies to a caesarean section that is recognized unequivocally as life-saving. The benefit conferred is well-known and far outweighs the risks of surgical delivery. The 'grey' zone is, thus, defined as caesarean section performed in the presence of clinical doubt and uncertainty about the best course of action. There is insufficient evidence that the maternal or neonatal benefits clearly outweigh the risks of surgical delivery. When clinical indications are ambiguous, non-clinical (social) factors also influence the decision to intervene surgically. The 'peripheral' zone is where there is no clinical indication for caesarean section and the benefit conferred is not likely to outweigh the potential harm. These operations are purportedly performed only for social reasons, including maternal or physician preference.

Table 12.1 summarizes the theoretical framework of three zones of clinical practice based on women's accounts of the main reason for their first caesarean section. The approach to decision-making by care givers and women also contributes to differentiating the three zones.

Central zone: life-saving surgery

Caesarean section undertaken for life-saving reasons operates predominately within a clinical framework, with little or no emphasis on women's social, informational or cultural needs. Any personal preference is suspended by the undisputed need to perform the surgery. When undertaken as a life-saving procedure, caesarean section invokes much greater benefit to mother and baby than the overall dangers of anaesthesia and surgical intervention. Preventing death, according to Sullivan (2003), is one of medicine's most important goals.

Williams (2005: 133–4) argues that, in undertaking life-saving interventions, patients' relationships with doctors are 'asymmetrical' because physicians have expert knowledge and are registered practitioners; their expertise is attained through years of education and clinical application. Decision-making is based on an entirely objective set of 'technical' facts.

We found few studies of theoretical perspectives on life-saving technology in maternity care. When views of medical technology were sought, in general, women placed high value on life-saving medical technology, such as heart transplant procedures, but were more critical of technology where the benefits were difficult to determine or doubtful (Gabe and Calnan, 1989). When caesarean section is performed in the central zone, or any life-saving intervention is undertaken, there is little controversy. Clinical staff and women are in agreement that there is no reasonable alternative action that will prevent loss of life or serious disability.

Grey zone: clinical uncertainty

In the grey zone of clinical practice, there is ambivalence about the necessity of surgical intervention and doubts about whether the benefits conveyed will outweigh the harm. The decision-making process is not clear-cut; physicians themselves may disagree about the best course of action. Women may or may not be encouraged by their care giver to become involved in the decision-making process; this is likely to depend on both the prevailing clinical circumstances and the individual characteristics of both physician and patient (as is discussed in the next section of this chapter). In the presence of clinical uncertainty, social factors begin to influence decision-making.

According to Parsons (1951), doctors are trained and motivated to reduce uncertainty in clinical practice. Uncertainty is usually managed by doctors taking some form of action, rather than adopting a 'wait and see' approach. Patients have been socialized into believing that medical action is better than watchful waiting. However, power imbalances operate in patients' and doctors' social roles. In the presence of uncertainty, patients have an opportunity to exert pressure on their doctor and to question medical knowledge. In reality, this is only likely when the patient's understanding of their illness differs from their doctor's, and they use their personal knowledge to contribute to decision-making.

Naylor (1995) argues that the growth of technology in medicine has outpaced our ability to appraise it, so that current data are not well able to guide clinical practice. When quality evidence does not exist, personal factors such as the experience, skill and knowledge of the physician, or reliance on the expert opinion of peers, are likely to inform practice. Some practitioners will act conservatively, while others tend to be more interventionist, which may differ according to training, individual skill base or personal experience.

Modern society, Alaszewski and Brown (2007) suggest, is characterized by both increased understanding of scientific knowledge and increased uncertainty. This is, in part, due to growing differences in expert and lay knowledge. Previously, doctors managed uncertainty by making decisions on behalf of the patient. However, since the 1960s, medical knowledge has been questioned and a burgeoning consumer culture has led to increased regulatory control of doctors, different approaches to decision-making, and the development of national standards and clinical guidelines. These changes may still be insufficient to enable women to make important health care decisions in stressful and uncertain times.

Some assert that, in maternity care, the introduction of medical technologies (such as electronic foetal monitoring in labour) has had the effect of adding to clinical uncertainty (Liamputtong et al., 2003; Possamai-Inesedy, 2006). Caesarean section, like other medical technologies, is sometimes used in times of clinical uncertainty. The increased use of this sophisticated and expensive surgical intervention has been attributed to a range of non-clinical factors, including a culture of risk, fear, consumerism and litigation in childbirth (Bastian, 1999; Wagner, 2000; Beckett, 2005; Bryant et al., 2007, Miesnik and Reale, 2007).

In the presence of uncertainty in a culture that is risk averse, obstetricians face the dilemma of multiple opinions for the same clinical situation, challenging their traditional monopoly of power (Lankshear et al., 2005). Feminist views suggest that the power imbalance between surgeon and patient can directly influence consent processes for caesarean section and other types of surgery. Women conform to their socially sanctioned position as patient, suggesting that the notion of patient autonomy is questionable, even 'illusionary' (Dixon-Woods et al., 2006; Goodall et al., 2009). According to Gabe and Calnan (1989), women have ambivalent views about non-life-saving medical technology. Their personal knowledge and experience is likely to influence their perceptions (Leone et al., 2008). Women are not passive recipients of medical power and actively participate in medicalization based on their own needs and motives (Gabe and Calnan, 1989; Liamputtong, 2005, 2007; Bryant et al., 2007).

In Brazil, Rocha and colleagues (1985) define the unnecessary use of finite public health resources in terms of the creation of a socially constructed phenomenon solved by the dominant influence of medicine. Social class, not ill health, determined the level of medical treatment one received, and, in the case of reproduction, women's social class determined the risk of caesarean section. Similar theories were being applied to the use of caesarean section in the United States at that time. According to Hurst and Summey (1984), more caesarean sections were being performed in the socio-economic group of women with the lowest medical risk. This was explained by non-medical factors such as low fertility rates and empty hospital beds. In order to maintain their income, obstetricians performed more caesarean operations and patients had longer hospital stays, defying hospital and governmental concerns regarding rising medical costs. Sakala (1993) also found a significant majority of caesarean sections were performed for ambiguous reasons where, in fact, the risk of surgery was likely to be greater than the benefit. When no clear-cut clinical indication existed, there was increased scope for non-medical factors to influence the use of caesarean section.

In Australia, the use of caesarean section has long been associated with private health insurance and the distribution of specialist obstetricians (Renwick, 1991; Johnston and Coory, 2006). When rates of obstetric intervention were examined among low-risk private and public maternity patients in New South Wales, Australia, private patients, whether cared for in private or public hospitals, were much more likely to have a caesarean section both before the onset of labour and after the onset of labour (Roberts *et al.*, 2000). National data shows a caesarean section rate of 41 per cent in 2006, up from 37 per cent in 2003, for women in private hospitals, compared with 27 per cent in 2006, an increase of only one per cent from 2003, for women in public hospitals. Of women aged 40 years or more, 55 per cent had a caesarean section in private hospitals, compared with 39.6 per cent in public hospitals in 2006 (Laws and Sullivan, 2005; Laws and Hilder, 2008).

Peripheral zone: the social construction of caesarean section

In the peripheral zone of clinical practice, caesarean section is undertaken primarily in the absence of medical indications. We restrict our discussion to situations were women actively request caesarean section, irrespective of any previous or existing clinical issues. Women might make the decision to have a caesarean section before they are pregnant, during pregnancy or after the onset of labour, depending on a number of factors. They might 'shop around' for a care giver who will agree to their request, or continue to negotiate with their care giver until such time as their request is accepted (Zadoroznyj, 2001). In this zone, caesarean section is socially constructed as a technical solution in times of distress.

Applying technical solutions in distressing social situations is not a new phenomenon. Figlio (1978, 1982) shows how, prior to the Second World War, miners in the United Kingdom developed 'miners' nystagmus' and, earlier, nineteenth-century housemaids developed chlorosis as a response to their compromised social circumstances. According to Graham and Oakley (1981), altered mood, labelled as 'depression', may be better explained as an identity adjustment to new motherhood, rather than as a disease state in need of medical treatment. Bury (1986) explains how, by naming an experience as 'medical', it provides significance in terms of place, meaning and shape in social life. However, medical knowledge and practice are viewed as contested terrains. Bury (1986:137) suggests that 'the stable realities of the human body and disease are "fabrications" or inventions rather than discoveries'. Caesarean section, when it is employed in the absence of medical indications, may be one such fabrication, constructed as normative birth.

The evidence supporting the notion that women choose caesarean section, asserts Beckett (2005), is premised on advice that this choice ensures the safe arrival of their unborn baby. Good mothers accept the risks associated with surgical childbirth if they believe it is best for their baby. However, Beckett is also concerned about the lack of equity in relation to the use of finite resources (such as maternal request caesarean section) in maternity care. This leads to a debate about the place of consumerism in health care. According to Elliot and Lemert (2006), Western society is increasingly characterized by consumerism and obsessed with quick fixes. Health is commonly viewed as a commodity, purchased to combat fear of ill-health and reduce anxiety. In the provision of health care, society has shifted responsibility from the nation to the individual. Individualism emphasizes freedom in personal choice. Choice is viewed as the opposite of social control, and a consumer society promotes the notion of free choice (Elliot and Lemert, 2006). Klein (2004) describes the caesarean section on demand debate as an example of this quick-fix culture.

Warde (1994) has noted that, far from reducing fear and anxiety, consumerism has increased it. Individualism and autonomy may lead to distrust in health care, creating additional vulnerability. This can have significant impact on childbearing women who are already feeling anxious and vulnerable. Responsible for two lives, pregnant women have to learn to juggle the competing needs of the unborn baby with their own needs. Martin (1994) argues that choices in childbirth are commonly framed as being in the best interests of the foetus/baby first and the mother/woman second. Women's unequal relationship with maternity care givers also contributes to vulnerability and anxiety. However, Zadoroznyj (2000, 2001) reminds us that childbearing women are both patients and consumers in the medical encounter.

Caesarean section has been reported to be a desirable commodity for women in some countries, irrespective of class status. "Too posh to push" was considered the dictum of the British middle-class celebrities who 'chose' caesarean section (Le Fanu, 2001). Cultural and social ideals of femininity and modernity are now sometimes viewed as more central than health risks. While women in Brazil value natural childbirth highly, they are also fearful of a lack of appropriate care and support in labour (Hopkins, 2000). Women in Brazil have also opted for caesarean section for practical reasons, such as having access to tubal ligation, and believing they will receive better care in the hospital setting. Elective caesarean section also enables doctors to schedule their working day more efficiently, and, until recently, there have been financial incentives in some health care systems (McCallum, 2005). Surgical birth becomes both a consumer item (an ideal birth), aesthetically pleasing for women and able to meet the self-interest of doctors (de Mello e Souza, 1994).

In the peripheral zone, the issue of individual choice is complex. The childbearing woman's status is just that – a woman with child – in a society that increasingly recognizes the rights of the child over the mother. Much of the literature on maternal-request caesarean section has not explored in detail the reasons why women choose or request surgical intervention. To date, the literature includes studies of women's preferences for caesarean section, sometimes hypothetically, and women's involvement in decision-making. Clearly, women do not choose caesarean section lightly. Instead, a number of factors inform their decisions and, commonly, they are heavily influenced by the opinion of their care givers (McCourt et al., 2007).

We now discuss how different theories of decision-making can be applied to help understand the relationship between doctor and maternity user within the three zones of clinical practice.

Different styles of decision-making

The contemporary literature describes multiple approaches, or styles, of decision-making in medical care. There are three common classifications of decision-making: paternalistic (also referred to as an authoritative approach); shared (also referred to as mutualistic); and informed choice (Cahill, 1996; Charles *et al.*, 1997; Elwyn *et al.*, 2000; Wirtz *et al.*, 2006). In traditional medical practice, a single approach to treatment decision-making was typical, with the physician (the paternalistic or authoritative figure) deciding on the patient's behalf (Sullivan, 2003; Wirtz *et al.*, 2006). Parsons' (1951) seminal work illustrated how the role of the doctor was to act kindly towards the patient, to have the patients' best interests at heart, and to make clinical decisions on their behalf.

We illustrate how the existing models of decision-making are able to offer limited application in relation to decision-making for caesarean section, and that new models are urgently needed to better guide clinical practice in maternity care. In this context, it should be noted that informed consent is different, and should not be confused with informed choice. Informed consent involves giving information, encouraging patient involvement, engendering realistic explanations of outcome, having sufficient understanding to weigh the ratio of risk and benefit in terms of personal life plans, and having the procedure or not having the procedure (Meredith, 1993).

Paternalistic approach

According to Meredith (1993), the paternalistic or authoritative approach to decision-making may be the only feasible model in emergency situations and life-threatening circumstances when patients are not in a physical state to participate. The role of doctors is as patient-guardians, argues Charles *et al.* (1997); they strive to protect their patients' best interests without first assessing patient preferences for treatment. The role of the patient is passive, usually confined to consenting to the essential intervention.

Thompson (2007) supports the notion that patients are unlikely to be involved in decision-making in times of psychological distress or emergency situations, suggesting that there is a place for a paternalistic approach. Thompson (2007) also believes that there can be two types of patient involvement within the paternalistic style: one, the patient is completely excluded from the decision-making process; the other, the patient is given information, but excluded from involvement in the treatment decision. In Western societies, the paternalistic approach tends to be viewed as an outmoded style of decision-making, emergency situations being the exception.

In urgent, life-threatening situations, caesarean section may be organized

and performed rapidly, with little opportunity to explain all the possible implications to the woman and/or her family before consent for surgery is obtained.
Ideally, every effort should then be made to ensure that appropriate information is given to the woman (and her partner) at a time convenient to the couple
after the surgery is completed. In extreme situations, where the woman is
unconscious or unable to sign, consent is sought from next of kin. In life-
threatening situations, the paternalistic approach to decision-making is appropriate because the need for surgical intervention is clear-cut; alternative
treatment options do not exist.

There are also times where it is clear that there is no alternative to
caesarean section, but maternal and foetal well-being are not likely to be
imminently compromised. While the clinical situation is carefully outlined to
the woman and her family, and informed consent for surgery obtained, the
decision and responsibility to intervene surgically remains with her care
givers. There is no doubt for any of those involved that the surgery is potentially life-saving and clinically warranted, as the benefits far outweigh the
potential harm.

Shared approach

According to Sullivan (2003), respect for patient autonomy, and recognition
of their preferences, values, and right to appropriate access to balanced information has gradually influenced medical decision-making since the Second
World War. A number of authors suggest that patient involvement in decision-
making can improve health outcomes (Cahill, 1996; Edwards *et al.*, 2005),
increase compliance and improve satisfaction (Ashworth *et al.*, 1992), and
promote self-responsibility and self-care (Pelkonen *et al.*, 1998). However,
challenges remain in determining how much involvement patients wish to have
in medical decision-making (Thompson, 2007) and how to measure the level
of involvement offered to them (Elwyn *et al.*, 2000). A shared approach to
decision-making is advocated from ethical standpoints of respect for patient
autonomy and pressure to respond to consumer demand for more involvement
(Elwyn *et al.*, 2000).

Shared decision-making (where information sharing is essential) in the
medical encounter has been suggested by Charles *et al.* (1997) to be the ideal
model of treatment decision-making. They argue, however, that power differ-
entials between doctors and patients influence treatment decision-making. Up
until the 1980s, both patients and doctors expected doctors to play a dominant role, due to status differences in education (medical training and expertise), income and gender. However, the legitimacy of doctors' knowledge came
into question with advances in the range of possible treatment options, the
complex nature of medical encounters (enhanced capacities to diagnose some
diseases) and increasing uncertainty about clinical care (Charles *et al.*, 1999).

A shared approach to decision-making includes the doctor recognizing a
duty to establish the values and preferences of the patient and to discuss their
relevance in light of the available treatment options. Shared decision-making
relies on an atmosphere of open communication and reflection (Wirtz *et al.*,

2006). In this approach, patients understand that involvement in decision-making is only to their preferred level; while their autonomy is respected, enforced choice is considered another version of paternalism (Elwyn *et al.*, 2000).

Shared decision-making, we argue, is contentious in childbirth when clinical uncertainty about the need for surgical intervention exists. To date, there is insufficient evidence about the harms and benefits of caesarean section for women to be able to make an informed decision about this mode of birth in the presence of doubt about the best course of action. Women are likely to be influenced by the subtle messages of health professionals that good mothers will do what is best for their baby; caesarean provides a safe and organized birth (Bryant *et al.*, 2007; Goodall *et al.*, 2009).

Informed choice

Informed choice or informed decision-making occurs when technical knowledge is transferred to the patient and they make the final decision (Thompson, 2007). Wagner (2000:1678) proposes that 'any woman consenting to any medical procedure must be given full, unbiased information on what is known about the chances that the procedure will make things better (efficacy) and worse (risks)'. He cautions that clinicians must first have the information before they can pass it on, which can be time consuming, and the information readily available to doctors is commonly influenced by commercial or institutional interests.

According to Thompson (2007), patient charters include the right to make informed choices and are explicit about involvement in personal health care decisions. They are usually couched in terms such as the consumerist model (where health service users mimic customers in market-style relationships), citizen involvement and individual freedom.

Informed decision-making takes place when the physician and patient share information and the patient decides the best course of action (Charles *et al.*, 1999). One of the limitations of the informed choice approach is that patients can feel abandoned when decision-making is left up to them. Having received information about treatment options, no guidance is given, and responsibility for decision-making rests entirely with the patient. This, according to Elwyn *et al.* (2000), is more typical in situations when medico-legal risks influence clinicians' decision-making styles. One of the negative consequences of the informed choice approach is patient anxiety as a result of uncertainty about the best course of action.

Wirtz *et al.* (2006) suggest one restriction to informed choice involves the dilemma of supporting patients to make treatment choices when the doctor is aware of options but has limited knowledge of the implications of various treatments. They argue that the social relations between patient and doctor most probably prohibit the patient from asking about options they have learnt about independently. However, doctors are held accountable for treatments, even if the patient has actively made the treatment decision, according to their legal and ethical professional standards. Wirtz *et al.* (2006) also argue that, in situations of informed choice, there should be an explicit increase in patient accountability for their treatment choices. Patients, they suggest, who choose options that are not professionally recommended should be required to forego rights of complaint or of legal action, with professionals bearing diminished responsibility in such circumstances.

The informed choice approach to decision-making does not adequately account for the situation where women request caesarean section when it is not medically indicated or recommended by their care giver. Hausman (2005) asserts that, as recipients of maternity care, women make choices over-determined by existing technologies, often with little insight about their efficacy. Ethical dilemmas include considering how far patients should be allowed to determine their own treatment, and at what cost to society or the individual (Sullivan, 2003; Beckett, 2005; Wirtz *et al.*, 2006). Nilstun *et al.* (2008) argue that, when considering the principles of beneficence and non-maleficence, and maternal autonomy, caesarean for maternal request, is unjustified.

Our concern is that there is literature on maternal request caesarean section framed as women's right to informed choice (Paterson-Brown, 1998); yet, a report from the US states there is insufficient evidence to recommend for or against maternal request caesarean section (National Institutes of Health, 2006). We argue that there is currently and historically a lack of good quality evidence available upon which women can make an informed choice regarding maternal request caesarean section. We believe that much of the debate about informed choice in maternity care has been misappropriated by proponents of elective caesarean section for personal reasons.

Maternal choice caesarean section: myth or reality?

Goffman (1959, 1968) theorizes that people are motivated in their social interactions to behave in particular ways. When they deviate from socially accepted standards, they are 'stigmatized' or singled out for their difference. Individuals do make personal sacrifices in order to impress others. A 'good' mother's sacrifice on behalf of her baby may include consenting to caesarean section because, in refusing it, a woman's choice might be perceived as selfish in denying her baby the best chance of a 'safe' birth (Beckett, 2005; Liamputtong, 2005, 2007). Reports of women choosing caesarean section are increasingly common, data suggest the rate to be anywhere between 0.3 per cent and 14 per cent (McCourt *et al.*, 2007). However, doctors have an ethical duty to 'do no harm' (Bewley and Cockburn, 2002; Penna and Arulkumaran, 2003) and, in acquiescing to women's requests for caesarean section, may be striving to maintain a good relationship with their patients in the short term only (Skene, 2007).

According to Beckett (2005), there are numerous issues surrounding maternal choice caesarean section. First, although caesarean section is now safer than previously thought, evidence on differences in safety between vaginal birth and caesarean section remain controversial. The second argument, she suggests, is that women should have the right to choose the kind of medical care they receive, including major surgery, if they are informed of the potential risks. However, women's choices for technology may be based on biased information, or information that overstates the risks to the foetus.

Wagner (2001) also argues against unnecessary caesarean section on ethical and economic grounds. He suggests that elective caesarean section requires multiple resources (for example, time, training, operating theatres and blood transfusions), creating huge pressure on institutional and government finances, even for wealthy countries. He believes women would not choose caesarean section if it were not medically indicated unless their doctor provided them with highly selective and limited information. Previously, however, Wagner (2000) suggested elective caesarean section offers many benefits for doctors, convenience being just one of them. Klein (2004) proposes that maternal request caesarean section is not a solution, but a symptom of a problem. Debates about the harms of elective caesarean section, in the absence of medical indication, centre on the ethical considerations of whether or not a doctor can accede or refuse an 'informed' woman's request. The agreed position suggests that the doctor acts in the woman's best interests. Policy documents such as the UK Government's 'Changing Childbirth' report recommended consumers of maternity services should have access to choice in place of birth, type of care giver and model of care, but not in choice of mode of birth (Department of Health, 1993).

Discourses of risk

According to Beck (1992), traditionally, risk was personal and hinted of bravery or adventure but, in modern societies, it has connotations of global dangers and threats to all life on earth. Traditional risks were discernible to the senses, sight and smell, whereas today's risks escape perception; for example, being located in physical and chemical formulas, such as radioactive waste or nuclear weapons.

Carter (1995) and Lupton (1995) suggest that assessing the 'risk' of a given situation should involve taking a neutral position to calculate the likelihood of gains or losses. However, in contemporary society, risk has assumed the same meaning as danger, to be avoided at all cost, rather than highlighting uncertainty of future harm or benefit, or the statistical likelihood of an event occurring. Lupton (1995) carries the risk discourse further, asserting that there are different ways in which risk is understood. One is that risks are consequences of life-style choices made by individuals. Typical examples of individual risk-engaging behaviours are smoking, drug misuse and excessive alcohol intake. Another relates to the social disadvantage (risk) experienced by those social groups with reduced access to health services. There is evidence of women who belong to different social groups having increased risk of exposure to unnecessary caesarean section (Sakala, 1993; Shearer, 1993). However, the essence of responding to risk is that it aims to 'tame uncertainty' (Lupton, 1995: 77).

Crawford (2006) theorizes that concerns about personal health have become a national preoccupation. An at-risk society produces at-risk individuals and behaviours. In earlier work, Crawford (1980) proposed that human behaviour needs to move beyond coping, to an ideology that enhances the individual's social capacity to control their social conditions. Further, in health, all emotions, behaviours and attitudes that put the individual 'at risk' tend to be medicalized; illness becomes a moral failing and the individual's fault; the ideology of victim-blaming is borne into popular culture. The 'imperative of health', according to Crawford (2006: 403), is a mandate to identify and control dangers, which is likely to require a life-long commitment to medical surveillance. Health is a state of constant jeopardy. The more important health becomes, the more insecure we feel. But, medicine is not risk-free; virtually all treatments involve some risk of possible harm.

Risk, uncertainty and fear in maternity care

The risk discourse of Western modern childbirth is contentious, in that all pregnant women are now described as having some risk, irrespective of their health status or foetal well-being (Lane, 1995; Hausman, 2005; Possamai-Inesedy, 2006). Hausman (2005) argues that risk is used as a threat to compel compliance with the norms of medicalized childbirth. In contrast, Zadorozynj (2001) contends that, even in the high-risk setting, women's views are sought regarding their pregnancy and childbirth care. Obstetricians view childbirth as a risky life-event, despite considerable reduction in perinatal and maternal mortality (Lankshear *et al.*, 2005), and assert that childbirth can only be judged to be safe in retrospect (Lane, 1995). Women's own sense of risk influences their acceptance or rejection of medical intervention, irrespective of their social class or background (Liamputtong, 2005, 2007). Wagner (2000) suggests that women and their babies bear the risks when a caesarean section is performed, while their doctors bear the risks if the surgery is not performed.

Juggling risks in pregnancy and childbirth creates anxiety for women, who will almost always have their babies' best interests at heart. Women may perceive technology such as caesarean section as the ideal way to give birth, if they believe it reduces risk of harm to their baby (Liamputtong, 2005, 2007; Liamputtong and Watson, 2006). In modern societies, where advanced technology is available and affordable, foetal and maternal surveillance has become routine and, paradoxically, so has increased uncertainty in maternity care (Possamai-Inesedy, 2006). Wagner (2001) suggests that risks increase, rather than decrease, with wider use of surgical interventions such as caesarean section. Giddens (1990) asserts that inaction is often risky, and Lupton (1995: 80) contends that 'the imperative to do something, to remove the source of a health risk, however tenuous, impels action'.

In childbirth, utilization of technological interventions is perceived both to reduce the risk of something going wrong and to increase iatrogenic risks to the mother and foetus (Lane, 1995; Possamai-Inesedy, 2006). By offering caesarean section in times of uncertainty, care givers might believe they are reducing their risk of litigation (Penna and Arulkumaran, 2003; Skene, 2007). Control over technical judgements and claims for the necessity of intervention and reliance on professionals ensures medicine maintains its dominant position in childbirth and as the arbiter of health and illness (Oakley and Richards,

1990). Perceptions, values and concerns about risk and uncertainty are important attributes differentiating trust according to patient or practitioner roles (Liamputtong, 2005, 2007; Riewpaiboon *et al.*, 2005).

Maternal fear, trust and confidence in childbirth

Giddens (1990) theorizes that feeling secure relies upon finding a balance between trust and acceptable risk. When calculating risk, it is necessary to know what threats might arise from each course of action. Danger is the known threat to desired outcomes. He further asserts that trust involves considering the alternatives and acknowledging the risks; when disappointment occurs, the individual accepts some of the blame and may regret being so trusting. In assessing risk status and ultimately making decisions based on the balance of the evidence available, honest and open communication and trust are essential (Giddens, 1990).

Whilst patient involvement may vary, there is mounting evidence of the importance of a good interpersonal relationship between doctor and patient, and this includes the development and maintenance of trust (Coulter, 2002). Patients' include trust, caring, concern and compassion as important features of the interpersonal skills of their health care practitioners (Mechanic and Meyer, 2000). Trust, however, does not equate to blind faith; patients do not want to be deceived about their illness or the risks and potential harms of treatment. Trust, Coulter (2002) suggests, has to be earned, and doctors should strive to ensure that patients' questions are answered honestly; they should allow time for listening and ascertaining patient views. Patients should be involved in decision-making as much or as little as they wish. Thompson (2007) hypothesizes that patients might want more, rather than less, involvement in treatment decision-making in situations where they feel that trust is abused or neglected.

According to Lane (1995), in a medically dominated maternity system, women's anxiety about safety may lead to the increasing normalization of caesarean section as a trusted obstetric procedure. Inner confidence, she asserts, as opposed to fear and anxiety, is a woman's greatest asset in childbirth, but medicalization of birth has reduced women's capacity to feel confident, comfortable and secure in labour. Lane (1995) also suggests women are influenced by their birth setting and their care givers' perceptions of risk. In order to feel supported without medical intervention, women need to feel safe, as fear erodes their capacity to give birth unassisted.

Conclusion

In this chapter, we have demonstrated how a range of different social theories help to inform understanding of contemporary caesarean section. Caesarean section is increasingly used despite concerns about its benefits, safety and costs. In many instances, since industrialization, maternity service provision has undergone incredible change. The rise of medicine, the increasing medicalization of childbirth and, more recently, emphasis on consumerism in health care within a political and economic focus on individualism have had a significant impact in the last 50 years. Medical and obstetric reasons are insufficient to explain the promotion of medical technologies such as caesarean section in maternity care.

We have developed three zones of clinical practice to provide a theoretical framework upon which to classify the range of reasons for caesarean section. In the central zone, caesarean section is essential for the preservation of the life of the foetus and/or the woman. When essential surgery is undertaken, an authoritarian approach to decision-making is appropriate, as a range of possible treatment options do not exist.

In the grey zone, the decision to perform a caesarean section is less certain in terms of clinical factors. Decision-making is often influenced by insufficient good-quality evidence, which creates doubt about the best course of action. Depending on the clinical situation and the individual care giver, there is opportunity for the maternity user to be involved in decision-making. Women's preferences and values regarding mode of birth may be considered.

The peripheral zone of clinical practice highlights how social factors determine the decision to have a caesarean section. Surgery is a solution imposed by the individual in the absence of clinical factors but often in the presence of fear, anxiety or distress. Decision-making takes a consumerist form, with the woman actively seeking caesarean section without initial input from care givers.

The existing ideologies of care – the medical model and the natural birth model – are insufficient to meet the needs of childbearing women. Women need access to the best of both models of maternity care: being supported to give birth safely with appropriate and timely use of carefully evaluated technology. We have shown how theories of risk, trust and uncertainty help to explain decision-making in pregnancy and childbirth. These social theories may help midwives, and the women they support in pregnancy and childbirth, to better understand the complexities of contemporary caesarean section in western societies.

ACTIVITIES

Undergraduate

Debate the pros and cons of the commentary as stated above (p. 276):

> Policy documents such as the UK Government's 'Changing Childbirth' report recommended consumers of maternity services should have access to choice in place of birth, type of care giver and model of care, but not in choice of mode of birth. (Department of Health 1993)

Postgraduate

It has been stated that caesarean birth decision-making can be theoretically mapped to fit within one of three zones: central, grey or peripheral. Design a research study to explore the theoretical assumptions presented in this chapter.

References

Alasuutari, P. (1995) *Researching Culture: Qualitative Method and Cultural Studies*. London: Sage Publications.

Alaszewski, A. and Brown, P. (2007) 'Risk, Uncertainty and Knowledge', *Health, Risk and Society*, 9(1): 1–10.

Ashworth, P., Longmate, M. and Morrison, P. (1992) 'Patient Participation: Its Meaning and Significance in the Context of Caring', *Journal of Advanced Nursing*, 17: 1430–9.

Barros, F., Vaughan, J. and Victora, C. (1986) 'Why So Many Caesarean Sections? The Need for a Further Policy Change in Brazil', *Health Policy and Planning*, 1(1): 19–29.

Bastian, H. (1999) 'Commentary: "Health has become Secondary to a Sexually Attractive Body" ', *British Medical Journal*, 319: 1402.

Beck, U. (1992) *Risk Society: Towards a New Modernity*. London: Sage.

Beckett, K. (2005) 'Choosing Cesarean: Feminism and the Politics of Childbirth in the United States', *Feminist Theory*, 6(3): 251–75.

Bewley, S. and Cockburn, J. (2002) 'The Unethics of "Request" Caesarean Section', *BJOG: An International Journal of Obstetrics and Gynaecology*, 109: 593–6.

Bloor, M. (1976) 'Bishop Berkeley and the Adenotonsillectomy Enigma: An Exploration of Variation in the Social Construction of Medical Disposals', *Sociology*, 10: 43–61.

Bryant, J., Porter, M., Tracy, S.K. and Sullivan, E.A. (2007) 'Caesarean Birth: Consumption, Safety, Order and Good Mothering', *Social Science and Medicine*, 64: 1192–201.

Bury, M. (1986) 'Social Constructionism and the Development of Medical Sociology', *Sociology of Health and Illness*, 8(2): 137–69.

Cahill, J. (1996) 'Patient Participation: A Concept Analysis', *Journal of Advanced Nursing*, 24: 561–71.

Carter, S. (1995) 'Boundaries of Danger and Uncertainty: An Analysis of the Technological Culture of Risk Assessment', in J. Gabe (ed.), *Medicine, Health and Risk: Sociological Approaches*. Oxford: Blackwell.

Chaillet, N. and Dumont, A. (2007) 'Evidence-Based Strategies for Reducing Cesarean Section Rates: A Meta-analysis', *Birth*, 34(1): 53–64.

Charles, C., Gafni, A. and Whelan, T. (1997) 'Shared Decision-Making in the Medical Encounter: What Does it Mean? (Or it takes at least two to tango)', *Social Science and Medicine*, 44(5): 681–92.

Charles, C., Gafni, A. and Whelan, T. (1999) 'Decision-Making in the Physician–Patient Encounter: Revisiting the Shared Treatment Decision-making Model', *Social Science and Medicine*, 49: 651–61.

Coulter, A. (2002) 'Patients' Views of the Good Doctor. Doctors have to Earn Patients' Trust', *British Medical Journal*, 325: 668–9.

Crawford, R. (1980) 'Healthism and the Medicalisation of Everyday Life', *International Journal of Health Services*, 10(3): 365–88.

Crawford, R. (2006) 'Health as a Meaningful Social Practice', *Health: An Interdisciplinary Journal for the Social Study of Health, Illness and Medicine*, 10: 401–20.

Cyr, R. (2006) 'Myth of the Ideal Cesarean Section Rate: Commentary and Historic Perspective', *American Journal of Obstetrics and Gynecology*, 194: 932–6.

Davis-Floyd, R. (1996) 'The Technocratic Body and the Organic Body: Hegemony and Heresy in Women's Birth Choices', in C. Sargent and C. Brettell (eds.), *Gender and Health: An International Perspective*. Upper Saddle River, NJ: Prentice Hall.

de Mello e Souza, C. (1994) 'C-Sections as Ideal Births: The Cultural Constructions of Beneficence and Patients' Rights in Brazil', *Cambridge Quarterly of Healthcare Ethics*, 3: 358–66.

Department of Health (1993) 'Changing Childbirth. Part 1: Report of the Expert Maternity Group'. London: HMSO.

Dixon-Woods, M., Williams, S., Jackson, C., Akkad, A., Kenyon, S. and Habiba, M. (2006) 'Why Do Women Consent To Surgery, Even When They Do Not Want To? An Interactionist and Bourdieusian Analysis', *Social Science and Medicine*, 62(11): 2742–53.

Edwards, A., Elwyn, G., Wood, F., Atwell, C., Prior, L. and Houston, H. (2005) 'Shared Decision Making and Risk Communication in Practice: A Qualitative Study of GPs' Experiences', *British Journal of General Practice*, 55: 6–13.

Elliot, A. and Lemert, C. (2006) *The New Individualism: The Emotional Costs of Globalization*. London: Routledge.

Elwyn, G., Edwards, A., Kinnersley, P. and Grol, R. (2000) 'Shared Decision Making and the Concepts of Equipoise: The Competences of Involving Patients in Healthcare Choices', *British Journal of General Practice*, 50: 892–7.

Figlio, K. (1978) 'Chlorosis and Chronic Disease in 19th Century Britain: The Social Constitution of Somatic Illness in a Capitalist Society', *International Journal of Health Services*, 8: 589–617.

Figlio, K. (1982) 'How Does Illness Mediate Social Relations? Workmen's Compensation and Medico-Legal Practices', in P. Wright and A. Treacher (eds), *The Problem of Medical Knowledge: Examining the Social Construction of Medicine*. Edinburgh: Edinburgh University Press.

Federation of International Gynecologists and Obstetricians (FIGO) (2007) FIGO Statement on Caesarean Section – 23/01/2007 (http://www.cngof.assoc.fr/ D_TELE/FIGO_cesar_230107 – accessed online 13 November 2009).

Francome, C. and Savage, W. (1993) 'Caesarean Section in Britain and the United States 12% or 24%: Is either the right rate?', *Social Science and Medicine*, 37(10): 1199–218.

Frost, J., Pope, C., Liebling, R. and Murphy, D. (2006) 'Utopian Theory and the Discourse of Natural Birth', *Social Theory and Health*, 4: 299–318.

Gabe, J. and Calnan, M. (1989) 'The Limits of Medicine: Women's Perception of Medical Technology', *Social Science and Medicine*, 28(3): 223–31.

Giddens, A. (1990) *The Consequences of Modernity*. Cambridge: Polity Press.

Goffman, E. (1959) *The Presentation of Self in Everyday Life*. New York, NY: Anchor Books.

Goffman, E. (1968) *Asylums: Essays on the Social Situation of Mental Patients and Other Inmates*. Harmondsworth: Penguin.

Goodall, K.E., McVittie, C. and Magill, M. (2009) 'Birth Choice following Primary Caesarean Section: Mothers' Perception of the Influence of Health Professionals on Decision-making', *Journal of Reproductive and Infant Psychology*, 27(1): 4–14.

Graham, H. and Oakley, A. (1981) 'Competing Ideologies of Reproduction: Medical and Maternal Perspectives on Pregnancy', in H. Roberts (ed.), *Women, Health and Reproduction*. London: Routledge & Kegan Paul.

Green, J. and Baston, H. (2007) 'Have Women Become More Willing To Accept Obstetric Interventions and Does This Relate to Mode of Birth? Data from a Prospective Study', *Birth*, 34(1): 6–13.

Hausman, B. (2005) 'Risky Business: Framing Childbirth in Hospital Settings', *Journal of Medical Humanities*, 26(1): 23–38.

Hopkins, K. (2000) 'Are Brazilian Women Really Choosing to Deliver by Cesarean?', *Social Science and Medicine*, 51(5): 725–40.

Hurst, M. and Summey, P. (1984) 'Childbirth and Social Class: The Case of Cesarean Delivery', *Social Science and Medicine*, 18(8): 621–31.

Johnston, T. and Coory, M. (2006), 'Increase in Caesarean Section Rates among Low-Risk Women in Queensland, 1990–2004', *Medical Journal of Australia*, 185(7): 404–5.

Kalish, R., McCulloch, L., Gupta, M., Thaler, H. and Chervenak, F. (2004) 'Intrapartum Elective Cesarean Delivery: A Previously Unrecognised Clinical Entity', *Obstetrics and Gynecology*, 103(6): 1137–41.

Kealy, M. (2007) 'Caesarean Section – A Response to Risk and Fear: An Australian Study of Women's Experiences', Unpublished PhD thesis, La Trobe University, Bundoora, Australia.

Kingdon, C., Baker, L. and Lavender, T. (2006) 'Systematic Review of Nulliparous Women's Views of Planned Cesarean Birth: The Missing Component in the Debate about a Term Cephalic Trial', *Birth*, 33(3): 229–37.

Klein, M. (2004) 'Quick Fix Culture: The Cesarean-section-on-demand Debate', *Birth*, 31(3): 161–4.

Kornelsen, J. (2005) 'Essences and Imperatives: An Investigation of Technology in Childbirth', *Social Science and Medicine*, 61: 1495–504.

Lane, K. (1995) 'The Medical Model of the Body as a Site of Risk: A Case Study of Childbirth', in J. Gabe (ed.), *Medicine, Health and Risk*. Oxford: Blackwell.

Lankshear, G., Ettorre, E. and Mason, D. (2005) 'Decision-Making, Uncertainty and Risk: Exploring the Complexity of Work Processes in NHS Delivery Suites', *Health, Risk and Society*, 7(4): 361–77.

Laws, P. and Sullivan, E.A. (2005) 'Australia's Mothers and Babies 2003', National Perinatal Statistics Unit, Australian Institute of Health and Welfare, Sydney.

Laws, P.J. and Hilder, L. (2008) 'Australia's Mothers and Babies 2006', National Perinatal Statistics Unit, Australian Institute of Health and Welfare, Sydney.

Lazarus, E. (1994) 'What Do Women Want? Issues of Choice, Control, and Class in Pregnancy and Childbirth', *Medical Anthropology Quarterly*, 8(1): 25–46.

Le Fanu, J. (2001) 'Doctor's Diary: Dr James Le Fanu Considers the Rise in Favour of Caesareans' ['Too Posh To Push?'], *Daily Telegraph*, 29 May.

Leone, T., Padmadas, S.S. and Matthew, Z. (2008) 'Community Factors Affecting Rising Caesarean Section Rates in Developing Countries: An Analysis of Six Countries', *Social Science and Medicine*, 67(8): 1236–46.

Liamputtong, P. (2005) 'Birth and Social Class: Northern Thai Women's Lived Experiences of Caesarean and Vaginal Birth', *Sociology of Health and Illness*, 27(2): 243–70.

Liamputtong, P. (2007) *The Journey of Becoming a Mother amongst Women in Northern Thailand*. Lanham, MD: Lexington Books.

Liamputtong, P., Halliday, J., Warren, R., Watson, L. and Bell, R. (2003) 'Why Do Women Decline Prenatal Screening and Diagnosis? Australian Women's Perspective', *Women and Health*, 37(2): 89–108.

Liamputtong, P. and Watson, L. (2006) 'The Meanings and Experiences of Cesarean Birth among Cambodian, Lao and Vietnamese Immigrant Women in Australia', *Women and Health*, 43(3): 63–82.

LoCicero, A. (1993) 'Explaining Excessive Rates of Cesareans and Other Childbirth Interventions: Contributions from Contemporary Theories of Gender and Psychosocial Development', *Social Science and Medicine*, 37(10): 1261–9.

Lupton, D. (2003) *Medicine as Culture: Illness, Disease and the Body in Western Societies*, 2nd edn. London: Sage.

Lupton, D. (1995) 'Taming Uncertainty: Risk discourse and diagnostic testing', in D. Lupton, *The Imperative of Health: Public Health and the Regulated Body*. London: Sage.

Mansfield, B. (2008) 'The Social Nature of Natural Childbirth', *Social Science and Medicine*, 6: 1088–94.

Martin, E. (1994) *The Woman in the Body: A Cultural Analysis of Reproduction*. Boston, MA: Beacon Press.

McCallum, C. (2005) 'Explaining Caesarean Section in Salvador da Bahia, Brazil', *Sociology of Health and Illness*, 27(2): 215–42.

McCourt, C., Weaver, J., Statham, H., Beake, S., Gamble, J. and Creedy, D. (2007) 'Elective Cesarean Section and Decision Making: A Critical Review of the Literature', *Birth*, 34(1): 65–79.

Mechanic, D. and Meyer, S. (2000) 'Concepts of Trust among Patients with Serious Illness', *Social Science and Medicine*, 51(5): 657–68.

Meredith, P. (1993) 'Patient Participation in Decision-Making and Consent to Treatment: The Case of General Surgery', *Sociology of Health and Illness*, 15(3): 315–36.

Miesnik, S.R., and Reale, B.J. (2007) 'A Review of Issues Surrounding Medically Elective Cesarean Delivery', *Journal of Gynecologic Neonatal Nurses*, 36: 605–15.

National Institutes of Health (2006) 'NIH State-of-the-Science Conference Statement on Cesarean Delivery on Maternal Request', *NIH Consensus and State-of-the-Science Statements*, 23(1): 1–29. National Institutes of Health.

Navarro, V. (2002) *The Political Economy of Social Inequalities: Consequences for Health and Quality of Life*. Amityville, NY: Baywood.

Naylor, C. (1995) 'Grey Zones of Clinical Practice: Some Limits to Evidence-based Medicine', *Lancet*, 345: 840–2.

Nelson, M. (1983) 'Working-Class Women, Middle-Class Women, and Models of Childbirth', *Social Problems*, 30(3): 284–97.

Nilstun, T., Habiba, M., Lingman, G., Saracci, R., Da Frè, M. and Cuttini, M. for the EUROBS study group (2008) 'Cesarean Delivery on Maternal Request: Can the Ethical Problem Be Solved by the Principlist Approach?', *BMC Medical Ethics*, 9: 11 (http://www.biomedcentral.com/1472-6939/9/11).

Oakley, A. (1980) *Women Confined: Towards a Sociology of Childbirth*. Oxford: Martin Robertson.

Oakley, A. and Richards, M. (1990) 'Women's Experiences of Caesarean Delivery', in J. Garcia, R. Kilpatrick and M. Richards (eds) *The Politics of Maternity Care*. Oxford: Clarendon Press.

Parahoo K (2006) *Nursing Research. Principles, Process and Issues*. 2nd edn. Basingstoke: Palgrave Macmillan.

Parsons, T. (1951) *The Social System*. London: Routledge & Kegan Paul.

Paterson-Brown, S. (1998) 'Should Doctors Perform an Elective Caesarean Section on Request? Yes, as long as the Woman is Fully Informed?', *British Medical Journal*, 317: 462–3.

Pelkonen, M., Perälä, M.-L. and Vehviläinen-Julkunen, K. (1998) 'Participation of Expectant Mothers in Decision Making in Maternity Care: Results from a Population-based Study', *Journal of Advanced Nursing*, 28(1): 21–9.

Penna, L. and Arulkumaran, S. (2003) 'Cesarean Section for Non-Medical Reasons', *International Journal of Gynecology and Obstetrics*, 82(3): 399–409.

Possamai-Inesedy, A. (2006) 'Childbirth Discourse in Risk Society', Unpublished PhD thesis, University of Western Sydney, Sydney.

Reiger, K. (2001) *Our Bodies, Our Babies: The Forgotten Women's Movement*. Melbourne: Melbourne University Press.

Renwick, M. (1991) 'Caesarean Section Rates, Australia 1986: Variations at State and Small Area Level', *Australian and New Zealand Journal of Obstetrics and Gynaecology*, 31(4): 299–304.

Riewpaiboon, W., Chuengsatiansup, K., Gilson, L. and Tangcharoensathien, V. (2005) 'Private Obstetric Practice in a Public Hospital: Mythical Trust in Obstetric Care', *Social Science and Medicine*, 61: 1408–17.

Roberts, C., Tracy, S. and Peat, B. (2000) Rates for Obstetric Intervention among Private and Public Patients in Australia: Population-based Descriptive Study', *British Medical Journal*, 321: 137–41.

Robson, S. and Ellwood, D. (2003) 'Should Obstetricians Support a "Term Cephalic Trial"?', *Australian and New Zealand Journal of Obstetrics and Gynaecology*, 43: 341–3.

Rocha, J., Ortiz, P. and Fung, Y. (1985) 'The Incidence of Caesarean Sections and Remuneration for Treatment during Childbirth', in K. White (ed.), *Health Services Research*. Washington, DC: Pan American Health Organization.

Sakala, C. (1993) 'Medically Unnecessary Cesarean Section Births: Introduction to a Symposium', *Social Science and Medicine*, 37(10): 1177–98.

Sandelowski, M. and Bustamante, R. (1986) 'Cesarean Birth outside the Natural Childbirth Culture', *Research in Nursing and Health*, 9: 81–8.

Shearer, E. (1993) 'Cesarean Section: Medical Benefits and Costs', *Social Science and Medicine*, 37(10): 1223–31.

Sinclair, M. and Gardner, J. (2002) 'Midwives' Perceptions of the Use of Technology in Assisting Childbirth in Northern Ireland', *Journal of Advanced Nursing*, 36(2): 229–36

Skene, L. (2007) 'Time for the Birth of a New Discussion', *The Age*, Melbourne: 15.

Sullivan, M. (2003) 'The New Subjective Medicine: Taking the Patient's Point of View on Health Care and Health', *Social Science and Medicine*, 56: 1595–604.

Thompson, A. (2007) 'The Meaning of Patient Involvement and Participation in Health Care Consultations: A Taxonomy', *Social Science and Medicine*, 64: 1297–310.

Treichler, P. (1990) 'Feminism, Medicine, and the Meaning of Childbirth', in M. Jacobus, E. Keller and S. Shuttleworth (eds), *Body/Politics: Women, Literature, and the Discourse of Science*. New York, NY: Routledge.

Wagner, M. (2000) 'Choosing Caesarean Section', *Lancet*, 356(9242): 1677–80.

Wagner, M. (2001) 'Fish Can't See Water: The Need to Humanize Birth', *International Journal of Gynecology and Obstetrics*, 75: S25–S37.

Warde, A. (1994) 'Consumption, Identity-Formation and Uncertainty', *Sociology*, 28(4): 877 898.

Waterstone, M., Bewley, S. and Wolfe, C. (2001) 'Incidence and Predictors of Severe Obstetric Morbidity: Case-control Study', *British Medical Journal*, 322: 1089–94.

Williams, S. (2005) 'Parsons Revisited: From the Sick Role to ...?', *Health: An Interdisciplinary Journal for the Social Study of Health, Illness and Medicine*, 9(2): 123–44.

Wirtz, V., Cribb, A. and Barber, N. (2006) 'Patient–Doctor Decision-Making about Treatment within the Consultation – A Critical Analysis of Models', *Social Science and Medicine*, 62: 116–24.

WHO (World Health Organization) (1985) 'Appropriate Technology for Birth', *Lancet*, 2: 436–7.

Zadoroznyj, M. (1999) 'Social Class, Social Selves and Social Control in Childbirth', *Sociology of Health and Illness*, 21(3): 267–89.

Zadoroznyj, M. (2000) 'Midwife-Led Maternity Services and Consumer 'Choice' in an Australian Metropolitan Region', *Midwifery*, 16(3): 177–85.

Zadoroznyj, M. (2001) 'Birth and the 'Reflexive Consumer': Trust, Risk and Medical Dominance in Obstetric Encounters', *Journal of Sociology*, 37(2): 117–39.

Developing a Theoretical Framework: Bullying in Midwifery

13

Patricia Gillen, Marlene Sinclair and George Kernohan

Key points

- Demonstrates theory development and testing using concept analysis and testing within a mixed method research study
- A mixed method research approach can enhance the quality and depth of understanding
- A formal approach to concept analysis is possible in a clinical setting yielding clarity over definition and characteristics of concepts
- The context of research is important as it contributes to the meaning and applicability of research in practice.

Theoretical assumptions

Research is: 'a systematic way of knowing' (Parahoo, 2006: 8) which may be further defined as: 'a systematic, formal, rigorous and precise process employed to gain solutions to problems and/or discover and interpret new facts and relationships' (Waltz and Bausell, 1981: 1).

It has been said that: 'theory without research and research without theory does little to advance knowledge in any meaningful way' (Fawcett and Downs, 1992: v). Theories are: 'abstractions created and invented by humans' (Polit *et al.*, 2001: 145) and, it has been argued, that theory generation involves constructing theory without being sure of its usefulness or accuracy (Walker and Avant, 2004). Theories are a tentative attempt to describe and explain a phenomenon as seen through the eyes of a particular person or researcher. It may not be possible to prove a theory, but it may be tested and evolve over time as a result of further research, or it may be discarded (Polit *et al.*, 2001).

When designing a research study, it is important to consider not only the design of the research in practical terms, but also the theory underpinning the research. Theory can be derived from a variety of sources (see Chapter 2). It may be possible to use a theory that has already been developed, but a theory may also be developed by the researcher drawn from their experience and reading about a particular subject.

From the outset, it was clear that when researching a phenomenon such as 'bullying in midwifery' an attempt had to be made to place the phenomenon within an appropriate context. Holloway (1997) stresses the importance of the context in which the research takes place, explaining that this includes the social and cultural system of the participants. So, in the case of bullying, an understanding of the context of the participants is a vital part of the research; a clearer understanding of the context of midwifery will promote a greater understanding of the phenomenon of bullying in midwifery.

Background

The first systematic description of the phenomenon of bullying is attributed to Heinemann (1972), who described bullying amongst schoolchildren. Adams (1992) was one of the first authors from the UK to write about bullying in the workplace, while research from European countries, Scandinavia in particular, highlighted the nature, extent and consequences of bullying in a variety of workplaces (Einarsen and Skogstad, 1996; Leymann, 1996; Niedl, 1996; Vartia, 1996). In the UK, the health service unions were amongst the first organizations to examine bullying amongst midwives (RCM, 1996; UNISON, 1997; RCN, 2002).

There are many terms that may be used as an alternative name for bullying (RCM, 1996; RCN, 2002). These include: 'psychological terror' (Leymann, 1990), 'work abuse' (Bassmann, 1992), 'harassment', 'intimidation', 'aggression', 'bad attitude', 'coercive management', 'personality clash', 'poor management style', 'brutalism' and 'working in a funny way' (Adams, 1992: 12–13).

As with many research topics, another issue that further confounds the true picture of bullying is the lack of consensus about the precise definition of bullying, with most researchers adopting a definition that best fits the needs of their research (Quine, 1999). In addition, most of the instruments used to measure the incidence or influencing factors have a weak theoretical basis, with little account being given to reliability and validity. A variety of time-related criteria are also applied without any firm basis for their inclusion (as evidenced in Hoel and Cooper (2000) and Quine (1999)).

Mackenzie Davey and Liefhooghe (2003: 453) suggested that bullying is an inevitable part of work and perceived it as: 'the legitimate exercise of power'. Bullying has been identified as the cause of more long-term sickness and trauma than all other forms of work-related stress (Wilson, 1991), with the suggested cost to UK businesses reported as being in the region of £2 billion pounds per annum (Chartered Institute of Personnel and Development, 2005).

Comparative international studies and statistics (Einarsen, 2000) suggest that the lowest incidence rates of bullying tend to come from the Scandinavian countries (between 2 per cent and 25 per cent). This may, in part, be explained by the fact that researchers apply strict criteria – such as duration and frequency of bullying behaviour – when measuring the nature and extent of bullying. For example, Leymann (1996) suggests that a person is bullied only if they have been subjected to a bullying behaviour once a week for a minimum of six months.

By contrast, two studies of National Health Service (NHS) Trust employees in Britain found a prevalence of between 11 per cent in a study using a definition of: 'self reported exposure to bullying in the preceding six months' (Hoel and Cooper, 2000) and 38 per cent where the criterion was exposure to one or more types of bullying behaviours during the previous year (Quine, 1999). In 2002, a survey of the RCN's membership revealed that 17 per cent (n = 670) of respondents said that they had been bullied at some time in the 12 months prior to the survey.

Bullying behaviours can be classified in many ways. One such classification is that of Rayner and Hoel (1997: 183), who place bullying under the following five categories:

- Threat to professional status – belittling opinion, public professional humiliation, accusation regarding lack of effort
- Threat to personal standing – name-calling, insults, intimidation, devaluing with reference to age
- Isolation – preventing access to opportunities, physical or social isolation, withholding information
- Overwork – undue pressure, impossible deadlines, unnecessary disruptions
- Destabilisation – failure to give credit when due, meaningless tasks, removal of responsibility, repeated reminders of blunders, setting up to fail.

Having set bullying within the context of the workplace generally, the focus will now turn to that of the midwifery workplace.

Bullying in midwifery

In 1996, the RCM undertook the first large-scale research into bullying in midwifery and surveyed 1,000 midwives and student midwives with a reported response rate of 46 per cent (n = 462). Almost half of the respondents (43 per cent; n = 197) reported experience of bullying. Although duration or frequency of bullying behaviours was not examined, a list of behaviours was identified as being closely associated with bullying:

- intimidation (67 per cent; n = 132)
- undervaluing of skills (67 per cent; n = 131)

- humiliation (66 per cent; n = 130)
- belittling of work (60 per cent; n = 119)
- undervaluing effort (57 per cent; n = 114)
- questioning of professional competence (51 per cent; n = 101)
- excessive criticism (51 per cent; n = 101).

Case studies by Hadikin and O'Driscoll (2000) further illustrate the culture of bullying, with midwives recalling occasions when they had been undermined, belittled, controlled, victimized, sent to Coventry, had work devalued and been passed over for promotion. Midwives were reported as having left their jobs as a way to escape the bully (Hadikin and O'Driscoll, 2000).

Manifestations of bullying in the midwifery workplace have emerged as findings from other midwifery research, including work by Begley (1999a, 1999b), Ball *et al.* (2002) and Curtis *et al.* (2003). Begley (2002) reported the feelings and views of student midwives who became more aware of the hierarchical environment and exposed: 'a subculture of nursing/midwifery subordination' as they progressed through their education programme in Ireland (Begley, 2002: 310). A study by Ball *et al.* (2002) into why midwives leave the midwifery profession included evidence that identified managers as bullies. Follow-up research by Curtis *et al.* (2003: 30) reported that, while managers accepted that certain types of behaviours did take place, they were keen to minimize the importance of these and blamed misinterpretation by colleagues, whom they described as being 'over-sensitive'.

There is much anecdotal evidence, but there is little recent empirical evidence beyond case study to support the existence of bullying in midwifery practice. From a review of the evidence to date, the definition of bullying is not clear; therefore, a study was undertaken in order to define and explore the nature and manifestations of bullying in midwifery (Gillen, 2007). This research was necessary, as the concept of bullying was unclear and poorly defined.

Aim

The aim of this study was to clarify a single concept in a single context: to define and examine the nature and manifestations of bullying in midwifery.

Methods

This was an exploratory descriptive study that used a mixed-method approach advocated by Tashakkori and Teddlie (2003). Ethical approval for the study was granted by the University of Ulster's Research Governance Ethics Filter Committee.

The research was carried out in four sequential phases (see Figure 13.1):

- Phase 1: exploratory telephone interviews with midwives (n = 3) from practice and academia

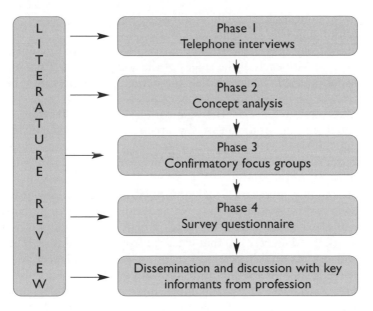

Figure 13.1   Four phases of the research design used qualitative and quantitative methods to define and examine the nature and manifestations of bullying in midwifery

- Phase 2: a concept analysis of bullying in the workplace using Walker and Avant's (2004) framework
- Phase 3: confirmatory focus groups with practising midwives, midwife managers, academic midwives and union representatives
- Phase 4: a questionnaire survey of student midwives to further validate and confirm the findings of the concept analysis.

Each of the four phases of the study contributed to the overall understanding of bullying in midwifery. It may be helpful to elaborate on Walker and Avant's (2004) concept analysis framework (see Box 13.1). Concept analysis

---

Box 13.1   Walker and Avant's Concept Analysis Framework

1   Select the concept of interest
2   Determine the aim of the analysis
3   Identify all uses of the concept
4   Determine the defining attributes
5   Construct a model case
6   Construct borderline, related, contrary and illegitimate cases
7   Identify antecedents and consequences
8   Define empirical referents

Source: Walker and Avant (2004).

is an important philosophical method of inquiry that facilitates knowledge and theory development. It is an eight-stage process.

While the stages are enumerated and written in sequential manner, it is an iterative process, with each of the stages of the analysis facilitating a progressive refocusing on the concept, so that the defining attributes may be identified.

The Walker and Avant (2004) framework provided a structured process that facilitated the identification of key attributes of bullying in midwifery (Gillen *et al.*, 2004). These attributes were then validated and confirmed by focus groups of midwives from practice, academia and trade unions, and tested in Phase IV of the study.

The underpinning literature review informed the four phases of the study by continually updating what was known about the concept of bullying in the workplace. It also contributed to the development of the preliminary theoretical framework (see Figure 13.2) that emerged from the lead researcher's (PG) personal and professional experience, from anecdotal evidence, and from a comprehensive review of the literature on bullying in the workplace. Three factors were considered to be the most influential in understanding the phenomenon of bullying in midwifery; these were drawn together to provide a tentative theoretical framework to guide the study.

Figure 13.2 shows a diagrammatic representation of the tentative theory of the three stages of bullying in midwifery: pre-bullying, bullying and post-bullying:

- pre-bullying relates to all that happens before bullying begins – those factors that, in some way, contribute to bullying in midwifery.
- bullying includes the definition, nature and manifestations of bullying in the workplace.
- post-bullying is where the effects of bullying may be seen with possible implications for the individual who has been bullied, but also for their profession and the organization in which they work.

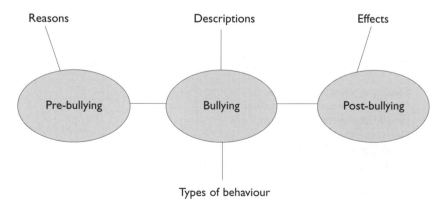

Figure 13.2   Initial theoretical framework for examining bullying in midwifery

This apparently simple framework was then developed into an explanatory model and tested through research and development. For deeper understanding, one might follow a series of cases through from stage to stage. Or, alternatively, each stage may be associated with a different exploration. Pre-bullying might be explored with neophytes, post-bullying with more experienced practitioners, and the centre stage might be directly observed.

Each of the phases of the research contributed to the refinement of the theoretical framework, crystallizing in a new definition of bullying in midwifery, and a description of the nature and manifestations of bullying in midwifery. The initial simplicity of the framework became a little more complex, reflecting the complexity that is found in the real world of practice, as the research progressed. The testing of the model need not necessarily follow the direction of the model: here, it was decided to explore the impact of the concept at Stage 3. Later, the other stages were explored and, indeed, most data collection provided support for the whole model: for example, the focus on Stage 3 illuminated the earlier stages as well.

Telephone interviews

Data collection began with three interviews in the post-bullying stage. The telephone interviews explored the phenomenon of bullying experienced by midwives in practice and within academia. Three midwives agreed to be interviewed. The telephone interviews were carried out using Rayner and Hoel's (1997) five categories of bullying behaviour (p. 287).

The midwives were all in the post-bullying stage and had left their jobs – in part, to escape the bully. Their stories provided compelling evidence of the existence of bullying in the lives of midwives working in clinical practice and academia (Gillen, 2002) and contributed to the theoretical framework (see Figure 13.3).

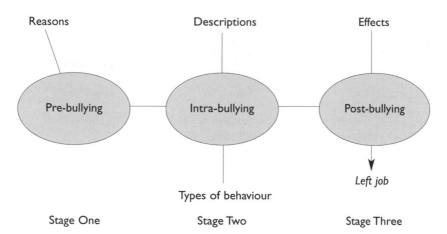

Figure 13.3   Modification of the framework following the telephone interviews.

(*Note: Italic* font indicates addition from telephone interviews.)

Concept analysis

Having confirmed the presence of bullying in midwifery and completed an initial literature review, it was apparent that there was a need for a deeper consensus regarding the definition of the concept of bullying. This meant placing the concept centre-stage and encompassing it as a whole. Concept analysis is a qualitative approach that facilitates knowledge and theory development. It provides clear definitions of concepts and terms prior to further research into the nature and manifestations of a phenomenon. Each of the stages of the analysis involves a progressive refocusing on the concept, so that the defining attributes can be identified (see Figure 13.4). However, one of the criticisms of concept analysis is that it removes the phenomenon that is under scrutiny from its context (Unsworth, 2000). One way in which this may be overcome is to undertake focus groups to confirm and validate the findings of the concept analysis. This context-intelligence (Holloway, 2005) is vital, so that the researcher may fully understand the participants' reality and, as a consequence, place the phenomenon in its most appropriate context.

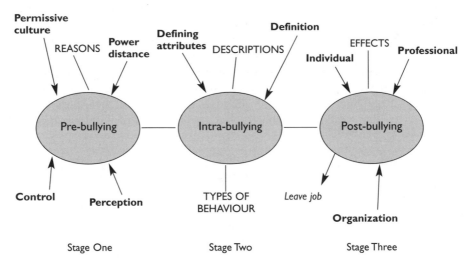

Figure 13.4   Diagrammatic representation of an emerging theoretical framework of the three stages of bullying in midwifery

Note: BLOCK capitals indicate literature sources; *italic* font was informed by Phase 1; concept analysis additions are presented in **bold**.

Confirmatory focus groups

The confirmatory focus groups were undertaken with practising midwives, midwife managers, academic midwives and union representatives with the purpose of validating and confirming the findings of the concept analysis.

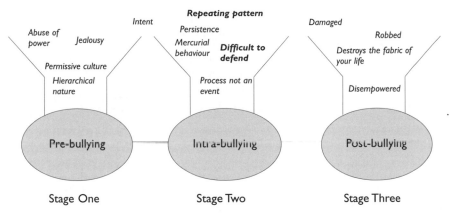

Figure 13.5   Diagrammatic representation of the three stages of bullying in midwifery with additions from the confirmatory focus groups.

Note: In this diagram, examples of the words used by the focus group members are used to confirm the findings of the concept analysis.

The definition of bullying in midwifery (see Box 13.2), and the critical (defining) attributes, antecedents and consequences, as identified within the concept analysis (Walker and Avant, 2004), were used as a framework for the discussion.

The focus groups were used as an inductive confirmatory process. They also provided a rich source of data that contributed to the theoretical framework (see Figure 13.5). The model informed the methodology, and the understanding and classification of qualitative data.

Student midwife survey

Having explored the three stages of bullying from a theoretical and conceptual perspective, and validated and confirmed the findings (within the context of midwifery) from the perspective of experienced midwives, it was necessary to test the defining attributes empirically. Therefore, in Phase IV a questionnaire was developed with specific items written to explore, define and test tentative attributes of bullying. The sample selected comprised novice midwives, because they were less likely to have been socialized and

---

Box 13.2   Definition of bullying

Bullying is persistent, offensive, abusive, intimidating, malicious or insulting behaviour, abuse of power or unfair penal sanctions that make the recipient feel upset, threatened humiliated or vulnerable, which undermines their self-confidence and which may cause them to suffer stress.

Source: RCM (1996: 3).

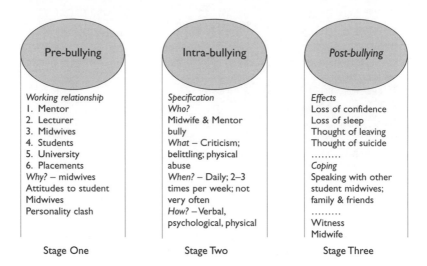

Figure 13.6   The three stages of bullying in midwifery, with contributions from the student midwife questionnaire

accustomed to accepting bullying behaviours. The student midwife survey was divided into three sections:

- Section 1: Profile of the student midwives
- Section 2: Working relationships
- Section 3: The nature and manifestation of bullying.

The questionnaire was completed by 164 student midwives. The findings from the questionnaire confirmed the phenomenon of bullying within midwifery and provided additional evidence to develop the theoretical framework. Figure 13.6 is a diagrammatic representation of how the findings from the questionnaire contributed to each stage of the theoretical framework.

Discussion of findings

Each phase of this study was necessary to build upon the tentative theoretical framework that was identified at the beginning of the research. Indeed, without that simple starting point, it would have been all too easy to become confused by terminology, experience and different emphasis given to different aspects by different informants. The findings of the research are important, as not only do they confirm the reality of bullying in midwifery, they also contribute to the development of theory.

Problems with the definition of bullying in the workplace were apparent from the plethora of words that are commonly used to mean bullying. The definition chosen for exploration and concept development in this study was the one used by the RCM (1996), as it is clear and succinct, and one that had been used in midwifery research before (see Box 13.2).

The eight-stage process of concept analysis facilitated the close examination of the concept and clarified the meaning of bullying in midwifery. However, in order that the concept remained within the context of practice and had real meaning for midwives, it was vital that it was subjected to a confirmatory and validation process. In this research, this was operationalized as focus groups, with midwives from a number of backgrounds, including practising midwives, midwife managers, academic midwives and union representatives. The three-stage model allowed this to proceed without losing track of the core purpose of the study: to illuminate the concept.

The focus group participants supported the key principles underpinning the RCM (1996) definition of bullying and considered the inclusion of the 'abuse of power' to be insightful, as it highlights subtle, and often unseen influences exerted by bullies. Abuse of power was not only manifest in treating someone badly, but also in showing favouritism. An equally important component of the definition was persistence, which was viewed as a crucial aspect of bullying behaviour – the ongoing and repeated nature of the behaviour that ultimately undermines and negatively affects the victim. There was a general consensus that bullying was often intentional.

Defining attributes

These attributes were what set bullying apart from the normal interpersonal interactions and organizational communication that exist within workplaces. These were identified as being:

- the repeated nature of the behaviour;
- the negative effect of the behaviour;
- difficulty in defending self and
- the intent of the bully.

This research provides rigorous evidence to describe and confirm the defining attributes, and this led to a clear re-definition of the concept.

Repeated nature

There are a number of behaviours that can be used by the bully to destabilize, undermine and negatively impact on the victim. The repeated nature of bullying was reflected by one of the focus group midwives:

> keeps you on edge all the time and it keeps you in a position where you are wanting to please all the time as well (4C).

The behaviours most often cited as bullying behaviour by the student midwives ranged from: intimidation, excessive criticism, and belittling of work to undervaluing skills and effort. These are recognized as behaviours that are frequently used by bullies (RCM, 1996; Einarsen and Raknes, 1997; Quine, 2001). While the majority of the behaviour to which the midwives and student midwives were subjected was non-physical, there were two occasions when these students were physically assaulted: one was 'pushed around' and the other had 'a bag of waste thrown' at her.

However, a perspective on bullying that is often overlooked and is relatively easy to access is that of the witness to bullying behaviour. It is acknowledged that as many bullying behaviours are subtle and take place behind closed doors, not all behaviour can be witnessed. Despite this, more than one third (36 per cent, n = 59) of these student midwives witnessed others being bullied. Witnessing bullying behaviour is considered an objective measure of the phenomenon, which acts as confirmation that bullying is not just a perception of the victim (Quine, 2003).

Negative effect of the behaviour

Some of the midwives suggested that it was the effect of the behaviour on the victim that was more important than the frequency of the behaviour. A variety of negative effects of the behaviour were indicated by the students, the majority indicating 'loss of confidence', a 'loss of self-esteem' and 'anxiety'. The detrimental effect of bullying on these students' physical and mental health was also apparent, with participants reporting 'disturbed sleeping patterns', and 'taking time off work and generally feeling unwell'. Similar effects were reported by members of the focus groups, who were aware of these effects either through personal experience or through second-hand accounts of victims who had confided in them. Other studies report similar effects, (RCM, 1996; Quine, 2001). Of great concern is the revelation by one of the student midwives that she had contemplated suicide as a consequence of being bullied. This effect was previously reported in the literature (Hastie, 1995; RCM, 1996).

Some of the student midwives also considered leaving the course (42 per cent, n = 25). This is a particularly common response to bullying behaviour by victims. Zapf and Gross (2001) reported that leaving their job is a final reaction from a victim of bullying. Victims may have tried to deal with the issue but, having been unsuccessful in resolving the problem – and, in some cases, having made it worse – they feel that their only option is to leave the profession.

Difficulty in defending self

Power imbalance can affect the victim's capacity to defend themselves, and the bully is dependent on this difficulty. Some of the midwives felt that the bully actually drew strength from the difficulties that the victim had, as they felt that they could get away with their behaviour. Therefore, as has been recognized by Zapf and Gross (2001), the longer the bully perpetuates the behaviour, the more likely they are to increase the frequency of the behaviour.

Many of the student midwives did try to defend themselves from the bullying behaviour by speaking with other student midwives and family and friends about their experience. This was recognized by some as a useful step in helping to work out how to react the next time the bully attacked. While some of the students tried to speak with the bully about the behaviour, this was found to be ineffective in getting them to change their behaviour.

It was apparent that, often, the student midwives put up with the behaviour because they did not want to jeopardize either their clinical or academic marks, or their job opportunities in the healthcare trust. This was also highlighted by Begley (2001) as a legitimate concern for student midwives. There was a clear power imbalance between student midwives and qualified staff; this was verbalized by the students in both clinical practice and the university setting. The students were often dependent on the very people who were bullying them for their academic and clinical assessments.

Intent of the bully

There is a general reluctance on the part of researchers into bullying to include the issue of intent (Rayner and Hoel, 1997). This may, in part, be due to the difficulty in measurement. However, the majority of these student midwives (53 per cent, n = 31) believed that the bully intended to bully them. They perceived intentional behaviour to be intricately woven into the culture of midwifery, and perceived their survival to be similar to an initiation test or a rite of passage. Begley (2002) suggests that there is a cyclical nature to hierarchy and bullying in midwifery, where successive generations of staff are taught, by the example of their senior colleagues, to behave in certain ways. In this study, the student midwives saw the intent of the bully as a need to take control and hold the power within the midwife–student relationship. If behaviour was intentional, it might continue and perhaps escalate. The escalation in the behaviour is associated with bullying behaviour that happens over a long period of time (Einarsen, 2000) when the bully feels above reproach.

Definition of bullying

In summary, the defining attributes of bullying have been identified and confirmed as:

- repeated nature of the behaviour
- negative effect on the victim
- difficulty in defending self
- intent of the bully.

Therefore, a new definition of bullying in midwifery has been developed as a result of this research (see Box 13.3).

Box 13.3   Definition, with amendments (in bold), following findings from research

Bullying in midwifery is the **often intentional, repeated,** persistent, offensive, abusive, intimidating, malicious or insulting behaviour, abuse of power or unfair penal sanctions **against which the victim finds it difficult to defend him/herself.** It **has a negative effect on the recipient** that makes them feel upset, threatened, humiliated or vulnerable; undermines their self-confidence and which may cause them to suffer stress.

This definition explicitly includes each of the defining attributes that have been confirmed and validated within the context of midwifery.

Antecedents

It is important to consider the antecedents to bullying because, as an event that must occur prior to the occurrence of a concept (Walker and Avant, 2004), it may be feasible to look at whether this can be changed in some way either to reduce or minimize the occurrence or impact of bullying. There were four antecedents that emerged from the literature which were confirmed by the research participants:

- perception of the behaviour by the victim
- lack of control (either perceived or actual)
- power distance
- permissive culture.

The antecedents are the first stage of the bullying process and, therefore, these informed the pre-bullying stage of the theory.

Perception of the behaviour by the victim: The bullying behaviour may be openly aggressive but, as reported by McKenna *et al.* (2003), it may also be subtle and covert. Ultimately, however, it is the victim's perception of the event that is important. While it is important to examine all factors that may, in some way, contribute to the phenomenon of bullying, it is important that the victim of the behaviour does not become further victimized by being made to feel that their perception of the world is the reason that they feel bullied, as opposed to an acceptance that they are being or have been bullied.

Lack of control, either perceived or actual: In the main, midwives work in the UK within the confines of large hierarchical health care trusts that are medically-dominated social institutions, within which many procedures and guidelines based on a medical model of care prevail (Hyde and Roche-Reid, 2004). This lack of control may reveal itself as frustration, which emerges as bullying behaviour to those over whom they have some control; that is, their midwifery colleagues and student midwives, in particular.

Power distance between the victim and the perpetrator: Power distance was first identified by Hofstede (1980) and is defined by Einarsen (2000) as the interpersonal power or influence difference between two persons as perceived by the less powerful of the two. The student midwives believed that much of the bullying behaviour that they experienced was the midwife exerting her control and power over the student. Power imbalances tend to be more prevalent in organizations where there is a reliance on hierarchy and power and control (Ashforth, 1994; Ireland, 2000); for example, prisons, the armed forces and the NHS.

Permissive culture within the workplace: The focus groups identified the culture within which midwives worked as being a contributory factor in bullying. The permissive role of the organization was highlighted, with no action being taken by the powers that be: thereby implying that bullying was an acceptable practice. There was little confidence expressed by midwives in this study of those support mechanisms put in place within the workplace. The belief was that the most senior person would be believed and, as this is most often the bully, the victim's point of view would be dismissed, leaving them feeling even more vulnerable. This may have a knock-on effect as bullies see that they get away with it and other victims are reluctant to come forward.

The socialization processes for new or potential members of the profession was seen as a major contributor to the perpetuation of bullying in midwifery. In essence, there was little opportunity for newcomers to influence; rather, there was an expectation that they would conform to the professional expectations and norms. The student midwives could clearly identify groups of notorious midwives who were well-known by the students for belittling and undermining student midwives. It is likely that their colleagues also knew who they were. Perhaps fear of losing experienced staff, as suggested by Curtis *et al.* (2003), goes some way to explain the inaction of colleagues and management.

Consequences

The consequences of bullying in the workplace have been shown to have a devastating impact on those affected by it. The impact is apparent at both the macro- and micro-levels of organizations, reducing their efficiency and effectiveness, and negatively influencing the working environment. These form Stage 3 of the bullying theory, and may have long-lasting consequences not only for the individual, but also the organization and the profession.

Participants were clear that the main consequence for some victims of bullying is to leave their job, which clearly impacts on the victim's professional and personal life. The consequences for the profession are clear, with union representatives witnessing midwives leaving the profession as a result of being bullied. Most often, these midwives leave on health grounds, which impacts on life outside the profession. Professional standards may also be affected by bullying. Midwives in this study indicated that the subsequent poor morale and lack of teamwork resulting from bullying has a detrimental effect on standards of care, impacting on the care that women receive.

The managers' focus group identified that many managers were fearful of being accused of bullying when they considered they were only trying to do their job. This included occasions where disciplinary actions were needed; the managers perceived themselves to be vulnerable in these situations and open to accusations of bullying.

It is clear that bullying in midwifery is a complex, multi-faceted problem. In an attempt to provide a structure for these complexities and provide a theoretical underpinning for the study, the three main areas that emerged were formulated into a three-stage theoretical framework of bullying in midwifery. The concept evolved throughout the duration of the study, and Figure 13.7 demonstrates the inductive and deductive processes that have led to the development of this model of bullying in midwifery.

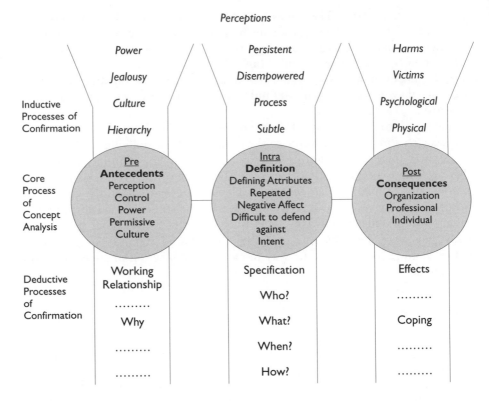

Figure 13.7 Diagrammatic representation of the refined theoretical framework

Note: The core work of concept analysis is shown in three circles with inductive (above) and deductive (below).

Conclusion

Bullying has been shown, in this study, to be rooted not only in the permissive culture of organizations in which midwifery care is provided, but also in the profession of midwifery itself. Further research needs to be undertaken to test the definition, the theoretical framework and questionnaire with trained midwives, in different cultures and within different models of care provision. An important aspect of this research is the theory that emerged from it. The theory has been built upon and developed through each phase of the research. It is practice-based and evidences the stages of bullying in midwifery within the context of the clinical and university settings in which midwifery practice and education take place. In addition to further testing and refinement of the concept, this work provides the basis for development of an intervention to address the attributes of bullying in midwifery. Indeed, an important next step is that an intervention is developed that builds on the validated and confirmed findings of this research.

ACTIVITIES

Undergraduate

This chapter provides a challenging picture of bullying behaviours within undergraduate education systems, and provides a description of a process that was undertaken to clarify the concept of bullying.

Read the paper by Gillen *et al.* (2004) and partially replicate the concept analysis using the eight-step approach advocated by Walker and Avant.

Gillen, P., Sinclair, M. and Kernohan, G. (2004) 'A concept analysis of bullying in midwifery', *Evidence Based Midwifery*, 2(2): 46–51.

Postgraduate activity

The final theoretical framework presented in Figure 13.7 has never been tested. Design a research study that will test this framework in your specialist area of practice.

References

Adams, A. (1992) *Bullying at Work: How to Confront and Overcome It.* London: Virago.

Ashforth, B. (1994) 'Petty Tyranny on Organizations', *Human Relations*, 47(7): 755–79.

Ball, L., Curtis, P. and Kirkham, M. (2002) *Why Do Midwives Leave?* London: Royal College of Midwives.

Bassman, E.S. (1992) *Abuse in the Workplace: Management Remedies and Bottom Line Impact.* Westport, CT: Quorum Books.

Begley, C.M. (1999a) 'A Study of Student Midwives' Experiences during their Two Year Education Programme', *Midwifery*, 15: 194–202.

Begley, C.M. (1999b) 'Student Midwives' Views of "Learning to be a Midwife" in Ireland', *Midwifery* 15: 264–73.

Begley, C.M. (2001) 'Knowing Your Place': Student Midwives' Views of Relationships in Midwifery in Ireland', *Midwifery*, 17: 222–33.

Begley, C.M. (2002) 'Great Fleas have Little Fleas': Irish Student Midwives' Views of the Hierarchy in Midwifery', *Journal of Advanced Nursing*, 38(3): 310–17.

Chartered Institute of Personnel and Development (2005) *Bullying at Work: Beyond Policies to a Culture of Respect.* London: CIPD.

Curtis, P., Ball, L. and Kirkham, M. (2003) *Why Do Midwives Leave? Talking to Managers.* London: RCM.

Einarsen, S. (2000) 'Harassment and Bullying at Work: A Review of the Scandinavian Approach', *Aggression and Violent Behaviour*, 5(4): 379–401.

Einarsen, S. and Raknes, B.I. (1997) 'Harassment at Work and the Victimisation of Men', *Violence and Victims*, 12(3): 247–63.

Einarsen, S. and Skogstad, A. (1996) 'Bullying at Work: Epidemiological Findings in Public and Private Organizations', *European Journal of Work and Organizational Psychology*, 5(2): 185–201.

Fawcett, J. and Downs, F.S. (1992) *The Relationship of Theory and Research*, 2nd edn. Philadelphia, PA: F.A. Davis.

Gillen, P. (2002) 'Bullies at Work: Midwives Memories', *Midwives Journal*, 5(9): 290–3

Gillen, P. (2007) 'The Nature and Manifestations of Bullying in Midwifery', Unpublished PhD, University of Ulster, Belfast, Northern Ireland.

Gillen, P., Sinclair, M. and Kernohan, G. (2004) 'A Concept Analysis of Bullying in Midwifery', *Evidence Based Midwifery*, 2(2): 46–51.

Hadikin, R. and O'Driscoll, M. (2000) *The Bullying Culture*. Oxford: Books for Midwives.

Hastie, C. (1995) 'Midwives Eat Their Young Don't They?', *Birth Issues* 4: 5–9.

Heinemann, P. (1972) *Mobbning. Gruppvåld mellan barn och vuxna* [*Bullying. Group Violence among Children and Adults*]. Lund: Natur och kultur. Cited in P.K. Smith, Y. Morita, J. Junger-Tas, D. Olweus, R. Catalano and P. Slee (1999) (eds), *The Nature of School Bullying: A Cross-National Perspective*. London: Routledge: 28–48.

Hoel, H. and Cooper, C.L. (2000) *Destructive Conflict and Bullying at Work*. Manchester School of Management: University of Institute of Science and Technology.

Hofstede, G. (1980) *Culture's Consequences: International Differences in Work Related Values*. Newbury Park, CA: Sage.

Holloway, I. (1997) *Basic Concepts for Qualitative Research*. Oxford: Blackwell Science.

Holloway, I. (ed.) (2005) *Qualitative Research in Health Care*. Buckingham: Open University Press.

Hyde, A. and Roche-Reid, B (2004) 'Midwifery Practice and the Crisis of Modernity: Implications for the Role of the Midwife', *Social Science and Medicine*, 58: 2613–23.

Ireland, J.L. (2000) ' "Bullying" among Prisoners: A Review of the Research', *Aggression and Violent Behaviour*, 5(2): 201–15.

Leymann, H. (1990) 'Mobbing and Psychological Terror at Workplaces', *Violence and Victims*, 5(2): 119–26.

Leymann, H. (1996) 'The Content and Development of Mobbing at Work', *European Journal of Work and Organizational Psychology*, 5(2): 165–84.

Mackenzie Davey, K. and Liefhooghe, A.P.D. (2003) 'Voice and Power: Critically Examining the Uses of the Term Bullying in Organizations', in A. Schorr, W. Campbell and M. Schenk, *Communication Research and Media Science in Europe*. Berlin: Walter de Gruyter, ch. 5.4: 441–57.

McKenna, B.G., Smith, N. A., Poole, S. and Coverdale, J.H. (2003) 'Horizontal Violence: Experiences of Registered Nurses in their First Year of Practice', *Journal of Advanced Nursing*, 42(1): 90–6.

Niedl, K. (1996) 'Mobbing and Well-Being: Economic and Personnel Development Implications', *European Journal of Work and Organizational Psychology*, 5(2): 239–49.

Olafsson, R.F. and Johannsdottir (2004) 'Coping with Bullying in the Workplace: The Effect of Gender, Age and Type of Bullying', *British Journal of Guidance and Counselling*, 32(3): 319–33.

Polit, D.F., Beck, C.T. and Hungler, B.P. (2001) *Essentials of Nursing Research Methods, Appraisal and Utilization*, 5th edn. Philadelphia, PA: Lippincott.

Quine, L. (1999) 'Workplace Bullying in NHS Community Trust: Staff Questionnaire Survey', *British Medical Journal*, 318: 228–32.

Quine, L. (2001) 'Workplace Bullying in Nursing', *Journal of Health Psychology*, 6(1): 73–84.

Quine, L. (2003) 'Workplace Bullying, Psychological Distress, and Job Satisfaction in Junior Doctors', *Cambridge Quarterly of Healthcare Ethics*, 12(1): 91–101.

Rayner, C. and Hoel, H. (1997) 'A Summary Review of Literature relating to Workplace Bullying', *Journal of Community & Applied Social Psychology*, 7(3): 181–91.

RCM (Royal College of Midwives) (1996) *In Place of Fear: Recognising and Confronting the Problem of Bullying in Midwifery*. London: RCM.

RCN (Royal College of Nursing) (2002) *Working Well?* London: RCN.

Tashakkori, A. and Teddlie, C (eds) (2003) *Handbook of Mixed Methods in Social and Behavioural Research*. London: Sage.

UNISON (1997) *UNISON Members' Experience of Bullying at Work*. London: UNISON.

Unsworth, J. (2000) 'Practice Development: A Concept Analysis', *Journal of Nursing Management*, 8(6): 317–26.

Vartia, M. (1996) 'The Sources of Bullying – Psychological Work Environment and Organizational Climate', *European Journal of Work and Organizational Psychology*, 5(2): 203–14.

Waltz, C. and Bausell, R.B. (1981) *Nursing Research: Design, Statistics and Computer Analysis*. Philadelphia, PA: F.A. Davis.

Walker, L.O. and Avant, K.C. (2004) *Strategies for Theory Construction in Nursing*, 3rd edn. Norwalk, CT: Appleton.

Wilson, C.B. (1991) U.S. 'Businesses Suffer from Workplace Trauma', *Personnel Journal*, 70(7): 47–50.

Zapf, D. and Gross, C. (2001) 'Conflict Escalation and Coping with Workplace Bullying', *European Journal of Work and Organizational Psychology*, 10(4): 497–522.

The Partnership Model

Rosemary Mander

> ### Key points
>
> - It is not possible to assume a common understanding of frequently used terms such as 'with woman'
> - Historical phenomena may be interpreted in a variety of ways, and the interpretation may be associated with the interpreter's intentions
> - There is a need for midwives to become politically astute, in order to practise optimally
> - Theory and models should be scrutinized critically by practitioners before being implemented.

Introduction

The meaning of the Old English word 'midwife' – we are all too frequently reminded – relates to the female companion who is 'with woman' around the time of childbearing (Page, 2003). This is a term that has been widely reinterpreted to refer to the companion 'being with' the childbearing woman in labour (Hunter, 2006, 2009). This concept has been taken on board by others, such as our nursing colleagues working in the field of palliative care, who have managed to transmogrify it into 'presencing' (Haraldsdottir, 2007).

In this chapter, I seek to explore the meaning of 'being with woman' in order to find out how this phrase is being used. I build on this to suggest that this relatively longstanding concept has become metamorphosed into the increasingly familiar 'partnership' model (Guilliland and Pairman, 1995). To comprehend its significance fully, it is essential to understand the context in which this model came into existence. I address its meaning at the time of its inception, and consider whether and to what extent this meaning may have changed. Because this model may have been elevated in some quarters to the level of dogma, I consider how this elevation has been achieved. I endeavour to evaluate the contribution of this model to midwifery in terms of its strengths, and any weaknesses that it may carry. To conclude this chapter, I probe the implications of 'partnership' for all those involved, with particular reference to the possibility of this model becoming a global reality.

With woman: rhetoric and reality

By virtue of its woman-centred orientation, midwifery has been shown to fit more appropriately into the social model of childbearing, as opposed to the biomedical model (van Teijlingen, 1994). Kitzinger (2003) recounts the domestic aspects of the social model and the midwife's original role in 'orchestrating' the activities and behaviours of those neighbourly women who were with the childbearing woman. These women became known by the then disparaging name of 'God's sibs' (God's sisters), condensed to 'gossips' by the disgruntled men who were excluded from the gathering. Kitzinger's account focuses on the support provided by the midwife for the childbearing woman in medieval societies, as well as in modern, less developed societies. In westernized cultures, childbearing has largely been moved out of its domestic, social setting into institutions; here, the role of women in providing supportive care has tended to be usurped by interventions offered by obstetricians, anaesthetists and surgeons. In spite of these more recent organizational changes in the orientation of care in childbearing, in many countries the term 'midwife' has survived. It may be necessary, though, to question whether this job title is anything more than a wishful mantra, reflecting a rosy-hued past, a kind of golden age, when the midwife was, in reality, 'with woman'. The resurrection of the philosophy of being 'with woman' has been tracked by Carolan and Hodnett (2007), who present this development as a groundswell originating with women's unhappiness with their birthing experiences in health systems featuring 'public hospitals' (2007: 140). These Canadian researchers continue by showing how this backlash supposedly resulted in the primacy of the midwife in the provision of 'woman-centred' care.

The reality or otherwise of the modern midwife's scope for being 'with woman' was demonstrated in an insightful and authoritative ethnographic study of midwives and midwifery students in Wales (Hunter, 2004; see Chapter 7). Tensions were shown to have arisen in view of the community midwife's ability to practise autonomously and to focus on relationships with clients. These tensions resulted from this midwife's organizational obligation to practise in the maternity unit. In these circumstances, this midwife found her autonomy diminished, her practice more medicalized and her relationships with clients threatened. Thus, the community midwife, who had been able to practise 'with woman' encountered the requirement to adopt a 'with institution' ideology (2004: 267). Hunter shows the emotion work required of the midwife obliged to practise within and between these two conflicting ideologies.

One possible result of the midwife finding herself practising in an over-whelmingly medicalized setting is that, as well as being 'with institution', she may transform herself into a 'medwife' (Davis-Floyd, 1999). This transformation happens as a result of the midwife being forced to choose between either being marginalized by the power structure, or becoming a part of it. If she chooses the latter, she becomes this chameleon-like practitioner who is able to cope with the patriarchal medical power structure only by ensuring that her practice and any decision-making accords with her hegemonic environment. The ability of the 'medwife' to be 'with woman' and to provide support for the childbearing woman is negligible to the point of ceasing to exist. In this way, both the midwife and the woman are disempowered and deprived of any autonomy.

It is becoming apparent, through research and observation, that the concept of the midwife being 'with woman' has been reduced in some practice environments to little more than an empty mantra. Its persistence may, in these environments, represent a form of rhetoric that verges on self-delusion. It was against this bleak background that, in one particular setting, the partnership model, came into being. In New Zealand, midwifery became defined in terms of the working relationship: 'Midwifery is the partnership between the woman and the midwife' (Guilliland and Pairman, 1994: 6); Pairman continues to maintain that this is still the case (2006: 73). In the next section, I analyze the contextual factors that provided the backdrop for the conception of this model.

The cultural context of the creation of the partnership model

In New Zealand, the concept of partnership is often claimed to provide a crucial underpinning to this vibrant, yet occasionally isolationist, society. The origin of partnership is not infrequently attributed to the Treaty of Waitangi (1840) between the British Crown and 500 Maori Chiefs (Orange, 1984; Pairman, 2006: 75), although Skinner disputes this (1999: 15). The *Pakeha*, which in this situation may be interpreted to mean the Europeans representing the British Crown, signed the document. It differed markedly, though, from the Maori language version, by the former offering different (that is, fewer) rights and privileges. New Zealanders' complacency about the benefits to all of the Treaty is sadly misplaced, having been described in terms of 'mythology' (Williams, 1940). Skinner (1999: 15) argues that, far from a partnership, the Treaty was a contract centred around 'sovereignty'. Benn (1999), on the other hand, suggests that this sovereignty was related not to European power, but to each group's potential for self-determination, while explaining that some New Zealanders feel less than comfortable with the concept of Maori sovereignty, due to it being linked by journalist Carol Archie (1995: 37) with 'tribalism'. Thus, there is not the total consensus that the cultural foundations on which the partnership model has been built carry the benign authority often claimed (Guilliland and Pairman, 1995).

As well as having been attributed to this long-standing myth, the partnership model emerged partly as a reaction to the more recent developments in the organization and practice of midwifery. These developments, recounted authoritatively by Mein Smith (1986) are summarized by Stojanovic (2008: 156–7) as: 'medicalisation, hospitalisation and nursification'. The partnership model also materialized out of the slipstream of a series of legislative changes introduced by the then Minister of Health, Helen Clark, who was to become New Zealand's Prime Minister in 1999. A further major influencing factor was the public enquiry into the non-treatment of women with cervical cancer in one major medical centre (Cartwright, 1988). All of these events served to strengthen the position of an already strong national population of women. It was into this tinder box of a cultural climate that new Obstetric Regulations (New Zealand Government, 1986) were introduced that threatened the midwife's role and, possibly, existence. The political activity that was ignited in the following cultural firestorm involved politicians, midwives and women, and resulted in the birth of the New Zealand College of Midwives (NZCOM) (New Zealand Nurses Association, 1989), followed in 1990 by the Nurses Amendment Act (Guilliland, 1999a). This ground breaking legislation was effortlessly enacted, much to the surprise of the medical fraternity: it separated midwifery from nursing, encouraged the childbearing woman to exercise choice of maternity service provider and the midwife to exercise autonomy. The passing of this legislation was greeted with euphoric triumphalism, quickly followed by bewilderment at this changed state of affairs. In this situation, NZCOM needed to establish itself by building on its high profile: the creation of the partnership model served to maintain the momentum which had been created.

The original meaning of 'partnership'

In the heady days, months and years after the successful enactment of the Nurses Amendment Act, New Zealand midwifery continued the process of reinventing itself. This novel persona took the form of a new professional image, which needed to distinguish itself from both nurses (its former dominatrices) and medical practitioners (an even longer-term threat). This newly autonomous professional persona was, thus, required to reject the traditional role of 'distant expert' in favour of a more egalitarian approach, in keeping with both professional and national aspirations. In order to operationalize this massive professional project, political action was required, involving not only midwives and childbearing women, but also the active support of women politicians, such as Helen Clarke, the then Minister of Health (Guilliland and Pairman, 1995: 12).

The approach chosen also featured the empowerment of the childbearing woman through the sharing of expert knowledges between midwives and women. Simultaneously, a new midwifery educational structure was developed, and the midwife's unique area of expertise – normal childbearing – was redefined to permit negotiation with the individual woman.

The partnership model provided the foundation on which this new professional persona would be built. As originally conceived by Guilliland and Pairman, the model comprised four philosophical underpinnings:

- pregnancy and childbirth are normal life events
- midwifery's primary professional role is with women experiencing a normal pregnancy, labour, birth and postnatal period.
- midwifery provides women with continuity of caregiver throughout her (*sic*) childbearing experience
- midwifery is women-centred. (Guilliland and Pairman, 1995: 34)

After the partnership model was originally published (NZCOM, 1990), it underwent its first major trial later the same year. This confrontation was not against either medical practitioners or nurses but, rather, against the International Council of Midwives (ICM) (Fleming, 2000: 197). The concept of partnership between the childbearing woman and the midwife in a clinical setting was considered quite acceptable to the ICM, and it may even have been familiar to some of the member states. The sticking point was quickly reached, though, when the concept of partnership was recommended to be applied at an organizational level – indeed, for the midwives' professional organization. This meant that NZCOM intended to include consumers and their representatives on their board of management. The ICM considered that such lay representation took the concept of partnership a step too far. The involvement of consumers at this level threatened the ICM's notion of what constituted a profession. Again, though, the political machinations of NZCOM's leading lights swung into action. On this occasion, they were successful in manoeuvring to ensure New Zealand's continuing membership of the ICM.

By 1993, at its meeting in Vancouver, the ICM was prepared to accede to New Zealand's position statement: 'Extending the midwifery partnership to the professional organisation' (NZCOM, 1993: 4). Applying this interpretation of partnership, however, to other states' midwifery professional organizations was too much for the ICM to take onboard and the position statement was not accepted.

The more refined version of the partnership model, which was published in 1995, is disconcertingly liberally sprinkled with references to autonomy, empowerment, responsibility and accountability (Guilliland and Pairman, 1995). In this monograph, the authors argue the balanced or reciprocal nature of the relationship between the partners. The cracks in the edifice start to become apparent, though, when the autonomy of the midwife is vetoed and is said to no longer apply within the partnership. In this situation, the woman is apportioned the role of primary decision-maker but, meanwhile, the midwife remains accountable – in spite of being denied autonomy (Guilliland and Pairman, 1995). Whether and to what extent this potentially fraught situation has been able to be put into practice to the mutual acceptability of both parties will emerge out of this chapter.

The partnership model monograph (Guilliland and Pairman, 1995) drew heavily on the ideas advanced by midwives in other countries, particularly in 'the old world', such as the Association of Radical Midwives (ARM) *The Vision in the UK* (ARM, 1986). The North American approaches to midwifery provided some input into the partnership model; however, certain shortcomings – such as the reality of partnership, the role of the midwife and the need for continuity of care – prevented more complete acceptance (Guilliland and Pairman, 1995).

The partnership model as it has evolved

The partnership model has been forced into the real world through further trials and tribulations. These include, for example, negotiations with the New Zealand Medical Association (NZMA) about the circumstances under which the woman's care may be or must be recommended to be transferred from the midwife to a medical practitioner (Daellenbach and Thorpe, 2007). These circumstances include the familiarly contentious situations, such as breech presentation in labour. The partnership model has evolved to take account of demands that the discussion and decision about the transfer of care requires the involvement of not only the woman and the midwife, but also the obstetric medical practitioner. Implicitly, Daellenbach and Thorpe recognize the transmogrification of the partnership, but go on to suggest that such three-way consultations serve to empower both woman and midwife; while, simultaneously, they paradoxically observe that: 'this has not put an end to obstetric coercion' (Daellenbach and Thorpe, 2007: 271).

As well as the obstetrician, the woman and the midwife's partnership has also been extended to include the general practitioner (GP) in those many situations where the GP has chosen to act as the lead maternity carer (LMC) in the place of the midwife or obstetrician. GP LMCs inevitably rely on having hands-on care provided by midwives during labour and in the postnatal period, which creates, in fact, a 'shared care' arrangement. Similarly, inevitably, the midwife allowing herself to be subcontracted to provide such care 'for less remuneration as the fees are divided between the two health providers' (Daellenbach and Thorpe, 2007: 271) is effectively reneging on the partnership concept. That the partnership, which is essentially a two-person relationship (Pairman, 2006), may change to involve others is recognized by Crabtree (2004) when she identifies the large proportion of women who are offered and accept referral. Despite such frequent and regular referrals being deprecated as medicalizing childbirth (Guilliland, 2002), a majority of child-bearing women in New Zealand experience at least one referral. Crabtree goes on to recognize that this, albeit temporary, introduction of a third 'partner' into the relationship brings with it dire implications for the woman-centred nature of the birth.

A serious criticism of the partnership model has always been its want of a sound basis in research (Surtees, 2003). For an occupational group or profession aspiring to evidence-based practice, this deficiency is a significant drawback and may render the model inapposite. An attempt was eventually made to remedy this shortcoming by one of the model's original creators (Pairman, 2000). The research was undertaken in 1996/7 and took the form of a study for a master's thesis. The study adopted a qualitative exploratory approach based on feminist philosophy (Pairman, 2000), using the 1995 model as the theoretical framework. The informants comprised six self-employed midwives who had volunteered to participate, and six of their clients selected at random.

The data collection was by individual semi-structured interviews, together with a final focus group to consider the emergent themes. Although the informants were clearly closely involved with the data analysis, a major publication provides limited detail of how this analysis was conducted (Pairman, 2000). Although Pairman protests the non-generalizability of the findings, such protestations carry little weight in such a well-acquainted occupational group in a country as small as New Zealand. The study supported tenets of the original partnership model (Guilliland and Pairman, 1995) and Pairman took the opportunity to employ the findings to further enhance certain aspects of it.

The redefined model sought to take account of the context of the New Zealand situation and, in particular, the dynamic developments in the relationships between midwives and their medical colleagues since the Nurses Amendment legislation of 1990. The input of women consumers into Pairman's study established the intention of childbearing women to assume not merely 'participation and self-responsibility', but also control over the childbearing experience (Pairman, 1999: 10). The extent of this control and the scope for negotiation does not appear to have been explored. Closely associated with control is the concept of being female, which is explained in terms of being fundamental to providing support in order to achieve 'being with' the childbearing woman (Pairman, 1999: 11). The anticipated outcomes of the midwifery partnership did not feature in the original diagram of the model. They were, however, elucidated clearly in the redefined model; the outcomes relate largely to the oppressive system within which midwives and childbearing women form their relationship. The expected outcomes are empowerment, emancipation, challenging the medical model and developing midwifery knowledge. In presenting the redefined model to the membership of NZCOM, Pairman endeavours to demonstrate its responsiveness to changing circumstances through its dynamic or evolutionary orientation. In this way, it is apparent that the partnership model – which had begun life as, essentially, a clinical practice model – had been transformed. Whereas it had begun life by applying to one woman and one midwife, it was subsequently converted into a 'go-anywhere' model. This meant that it could also be applied at an organizational level, in midwifery regulation and in midwifery education (Pairman, 2006).

Critique: questioning the unquestionable

In analyzing the contribution of any theoretical material, the analyst's task cannot but be affected by the degree of acceptance of that theory. Thus, a popular and widely-known concept may be less easily examined than one the status of which is less certain. This caveat certainly applies to the concept of 'partnership', which has become seriously fashionable in health care. A search engine showed me in January 2010 that, in 1990, there were only 13 scholarly publications mentioning 'partnership' and 'health' in their titles. By 2000, though, that figure had risen to 101 and, since that date, the number of such publications has continued to fluctuate at around 90 per annum. Thus, my introductory observation – that the concept of the midwife being 'with woman' may have been reduced to rhetoric – may also apply to 'partnership'; in support of this, in partnership's application to midwifery the term 'dogma' (Surtees, 2003: 38) has been applied and its use described as 'ritualistic' (Calvert, 2002: 135).

Of fundamental importance to the partnership model, and as has always been emphasized, is the balanced nature of the inputs from the childbearing woman and the midwife. Guilliland and Pairman discussed this aspect in terms of 'equality' and 'shared responsibility' (1995: 45). It should come as no surprise that this is the basis of what 'partnership' is all about. The achievement of such equal inputs is, according to Daellenbach (1999), easier when midwives choose to ignore the inevitable differences between them and their clients. The possibility of such equality has been questioned relatively recently, though, by Canadian researchers (Carolan and Hodnett, 2007). Their argument, though, relies too heavily on a pathological orientation, which calls into question the midwifery focus on healthy childbearing, to allow it to make a genuine challenge on the partnership model.

More authoritative criticisms of this aspect of the model have been articulated on the grounds that equality is not possible when midwives are so 'differently positioned' (Surtees, 2003: 37). These differences do not merely refer to the contrasts in aspects such as knowledge, power, social status, ethnic origin and access to resources between the midwife and the woman who is her client. The differences also apply between midwives, giving rise to the question of whether and how all midwives are able to offer equality. This point relates to some midwives, such as those who are self-employed and Lead Maternity Carers having considerable autonomy to decide what they are able to offer. Other midwives, such as those who are employed in maternity units, may find themselves working within a less flexible framework or environment, and are less able to offer, for example, equal services.

As well as equality being fundamental to it, the term 'partnership' has itself proved somewhat problematic. This term is an example of one of many that have become used so widely that their original meaning has become lost in mists and myths. The shifting nature and slipperiness of this term has been noted by both its critics and its advocates (Daellenbach, 1999; Calvert, 2002; Surtees, 2003). While certain advocates appear to regard the flexibility of the partnership model as one of its strengths (Daellenbach, 1999; Pairman, 1999), this interpretation is clearly not shared universally. The interpretation of such models is often determined by the context in which the model is applied, as shown by the misinterpretation of partnership by the Queensland Government (2008), where the maternity partnership includes not only general medical practitioners and specialist medical services, but also the Child Health services.

Although, as mentioned already, an attempt has been made to address the problem of the model's lack of a research basis (Pairman, 2000), the extent to which this has been achieved is less than certain. Calvert (2002) draws attention to the small sample sizes featuring in partnership and other midwifery model research. Whether such small samples would provide a sufficiently strong evidence base for a midwife to implement research findings in her clinical practice is highly questionable. But a multitude of midwives appear to have implemented the partnership model on what is, to say the least, flimsy evidence.

The most authoritative and significant onslaught on the partnership model was published, perhaps surprisingly, in the issue of the NZCOM Journal celebrating the tenth anniversary of the College (Skinner, 1999). This critique met with, marginally less than convincing, ripostes (Benn, 1999; Daellenbach, 1999). One aspect of the partnership model that was articulated and demonstrated was its limited relevance to the woman who is underprivileged and/or dispossessed (Skinner, 1999). On the basis of a heart-rendingly familiar account of her clinical practice, involving a 'morose, uncooperative and uninterested' (1999: 14) young woman, Skinner explained her rationale for rejecting the partnership model as the philosophical framework for her clinical practice. Although not stating it explicitly, it is clear that introducing the idea of partnership to this young woman would have been one imposition too far. Skinner argues, as has been suggested before (Mander, 1993), that some women may not wish to participate in making decisions about their childbearing experience. This wish constitutes a decision *per se* by the woman and, as with any other, deserves to be respected and accepted. Thus, women have every right to decline the opportunities for involvement that are presented to them by models such as partnership.

Drawing on organizational theory relating to the concept of 'contractualism', which is familiar to all who work in health care, Skinner goes on to argue that the partnership model may be construed as a contract (1999: 16). As such, the model operates optimally when both parties involved in the contract are comfortable to adhere to its conditions. Skinner purports, however, that under certain circumstances, such as a less than ideal outcome, the woman and/or those who influence her thinking may renege on the contract because it is not equally binding on the woman. In such a situation, the midwife will, effectively, find herself 'hung out to dry', and her vulnerability to accusations of malpractice or negligence becomes obvious. Thus, rather than supporting her, Skinner maintains that the partnership model may actually serve to expose the midwife to immense and unforeseen risks.

A further criticism, levelled by Skinner, relates to one of the many assumptions inherent, but not always explicitly recognized, in the partnership model. One example of these unstated assumptions relates to the gender of the midwife (Pairman, 2000), but the assumption in question is concerned with the homogeneity of the population of midwives. The widespread application of the model by NZCOM members anticipates its general use (Guilliland, 1999a: 4). Skinner questions, though, both the willingness and the ability of every midwife to enter into a partnership with the childbearing woman. Although the midwife's midwifery education may enable her to relate to her client, there is a wealth of other personal and occupational factors that may inhibit the development of such a partnership. Thus, the: 'imposition of particular philosophies onto the practices of others' (Surtees, 2003: 38) has clearly not been met with universal or unalloyed pleasure. Skinner goes on to report that she has adopted a post-modern approach to identify and implement other, more individualized and culturally appropriate ways of being 'with woman' in her midwifery practice.

Evaluation of the partnership model

The evaluation of theoretical models is a crucial step in their assessment prior to general acceptance. Stevenson *et al*. (2002) identify the reluctance of one particular occupational group to test and to apply theoretical models. This occupational group and its reluctance appear to have much in common with midwives and midwifery. In a highly respectable edited account of organizational systems for the delivery of midwifery care, *Birth Models that Work* (Davis-Floyd *et al*., 2009), it is unsurprising that the New Zealand maternity system features prominently (Hendry, 2009). What is surprising, though, is that the partnership model is only mentioned in passing, in terms of partnership being: 'the underlying philosophy of the College [NZCOM]' (Hendry, 2009: 85). The rationale for this omission, and for Hendry's cursory attention to the model, is uncertain. While the success of the revitalized midwifery input into this admirable maternity service is undisputed, the nature of the model's contribution is not clear and has yet to be fully evaluated. In spite of this, by focusing on published material, I attempt here to address the question of what difference the model has made.

While Guilliland claimed that the model 'has achieved so much for women and midwives' (1999a: 4); the details of the nature of that achievement were demonstrated in a conference presentation (1999b). Guilliland emphasized the hugely beneficial outcomes to Maori women, often regarded as a vulnerable population. These data showed the familiar and continuing gradual decline in perinatal mortality since the legislation changed, and a lower caesarean rate than neighbouring states, although a higher forceps/ventouse rate may have balanced this. In spite of these encouraging evaluative data, concern continues about New Zealand's persistently increasing caesarean rate (Davis and Walker, 2009).

A further, although less clearly demonstrable, benefit of the partnership model is advanced by Daellenbach (1999). Taking a wide and a long-term view of the evolution of the New Zealand maternity services, she contemplates the challengingly patriarchal social, political and legislative background against which the Nurses Amendment legislation (1990) was enacted. She regards the struggle as ongoing in order to emancipate women, and that consumer activists are in the forefront of this continuing conflict. The partnership model, Daellenbach argues, is one of the major weapons in the armoury needed in the effort to achieve the acceptance of midwifery.

A somewhat dissimilar evaluation of the partnership model resulted from a qualitative study investigating the relationships between childbearing women and the midwives attending them (Fleming, 1998a). This study showed the differing understandings of their relationship held by the women and the midwives. While the midwives were generally fully 'signed up' to the model of partnership and viewed it as fundamental and central to their practice, the women's views were at variance. The women regarded the midwife's role as limited to responsibility for the 'medical things' (1998a: 10). This focus on the midwife's medical function was echoed by women, who perceived midwifery practice in this context as comparable with that of a GP. Fleming's study showed that the balance of power, far from being equal (as intended by the partnership model), tended to be held by one 'partner' to the disgruntlement of the other. The traditionally oral culture on which midwifery has long been based is, Fleming argues, under threat from the medical values to which she indicates that the midwives were aspiring. She goes on to suggest that the midwives had been unwilling or insufficiently able to dispense with their firmly-held professional attitudes to take onboard not only the letter, but also the spirit of the model. In this way, she explains how midwifery practice seems to be in conflict with the partnership model.

Conclusion

It is clear that the model of partnership has been changed markedly since it was first introduced. The original 'one-to-one' focus has been modified to move in the direction of becoming, probably more realistically, one-to-two or one-to-three (Pairman, 1999: 7). Further, the model originally applied to the midwife being with the woman, invariably assumed to be at a clinical or inter-personal level (Pairman, 1999: 7). This has been amended and extended so that partnership, if it is to be more than rhetoric, needs to operate at a range of levels. As well as its clinical or interpersonal functioning, in order to become a reality, partnership needs to operate at a higher, organizational level. As Skinner (1999) astutely observes, consumers may appropriately provide an effective input into unit policy-making, such as through maternity services liai-son committees (MSLCs) (Edwards, 1996; Smith, 2005). In the same way, women's consumer voices need to be heard more clearly at the level of govern-mental policy-making.

The long-standing thorny issue, though, and one that remains unresolved, is related to the problem of autonomy. This problem may be ascribed the status of a sticking-point. Although Pairman avoids the 'A-word' by arguing the 'self-determination' of the woman (1999: 10), her re-interpretation of midwifery autonomy as being held collectively by the profession may be less than helpful in a clinical situation. Similarly, although Pairman (1999: 10) advocates 'negotiation' and 'listening and talking about working things out', the issue of autonomy represents a deep fault line in the model. This fault line may be the impediment on which relationships may founder.

In examining the value of the partnership model, it is necessary to bear in mind that the model is just that. It is one of many theoretical approaches from which the midwife may choose. There are a variety of other models available; some of them are equally relevant to midwifery and some of them have New Zealand origins, making them doubly appropriate for midwives in that and other countries. For example, these include Fleming's research-based model, which features reciprocity and interdependence (1998b). Another very relevant possibility would be Skinner's practice-based post-modern 'non-model' (1999: 17). A further distinct possibility, recommended by Skinner (1999), is found in the WHO model of 'Health for All', as propounded by Bryar (1995).

In summary, I would argue that the maturity of an occupational or professional group may be measurable by the members' ability to select an appropriate model for the situation, the locality, the clientele and the midwife's philosophy. I suggest that the force-feeding of one particular midwifery model, irrespective of its strength, to a population of midwives is inconsistent with an occupational group's aspiration to professional status.

Acknowledgement

I would like to acknowledge the kind help of Jane Stojanovic.

ACTIVITIES

Undergraduate

Is there sufficient evidence to support the adoption of the partnership model?

Postgraduate

Critically appraise Fleming's (1998b) research-based model featuring reciprocity and interdependence.

References

Archie, C. (1995) *Maori Sovereignty. The Pakeha Perspective*. Auckland: Hodder Moa Beckett.

ARM (1986) *The Vision – Proposals for the Future of the Maternity Services*. London: ARM.

Benn, C. (1999) 'Midwifery Partnership: Individualism Contractualism or Feminist Praxis?', *New Zealand College of Midwives Journal*, 21: 18–20.

Bryar, R. (1995) *Theory for Midwifery Practice*, 1st edn. London: Macmillan.

Calvert, S. (2002) 'Being With Women: The Midwife–Woman Relationship', in R. Mander and V. Fleming (eds), *Failure to Progress: The Contraction of the Midwifery Profession*. London: Routledge, ch. 8: 133–49.

Carolan, M. and Hodnett, E. (2007) ' "With Woman" Philosophy: Examining the Evidence, Answering the Questions', *Nursing Inquiry*, 14(2): 140–52.

Cartwright, S. (1988) *Report of the Committee of Enquiry into Allegations concerning the Treatment of Cervical Cancer at the National Women's Hospital and into Other Related Matters*. Wellington: Government Printing Office.

Crabtree, S. (2004) 'Midwives Constructing "Normal Birth" ', in S. Downe (ed.), *Normal Childbirth; Evidence and Debate*, 2nd edn. Edinburgh: Churchill Livingstone Elsevier, ch. 6: 85–100.

Daellenbach, R. (1999) 'Midwifery Partnership – A Consumer's Perspective', *New Zealand College of Midwives Journal*, 21: 22–3.

Daellenbach, R. and Thorpe, J. (2007) 'Independence in Practice: New Zealand Case Study of Midwives in Partnership', in L. Reid (ed.), *Freedom to Practise*. London: Routledge, ch. 14: 261–81.

Davis, D.L. and Walker, K. (2009) 'Case-loading Midwifery in New Zealand: Bridging the Normal/Abnormal Divide "with Woman"', *Midwifery*, in press (doi:10.1016/j.midw.2009.09.007 – accessed 26 July 2010).

Davis-Floyd, R. (1999) 'Some Thoughts on Bridging the Gap Between Nurse- and Direct-Entry Midwives', *Midwifery Today*, March (www.davis-floyd.com – accessed 6 August 2010).

Davis-Floyd, R.E., Lesley Barclay, L., Daviss, B.-A. and Tritten, J. (2009) *Birth Models that Work*. Berkeley, CA: University of California Press

Edwards, N. (1996) Is Everything Rosy in the MSLC Garden? Part 1. *AIMS Journal*, 8 (3) 6–9.

Fleming, V. (1998a) Women and Midwives in Partnership: A Problematic Relationship? *Journal of Advanced Nursing*, 27 (1) 8–14.

Fleming, V. (1998b) Women-with-midwives-with-women: A Model of Interdependence. *Midwifery*, 14 (3) 137–43.

Fleming, V. (2000) 'The Midwifery Partnership in New Zealand: Past History or a New Way Forward?', in M. Kirkham (ed.), *The Midwife–Mother Relationship*. Basingstoke: Palgrave Macmillan, ch. 9: 193–205.

Guilliland, K. (1999a) 'Editorial: Towards a New Millennium in Partnership', *New Zealand College of Midwives Journal*, 21: 4.

Guilliland, K. (1999b) 'Midwifery in New Zealand: The New Zealand Experience Future Birth', The Place to be Born Conference, February New South Wales, Australia (www.birthinternational.com – accessed 6 August 2010).

Guilliland, K. (2002) 'The New Zealand Context: Similarities and differences', *New Zealand College of Midwives Journal*, 26: 12.

Guilliland, K. and Pairman, S. (1994) 'The Midwifery Partnership – A Model for Practice', *New Zealand College of Midwives Journal*, 11: 5–9.

Guilliland, K. and Pairman, S. (1995) 'The Midwifery Partnership A Model for Practice', Department of Nursing and Midwifery, Victoria University of Wellington, *Monograph Series 95/1*. Wellington: Victoria University of Wellington.

Haraldsdottir, E. (2007) 'The Constraints of the Ordinary: "Being with" Patients in a Hospice in Scotland', Unpublished PhD Thesis, University of Edinburgh, Edinburgh.

Hendry, C. (2009) 'The New Zealand Maternity System', in R.E. Davis-Floyd, L. Barclay, B.-A. Davis and J. Tritten, *Birth Models That Work*. Berkeley, CA: University of California Press, ch. 2: 55–88.

Hunter, B. (2004) 'Conflicting Ideologies as a Source of Emotion Work in Midwifery', *Midwifery*, 20(3): 261–72.

Hunter, L.P. (2006) 'Being With Woman: A Guiding Concept for the Care of Laboring Women', *Journal of Obstetric Gynecologic and Neonatal Nursing*, 31(6): 650–7.

Hunter, L.P. (2009) 'A Descriptive Study of "Being with Woman" during Labor and Birth', *Journal of Midwifery and Women's Health*, 54(2): 111–8.

Kitzinger, S. (2003) *A Cross-Cultural View of Birth at Forum on Maternity and the Newborn*. London: Royal Society of Medicine. (http://www.btinternet.com/~basil_lee/eth4.html – accessed 26 July 2010).

Mander, R. (1993) 'Who Chooses the Choices?', *Modern Midwife*, 3(1): 23–5.

Mein Smith, P. (1986) 'Maternity in Dispute: New Zealand, 1920–1939', Wellington: New Zealand Historical Publications Branch, Department of Internal Affairs.

New Zealand Government (1986) *Obstetric Regulations*. Wellington: Government Printing Office.

New Zealand Government (1990) Nurses Amendment Act 107, Commenced: 28 August 1990. Wellington: Government Printing Office.

NZCOM (1990) 'Constitution', Unpublished, New Zealand College of Midwives. Christchurch: NZCOM.

NZCOM (1993) 'Remit to ICM on Partnership', National Newsletter, April/May: 9, New Zealand College of Midwives.

New Zealand Nurses Association (1989) 'Midwifery Policy Statement'. Wellington: New Zealand Nurses Association.

Orange, C. (1984) 'The Treaty of Waitangi: A Study of its Making, Interpretation and Role in New Zealand History', Unpublished PhD thesis, University of Auckland, Auckland.

Page, L. (2003) 'One-to-One Midwifery Restoring the "With Woman" Relationship in Midwifery', *Journal of Midwifery and Women's Health*, 48(2): 119–25.

Pairman, S. (1999) 'Partnership Revisited: Towards Midwifery Theory', *New Zealand College of Midwives Journal*, 21: 6–12.

Pairman, S. (2000) 'Woman-Centred Midwifery: Partnerships or Professional Friendships', in M. Kirkham (ed.), *The Midwife–Mother Relationship*. Basingstoke: Palgrave Macmillan, ch. 10: 207–26.

Pairman, S. (2006) 'Midwifery Partnership: Working "with" Women', in L.A. Page and R. McCandlish, The New Midwifery: Science and Sensitivity in Practice. Edinburgh: Churchill Livingstone, ch. 4: 73–96.

Queensland Government (2008) 'Midwifery Models of Care: Implementation Guide'. Queensland Health. (http://www.papsmear.qld.gov.au/ocno/content/middy_models. pdf – accessed 26 July 2010).

Skinner, J. (1999) 'Midwifery Partnership: Individualism Contractualism or Feminist Praxis?', *New Zealand College of Midwives Journal*, 21: 14–7.

Smith, K. (2005) 'Consuming Passion: Life as an MSLC Rep', *Practising Midwife*, 8(8): 40–1.

Stevenson, C., Barker, P. and Fletcher, E. (2002) 'Judgement Days: Developing an Evaluation for an Innovative Nursing Model', *Journal of Psychiatric and Mental Health Nursing*, 9(3): 271–6.

Stojanovic, J. (2008) 'Midwifery in New Zealand 1904–1971', *Advances in Contemporary Nursing: History of Nursing and Midwifery in Australasia*, 30(2): 156–67.

Surtees, R.J. (2003) 'Midwifery as Feminist Praxis in Aotearoa/New Zealand', Unpublished PhD thesis, University of Canterbury, Christchurch, New Zealand. (http://ir.canterbury.ac.nz/bitstream/10092/1662/1/Thesis_fulltext.pdf – accessed 26 July 2010).

van Teijlingen, E. (1994) 'A Social or Medical Model of Childbirth? Comparing the Arguments in Grampian (Scotland) and the Netherlands', Unpublished PhD thesis, University of Aberdeen, Aberdeen.

Williams, E.T. (1940) 'The Treaty of Waitangi', *History*, 25(9): 237–51.

Index

Note: page numbers in **bold** refer to the more important references.